Y0-EDE-627

3 0000 003 421 207

DATE DUE

FEB 2 6 2002			

Demco, Inc. 38-293

ACS SYMPOSIUM SERIES 661

Wine

Nutritional and Therapeutic Benefits

Tom R. Watkins, EDITOR
Kenneth L. Jordan Heart Foundation

Developed from a symposium sponsored
by the Division of Agricultural and Food Chemistry

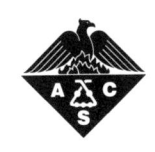

American Chemical Society, Washington, DC

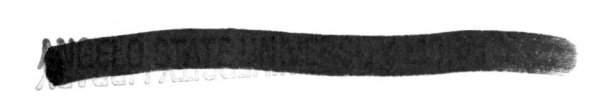

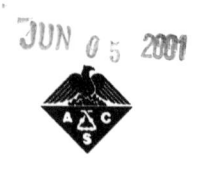

Library of Congress Cataloging-in-Publication Data

Wine: nutritional and therapeutic benefits / Tom R. Watkins.

　　p.　cm.—(ACS symposium series, ISSN 0097–6156; 661)

"Developed from a symposium sponsored by the Division of Agricultural and Food Chemistry at the 210th National Meeting of the American Chemical Society, Chicago, Illinois, August 20–24, 1995."

Includes bibliographical references and indexes.

ISBN 0–8412–3497–3

1. Wine—Therapeutic use—Congresses. 2. Wine—Health aspects—Congresses. 3. Antioxidants—Congresses.

I. Watkins, Tom R. II. American Chemical Society. Division of Agricultural and Food Chemistry. III. American Chemical Society. Meeting (210th: 1995: Chicago, Ill.) IV. Series

RM256.W64　　1997
615.8′54—dc21　　　　　　　　　　　　　　　　96–52456
　　　　　　　　　　　　　　　　　　　　　　　　CIP

This book is printed on acid-free, recycled paper.

Copyright © 1997 American Chemical Society

All Rights Reserved. Reprographic copying beyond that permitted by Sections 107 or 108 of the U.S. Copyright Act is allowed for internal use only, provided that a per-chapter fee of $17.00 plus $0.25 per page is paid to the Copyright Clearance Center, Inc., 222 Rosewood Drive, Danvers, MA 01923, USA. Republication or reproduction for sale of pages in this book is permitted only under license from ACS. Direct these and other permissions requests to ACS Copyright Office, Publications Division, 1155 16th Street, N.W., Washington, DC 20036.

The citation of trade names and/or names of manufacturers in this publication is not to be construed as an endorsement or as approval by ACS of the commercial products or services referenced herein; nor should the mere reference herein to any drawing, specification, chemical process, or other data be regarded as a license or as a conveyance of any right or permission to the holder, reader, or any other person or corporation, to manufacture, reproduce, use, or sell any patented invention or copyrighted work that may in any way be related thereto. Registered names, trademarks, etc., used in this publication, even without specific indication thereof, are not to be considered unprotected by law.

PRINTED IN THE UNITED STATES OF AMERICA

Advisory Board

ACS Symposium Series

Mary E. Castellion
ChemEdit Company

Arthur B. Ellis
University of Wisconsin at Madison

Jeffrey S. Gaffney
Argonne National Laboratory

Gunda I. Georg
University of Kansas

Lawrence P. Klemann
Nabisco Foods Group

Richard N. Loeppky
University of Missouri

Cynthia A. Maryanoff
R. W. Johnson Pharmaceutical
   Research Institute

Roger A. Minear
University of Illinois
   at Urbana–Champaign

Omkaram Nalamasu
AT&T Bell Laboratories

Kinam Park
Prudue University

Katherine R. Porter
Duke University

Douglas A. Smith
The DAS Group, Inc.

Martin R. Tant
Eastman Chemical Co.

Michael D. Taylor
Parke-Davis Pharmaceutical
   Research

Leroy B. Townsend
University of Michigan

William C. Walker
DuPont Company

Foreword

THE ACS SYMPOSIUM SERIES was first published in 1974 to provide a mechanism for publishing symposia quickly in book form. The purpose of this series is to publish comprehensive books developed from symposia, which are usually "snapshots in time" of the current research being done on a topic, plus some review material on the topic. For this reason, it is necessary that the papers be published as quickly as possible.

Before a symposium-based book is put under contract, the proposed table of contents is reviewed for appropriateness to the topic and for comprehensiveness of the collection. Some papers are excluded at this point, and others are added to round out the scope of the volume. In addition, a draft of each paper is peer-reviewed prior to final acceptance or rejection. This anonymous review process is supervised by the organizer(s) of the symposium, who become the editor(s) of the book. The authors then revise their papers according to the recommendations of both the reviewers and the editors, prepare camera-ready copy, and submit the final papers to the editors, who check that all necessary revisions have been made.

As a rule, only original research papers and original review papers are included in the volumes. Verbatim reproductions of previously published papers are not accepted.

ACS BOOKS DEPARTMENT

Contents

Preface ix

WINE COMPOSITION

1. Wine: Yesterday's Antidote for Today's Oxygen Stress 2
   Tom R. Watkins

2. Chromatography of Phenolics in Wine 6
   Jean-Pierre Roggero, P. Archier, and S. Coen

3. Levels of Phenolics in California Varietal Wines 12
   Andrew L. Waterhouse and Pierre-Louis Teissedre

4. Identification and Assay of Trihydroxystilbenes in Wine
   and Their Biological Properties 24
   David M. Goldberg, G. J. Soleas, S. E. Hahn, E. P. Diamandis,
   and A. Karumanchiri

5. Resveratrol in Wine 44
   Kenneth D. McMurtrey

6. Resveratrol and Piceid Levels in Wine Production and
   in Finished Wines 56
   Rosa M. Lamuela-Raventós, A. I. Romero-Pérez,
   Andrew L. Waterhouse, M. Lloret,
   and M. C. de la Torre-Boronat

7. The Content of Catechins and Procyanidins in Grapes and
   Wines as Affected by Agroecological Factors and Technological
   Practices 69
   Eugenio Revilla, E. Alonso, and V. Kovac

8. The Structures of Tannins in Grapes and Wines and Their
   Interactions with Proteins 81
   Véronique Cheynier, Corine Prieur, Sylvain Guyot,
   Jacques Rigaud, and Michel Moutounet

9. Enantiomeric Analysis of Linalool for the Study of the Muscat Wine Flavorings Composition 94
   Fernando Tateo, E. Desimoni, and M. Bononi

10. Monitoring Authenticity and Regional Origin of Wines by Natural Stable Isotope Ratios Analysis 113
    Giuseppe Versini, A. Monetti, and F. Reniero

HEALTH BENEFITS

11. The Epidemiology of Alcohol and Cardiovascular Diseases 132
    Arthur L. Klatsky

12. Wine Antioxidants and Their Impact on Antioxidant Activity In Vivo 150
    Simon R. J. Maxwell

13. The Relative Antioxidant Potencies of Some Polyphenols in Grapes and Wines 166
    Alessandro Baldi, Annalisa Romani, Nadia Mulinacci, Franco F. Vincieri, and Andrea Ghiselli

14. Metabolic Syndrome X and the French Paradox 180
    Linda F. Bisson

15. Wine Phenolics and Targets of Chronic Disease 196
    J. Bruce German, Edwin N. Frankel, Andrew L. Waterhouse, Robert J. Hansen, and Rosemary L. Walzem

16. An In Vivo Experimental Protocol for Identifying and Evaluating Dietary Factors That Delay Tumor Onset: Effect of Red Wine Solids 215
    Susan E. Ebeler, Andrew J. Clifford, John D. Ebeler, Nathan D. Bills, and Steven H. Hinrichs

17. The Role of Wine in Ethyl Carbamate Induced Carcinogenesis Inhibition 230
    Gilbert S. Stoewsand, J. L. Anderson, and L. Munson

18. Endothelium-Dependent Vasorelaxing Activity of Wine, Grapes, and Other Plant Products 237
    David F. Fitzpatrick, Ronald G. Coffey, and Paul T. Jantzen

19. Antithrombotic Effect of Flavonoids in Red Wine 247
    N. Maalej, H. S. Demrow, P. R. Slane, and John D. Folts

20. California Wine Use Leads to Improvement of Thrombogenic and Peroxidation Risk Factors in Hyperlipemic Subjects................ 261
Tom R. Watkins and Marvin L. Bierenbaum

INDEXES

Author Index 276

Affiliation Index 276

Subject Index 277

Preface

IN HIS FAMOUS OATH, HIPPOCRATES said that he would use food first to treat disease and alleviate suffering in his patients. Natural products still serve as models for therapeutic substances. No wonder that wine has enjoyed a renaissance as an important part of the diet in recorded history. Wine has received considerable attention in the past decade because of its potential value in tempering risk factors for cardiovascular and other diseases. Which constituents in wine may confer such protection? Phenolics, which are abundantly present, may be important as antioxidants.

Exposure of food to oxygen leads to premature aging of the food in the form of peroxidized lipid and other compounds. Food quality generally deteriorates upon exposure to oxygen (under appropriate environmental conditions), resulting in a loss of palatability and eventually consumer rejection. To prevent food deterioration, antioxidants such as phenolics (e.g., butylated hydroxytoluene) are added to items such as breakfast cereals.

Both grape juice and wine are naturally endowed with abundant amounts of phenolics and other reducing substances. Better analytical tools now enable us to analyze the phenolic composition of foods and beverages such as fruit, juice, and wine in great detail.

The tissue damage and deterioration of food quality by toxic forms of oxygen, such as peroxy fatty acids, have received wide attention recently, especially with the popularity of Steinberg's hypothesis of risk associated with the oxidized low-density lipoprotein (LDL) lipid particle. Newer packaging strategies have been developed to protect food from oxygen-induced damage to lipids. Aluminum foil has been replaced with laminated polyester films to preclude oxygen interaction with food, thus enhancing product stability and safety for the consumer. Potato chips, for example, are now packaged to prevent oxygen exposure and damage.

On another front, in about 1920 Bishop and Evans in Berkeley learned of the importance of substances in lettuce, now known as antioxidants, in protecting virility in the male laboratory rat and reproductive capacity in the female. When semipurified diets lacked a lettuce addendum, the male became sterile and the female resorbed her pups. Soon thereafter, Alcott isolated phenolic substances with reducing potential from lettuce and identified them as the protective factors. A diet without these reducing substances led to sterility and resorption of pups, while restoration of them led to virility and restoration of fertility in the female. They were aptly named "tocopherols", derived from the Greek for childbearing (τοκοσ + φερειν). Their role in protecting polyunsaturated tissue lipid from oxygen damage is now better understood.

Gey observed some fifty years later that the phenolic content of the blood, in particular the α-tocopherol level, has more predictive power for cardiovascular disease risk than the classic risk factors smoking, hypertension, or serum cholesterol. This still startles some. One may wonder what phenolic-like substances other than tocopherols the diet provides.

Renaud's observation that the residents of southern France have a much lower incidence of cardiovascular disease than their age-matched Irish counterparts, in spite of the fact that more of the French smoke cigarettes, eat fat-rich diets, and generally have higher serum cholesterol levels than the Irish, has seemed contradictory. He termed this contradiction the French Paradox. Because French alcohol consumption, especially wine, is about twice as great as Irish alcohol consumption, attention is focused on the composition of wine and other alcoholic beverages. Which factors in wine, if any, might confer protection against such known risks?

It is within this context that we have investigated wine composition and some of its potential health benefits. What are some of the key components in wine that may decrease the damage associated with oxygen that eventually leads to increased cardiovascular risk, even death?

The symposium on which this book is based was sponsored by the ACS Division of Agricultural and Food Chemistry at the 210th National Meeting of the American Chemical Society, which took place in Chicago, Illinois, August 20–24, 1995. The papers in this volume explore the composition of wine and its potential health benefits when consumed regularly.

Chromatographic and other problems associated with measuring phenolics, stilbenes and other reducing substances in wine are discussed, with special attention given to stilbenes and piceids.

Ecology and agronomic practice may influence crop yield and quality. These factors are reviewed here, especially in terms of catechins and procyanidins. Tannin composition, structure, and protein interaction in wine are also discussed.

Economic pressure often leads to deception in the marketplace. In the case of the wine trade, we have included papers about evaluating adulterants in wine. Labeling misrepresentation of the origin of wines as revealed by appropriate isotope ratio analysis is also addressed.

Once imbibed, does the human digestive system actually take up these reducing substances in wine intact? Data are presented showing the uptake—and its kinetics—of usable reducing power from wine by the digestive system. A review of epidemiological evidence shows the correlation between consumption of beverage alcohol and protection from cardiovascular risk factors.

Antioxidants may confer detoxifying potential in the diet in terms of several chronic diseases, and this concept is reviewed in an orderly fashion. Further detailed questions are evaluated, such as the role of wine as a source of ethanolic energy and its implication in metabolic syndrome X. Two papers present evidence about wine antioxidants and inhibition of cancer in animal models, more specifically tumor onset in a transgenic mouse model and ethyl carbamate induced carcinogenesis.

Wine antioxidants have been shown to temper thrombogenic risk factors in animal models and human subjects. In terms of cardiovascular risk factors, wine and grape components have been shown to induce endothelial-dependent vasorelaxing activity. The importance of French red wine in inhibiting platelet aggregation and prolonging bleeding time is discussed. The potential benefit to the hyperlipemic subject, the person presumed at very high heart risk, of regular California wine use in modest quantity—both red and white—was evaluated in terms of decreased thrombogenic risk.

Evidence presented by these experts has shown that the composition of wine can afford the user with many antioxidant compounds. Facts are also presented demonstrating that the body will use these reducing substances in wine for protection against cardiovascular and other risk factors when taken daily, even in modest amounts.

No book can be compiled without the cooperation of many people. This book is truly international in flavor. I thank the contributors for their expert and timely contributions. To the many reviewers I also extend a thank you. I gratefully acknowledge the support of Elisabeth Holmgren and the Wine Institute (California); C. T. Ho and the American Chemical Society; and Marvin Bierenbaum and the Kenneth L. Jordan Heart Foundation. I especially appreciate the constructive criticism of Marvin Bierenbaum, the Director of the Jordan Foundation.

We commend this volume to you with the hope that wine, the "fruit of the vine", will be given due recognition for its social and wellness benefits. Let us give Hippocrates his due respect. King Solomon said, "A little wine makes the heart glad." St. Paul advised his protege Timothy, "Take a little wine instead of water for your frequent infirmities." We offer more evidence here that their advice was sound. Indeed, in moderation wine may lead to a glad and healthy heart.

TOM R. WATKINS
Kenneth L. Jordan Heart Foundation
48 Plymouth Street
Montclair, NJ 07042

December 2, 1996

WINE COMPOSITION

Chapter 1

Wine: Yesterday's Antidote for Today's Oxygen Stress

Tom R. Watkins

Kenneth L. Jordan Heart Foundation, 48 Plymouth Street, Montclair, NJ 07042

Health and vitality rests on more than good genes. Good food and 'accessory food factors' must be available to maintain the internal milieu of the cell, to provide inputs capable of supporting life, balanced for a state of optimal health. The balanced inputs we call good nutrition. Formerly, the 'accessory food factors', now called vitamins and minerals, were typically associated with alleviation of specific disease symptoms. Lack of adequate ascorbic acid led to the scorbutic condition. Thus, we have a list of 'recommended dietary allowances' (RDA's), recommended levels of intake designed to promote health and vitality in most of the population. Each of these has been defined by a one-to-one correspondence established by demonstrating that the absence of a nutrient results in the presentation of a set of particular symptoms. Now, other benefits have been associated with risk modification for many chronic diseases when levels of key essential nutrients have been added above and beyond the RDA's. This can be illustrated by vitamin E, one of the antioxidant nutrients. To protect against hemolytic anemia, 30 milligrams of vitamin E would suffice, whereas several hundred would be needed to protect against cardiovascular risk factors.

Toxic forms of oxygen have been implicated in the causation of chronic disease, such as cardiovascular disease, cancer, viral disease and arthritis. The toxicity may be mediated by superoxide anion. According to this notion, a metabolic imbalance between reducing substances and toxic oxygen stress as free radicals, such as superoxide and hydroxyl, heavily favoring toxic oxygen species leads to disease, as postulated by Gerschman and Gilbert (1). Later, McCord and Fridovich (2) pointed out the nature and danger of the superoxide anion and the presumed importance of the superoxide dismutase enzymes (SOD's). The SOD's detoxify superoxide in affected tissue by dismutation. He and his co-workers then formulated the superoxide theory of disease. The healthy body maintains defenses against superoxide and other toxic oxygen radicals in the form of vitamins and enzymes with reducing potential. If (and when) the level of such

© 1997 American Chemical Society

oxygen radicals exceeds the available reducing capacity, i. e. antioxidant reserve, such toxic oxygen stress will lead to tissue damage. Damaged tissue unrepaired leads to debilitating disease.

Further, in the presence of certain transition metals, superoxide accumulation can lead indirectly to more serious tissue damage via metal catalyzed oxidation reactions. Hydrogen peroxide and hydroxyl radical will be formed from superoxide in the presence of ferrous ion as originally described by Fenton (3). Hydroxyl radical (·OH), perhaps the most reactive oxygen based radical, can damage any organic substance near the site where it is generated. For example, fats--particularly polyunsaturated ones--readily react to yield carbon centered radicals and peroxy radicals form once oxygen has been attached. These intiate chain reactions that perpetuate tissue damage. Such damage to tissue lipids has been implicated in the development of chronic disease.

In cardiovascular disease, lipid peroxy radicals have been identified as a risk factor in both atherosclerosis and thrombosis, the increased tendency of platelets to clump together so obstructing normal blood flow. These cells, a fraction the size of the red blood cell, normally protect against internal hemorrhage by clumping. In the presence of peroxy radicals, their clumping tendency increases, thus increasing thrombogenic risk. [The well known effect of aspirin counters such thrombogenic risk.] Gey (4) has reported epidemiologic evidence showing that serum antioxidant vitamin levels have greater forcasting power in predicting risk than the classical risk factors serum cholesterol, smoking status and elevated blood pressure. Antioxidant vitamins such as vitamin E--when provided in the diet in adequate amounts, amounts considerably larger than RDA levels--can attenuate the risk of cardiovascular disease by detoxifying such oxygen radicals.

The DNA polymer in the nucleus of each cell, the genetic blue print for cell growth and reproduction, may also be seriously damaged by oxygen radicals. Hydroxyl radical attacks guanine, one of the four chief bases in DNA, yielding 8-OH-guanine. Available dietary antioxidant reserves can sacrifice themselves, 'take the free radical hit', thus protecting the DNA. In due course this oxygen damaged base may be excised so that the DNA will be a faithful template for the reproducing cell. However, in conditions of insufficient antioxidant supplies, when so many of these bases have been damaged that the antioxidant and repair defenses have been exceeded, an erroneous DNA template exists. When the cell begins to divide, transformed cells will be produced. Thus, cancer is a possible outcome, as has been discussed by Ames and his colleagues (5).

Fruit, such as the grape and wine, and vegetables are major sources of anitoxidants in the diet. Presently, according to Block (6) only 9% of Americans eat enough fruits and vegetables each day to obtain and maintain sufficient antioxidant reserves to thwart the level of radiation damage to which the body is subjected each day. The consequences in terms of chronic disease are dire.

Cardiovascular disease alone leads to one million deaths annually in the United States. More than 59 million Americans actually suffer from this disease (7). Oxidation of the LDL particle, a major cholesterol carrying lipoprotein structure in the blood, greatly enhances its atherogenicity (8). Once peroxidized, this toxic form of this cholesterol and fatty acid laden particle proceeds to injure the arterial wall, leading to a compensatory emergency response there to remove the toxic, damaging particle from the circulation. The oxidized LDL particle by its nature may attract monocytes to the site of arterial injury, leading to accumulation of macrophages now fat-laden and unable to leave the site of injury. This ultimately leads to accumulation of much oxidized (toxic) lipid there. Oxidized LDL may also stimulate the monocyte to release chemoattractant proteins, thereby recruiting more monocytes. As this debris builds up, constricting the arterial diameter, the site is ripe for trapping a cluster of sticky platelets coursing through the artery. When platelets are thus trapped, an infarction occurs, killing local tissue by oxygen starvation (ischemia). Unoxidized LDL does not thus attract the monocyte.

What sort of protection could effectively thwart a foe such as toxic oxygen, be it superoxide, hydroxyl radical, hydrogen or fatty peroxide or some other? The ideal candidate would be a substance readily oxidizable, *i. e.*, a reducing substance, able to sacrifice itself to save the LDL particle (DNA, protein, etc.), and ultimately the artery. Such reducing substances have been styled *anti*oxidants.

The therapeutic potential of wine has been touted since ancient days. Paul's advice (9) in scripture to an oft ailing assistant named Timothy included the exhortation, "No longer drink only water, but use a little wine for the sake of your stomach and your frequent ailments." Various substances in wine other than the alcohol may indeed temper, even decrease one's peroxidation potential, one's risk for succumbing to a chronic disease such as heart disease or cancer.

Renewed interest in wine and its nutritional and therapeutic benefits has arisen from Renaud's observation (10). He observed that the folk in Toulousse, France, people eating fat-rich diets, smoking cigarettes, and avoiding much exercise, have a remarkably low incidence of heart disease morbidity and mortality, in comparison with age matched folk in Belfast, Ireland, who share all of these common risk factors. The major difference in their habits was noted to be that the French consumed about twice as much alcohol--most of it wine--as the Irish (45 vs. 20 grams/day). This observation has been styled the 'French paradox'.

Wine is a rich source of flavonoids and other polyphenolic antioxidants. Taken on a regular basis as part of a varied diet, could wine (even grape juice) provide sufficient amounts of these antioxidants to alter cardiovascular and other risk factors significantly? We have presented considerable evidence herein about the identity, nature and concentration of several polyphenols, resveratrols and some resveratrol glycosides, as well as information about signs of adulteration of wine, and some chemical signatures useful as 'ID cards' in documenting origin and fraudulent labelling of wine. Environmental and soil factors modulate crop quality. On this basis, we have examined the content and quality of numerous antioxidants in wine as modulated by agronomic and ecologic stresses.

Wine, the aged 'fruit of the vine', indeed provides a wide spectrum of antioxidants. Incorporation of these reducing substances into test rations for animals in model studies has conferred protection against carcinogenesis and transformation. Were they similarly included in human dietaries would they be absorbed and confer health benefits?

A large and growing body of evidence supports the nutritional value and therapeutic potential of wine in human diets, both as a source of energy and antioxidants. Epidemiologic data shows that both alcohol and wine confer protection against cardiovascular disease, affording protection against both atherogenic and thrombogenic risks. Substances in wine also enhance blood flow by promoting vasodilation, inhibiting peroxidation processes thereby conferring antioxidant protection (measured by various and sundry methods of detecting toxic oxygen species), prolonging bleeding time (thinning the blood), and preventing the platelet aggregation which immediately precedes a possibly fatal heart attack (myocardial infarction) or stroke (cerebral infarction).

The toxic oxygen radical, unfettered and unchecked in the body, has been recognized as an important risk factor in the etiology of chronic, killer disease. The hazard of the oxygen radical can be countered by various antioxidants. Wine, rich in reducing substances, certainly offers therapeutic potential for many chronic diseases, such as cardiovascular disease and cancer, which account for about 75% of the deaths in America. In the papers that follow, several of the benefits will be documented and mechanisms offered for your edification. The evidence presented suggests that we may be wise to look back in time to wine, one of the older, natural beverages, in order to step into a future of safe and effective nutritional therapy.

References

1   Gerschman, K., Gilbert, D. L., Nye, S. W., Dwyer, P. and Fenn, W. O. *Oxygen poisoning and X-irradiation: a common mechanism.* Science 1954, 119: 623-626.
2   McCord, J. M. and Fridovich, I. Superoxide dismutase. An enzymatic function for erythrocuprein (hemocuprein). *J. Biol. Chem.* **1969**, *244*, 6049-6055.
        Fridovich, I. Superoxide radical: an endogenous toxicant. *Ann. Rev. Pharmacol. Toxicol.* **1983**, *23*, 239-247.
        _____. Superoxide dismutases. *Meth. Enzymol.* **1986**, *58*, 61-97.
3   Gutteridge, J. M. C. and Halliwell, B. Iron toxicity and oxygen radicals, In *Iron Chelating Therapy*, Vol 2; Ed. C. Hershko; Bailliere Tindall: London, 1989; pp. 195-256.
4   Gey, K. F., Puska, P., Jordan, P., and Moser, U. Inverse correlation between plasma vitamin E and mortality from ischemic heart disease in cross-cultural epidemiology. *Am. J. Clin. Nutr.* **1991**, *53*, 326S-334S.
5   Ames, B. N. Endogenous oxidative DNA damage, ageing and cancer. *Free Rad. Res. Comm.* **1989**, 7: 121-128.
        _____, Shigenaga, M. K., and Hagen, T. M. Oxidants, antioxidants and the degenerative diseases of aging. *Proc. Natl. Acad. Sci. USA* **1993**, *90*, 7915-7922.
6   Block, G. Epidemiological evidence regarding vitamin C and cancer. *Am. J. Clin. Nutr.* **1991**, *54*, 1310S-1314S.
7   American Heart Association statistics, 1992.
8   Steinberg, D. Beyond cholesterol: modifications of low density lipoprotein that increase its atherogenicity. *New Engl. J. Med.* **1991**, *328*, 1427-1429.
9   1 Tim. 5:23, Revised Standard Version, Grand Rapids, Zondervan, 1971.
10 Renaud, S. and de Lorgeril, M. Wine, alcohol, platelets, and the French paradox for coronary heart disease. *Lancet* **1992**, *339*, 1523-1526.

Chapter 2

Chromatography of Phenolics in Wine

Jean-Pierre Roggero, P. Archier, and S. Coen

Laboratoire de Chimie Organique et Analytique, Faculté des Sciences de l'Université d'Avignon, 33 rue Louis Pasteur, 84000 Avignon, France

In wine phenolics analysis, extraction induces many artefacts due to oxidation, isomerization or hydrolysis. Moreover, extraction is never exhaustive as wine is actually a partially colloidal solution; as a consequence, the recovery of many substances is low. The assay of many phenolics, based upon a recovery ratio determined from the extraction of an artificial mixture, is then generally wrong. The analysis via direct injection of wine into the chromatographic column avoids most of these difficulties, but requires an efficient and thermostated column, a perfectly adapted gradient and the use of a diode array detector. In some cases confirmation may be obtained by electrochemical or fluorometric detection. Up to 30 compounds may be identified and assayed including catechins and proanthocyanidins, caffeic, p-coumaric and ferulic acids and their combinations with tartaric acid, vanillic, gallic, protocatechuic, p-hydroxybenzoic, syringic acids, tyrosol, tryptophol, flavonols and flavonol glycosides, resveratrol, etc.

The growing interest in chromatography of phenolics in wine has arisen for several reasons some of which are taxonomic, as the concentrations of the various phenolics, which depend on the variety and on the age of the wine, permit one to distinguish the vintage. Better chromatography serves sanitary purposes, because the phenolic composition may be altered by illness and so reveal an unhealthy crop. Good chromatography has also been used to document changes during aging.

Owing to the presence of a considerable quantity of various compounds, these analyses are difficult, and the analyst always chose to extract the compounds of interest, in order to obtain a clear chromatogram. Some of them require two extractions of the wine, the first at pH 7.0 to extract neutral phenolics, and the second at pH 2.0 for phenolic acids. They generally use ethyl acetate or ethyl ether as solvents. Others choose the percolation upon a column of Polyclar AT or a C-18 cartridge and wash it with various buffers or solvents before recovering the compounds. Unfortunately, many artefacts result from these manipulations:

-1) Many phenolics are easily oxidized, especially in basic medium, and, even when extraction is done under nitrogen, the risk remains evident.

-2) Another possibility is hydrolysis of esters in basic solution and of ethers in acidic medium, and so, many glycosidic bonds may be broken.

-3) Moreover some isomerization may occur, and particularly upon caffeic and p-coumaric acids or esters which are frequently detected in the *cis*-form, which is not apparent in our analyses.

The main feature of any wine extraction is not to be exhaustive or reproducible, because of the important and variable associations between the different phenols. This explains why quercetin, whose solubility is zero in water and very low in ethanol, may be detected in large quantities in some wines. Consequently, all the authors who calculate the recovery ratios of various phenolics by extracting them from a synthetic wine, constituted of ethanol, water and potassium hydrogen tartrate, and which lacks the colloidal properties of a real wine, obtain very low results for many compounds.

For all these reasons, and despite the difficulties, we tried several years ago to develop a method for analysis of wine phenolics via direct injection of the filtered sample into the chromatographic column.

Setup of the method

The first analyses via direct injection were performed using a binary gradient G-1 between a 5% acetic acid solution and a mixture of water, acetic acid and acetonitrile (*1*). In that confusing analysis, the first difficulty we encountered was detection, as several compounds being very close in the chromatogram it became apparent that a double detection at 280 and 313 nm was insufficient. Moreover, we noted a large hump in which the condensed tannins were not separated. The problem was partially solved by use of a diode array detector, which gave a plot at any wavelength and the uv spectra of all compounds, which was essential in these analyses. It was also noteworthy that some columns, even very efficient, were not able to separate some critical pairs. We finally chose the Merck Superspher RP18, 250x4 mm.

Owing to the large number of compounds we detected, the gradient was extended to 150 minutes. Still, some separations remained difficult. We tried a ternary gradient G-2 between 1% and 5% acetic acid solutions and water-acetic acid-acetonitrile 65/5/30, beginning with only 1% of acetic acid and slowly increasing it before introducing acetonitrile into the elution solvent (*2*). This modification permitted separation of the peaks of catechins and proanthocyanidins which are very sensitive to acetic acid concentration and then to improvement of their separation from other compounds. The result was further enhanced by a slight change in the gradient shape (G-3). See Table.

Time (min)	A%	B%	C%
0	100	0	0
15	0	100	0
30	0	100	0
50	0	90	10
60	0	80	20
80	0	70	30
120	0	0	100

The last modification we have done was required by the long time of analysis which results in sensitivity to variations in temperature. After a series of trials, we chose to maintain the temperature at 22.5°C by water circulation, and to accomplish that we used a continuously acting cryogenic coil and a regulated heating coil (3). Thus, no variation above one-half a minute was ever noted. Nevertheless, we observed that, for some critical pairs, separation was obtained only when the second solvent B is a 5% acetic acid solution; for others it was necessary to use a 6% solution. Using 5% acetic acid p-hydroxybenzoic acid was separated, but proanthocyanidin B1 and coutaric acid were not separated. In the chromatogram obtained using a 6% acetic acid solution, these compounds were well resolved but three other minor compounds, namely, p-coumaroyl-tartaric acid glucosidic ester, GRP (Grape Reaction Product, or 2-S-glutathionyl caftaric acid), and di-caffeoyl-tartaric acid were not separated, and p-hydroxybenzoic acid lay under the large peak of coutaric acid. We generally prefer this second analysis to the first.

The separations obtained with our method were then excellent, and permitted us to survey the changes in the content of many phenolics during wine making (4). Nevertheless, the presence of acetic acid in the elution solvent did not permit the detector to be used below 240 nm. So, we are now trying a gradient using phosphoric acid. Unfortunately, an increase in phosphoric acid concentration gave no real effect upon retention and we could only perform a binary gradient. However, the use of phosphoric acid permitted us to obtain uv spectra at low wavelengths, and therefore to distinguish two very closely related compounds like resveratrol and piceid.

The gradient modifications we have done also moved the hump for condensed tannins to a part of the chromatogram where few compounds of interest were detected.

Results

In a single analysis most of the phenolics may be detected including:

Phenolic acids and esters: Gallic, protocatechuic, vanillic, caffeic, p-coumaric and syringic acids, tartaric acid caffeate and tartaric acid p-coumarate (often named caftaric and coutaric acids) are easily detected and assayed. Ferulic acid was usually present in low concentration and p-hydroxybenzoic acid was difficult to detect because it was co-eluted with the abundant coutaric acid. Nevertheless, the slight modification, which consisted of use of a 5% solution of acetic acid as second solvent instead of a 6% solution, permitted its detection, as previously noted. Its concentration was usually below 1 mg/litre. The ethyl esters of caffeic and coumaric acids were also present in old wines.

Catechins and proanthocyanidins: Catechin gave a clean and important peak that was easily assayed, but epicatechin appeared in a confusing part of the chromatogram where several other compounds, some of them giving peaks whose uv spectra were very close one with another, were also present. We found that an electrochemical detector was very useful in identifying epicatechin when the content of that phenol was low, because it easily detects the ortho-diphenols, even at low potential. That instrument also distinguished caffeic and p-coumaric acid derivatives.

Three proanthocyanidins, namely B1, B2 and B3, the latter in very low abundance, were also detected. The peak for B2 was close to caffeic acid, but was too large to be easily assayed. Several other proanthocyanidins, although evident, were not identified.

Flavonols and flavonol glycosides: These compounds appeared in the last part of the chromatogram, between 100 and 130 minutes of analysis, and some of them co-eluted with anthocyanins. Fortunately, anthocyanins lack absorbency between 330 and 450 nm, whereas flavonols and flavonol glycosides absorb respectively at 370 and 355 nm. That feature permitted us to detect and assay these compounds, and to record their spectra, although the part between 240 and 300 nm may have been distorted in some cases by anthocyanin's absorbency. Anthocyanins themselves could not be clearly separated and identified in that analysis because of the very high pH value of the mobile phase. They may be analysed separately using a water, formic acid and acetonitrile mixture of pH 1.6 (4).

Discussion

The relative percentages of flavonols and flavonol glycosides are important in taxonomic studies. They allow distinction of some varieties. For instance, the wines from Cabernet-Sauvignon are rich in flavonols (myricetin and quercetin, max 372 nm) and relatively poor in glycosides and those from Mourvèdre pre- sent an exceptional content in flavonol glycosides (max 355 nm).

Quercetin is the most abundant flavonol in wine; two of its glycosides are also present, one of them is isoquercitrin, the other perhaps rutin. Myricetin is less important, but a large peak, not yet identified, is very likely a myricetin glycoside. Kaempferol is absent, or in very low quantity.

Other compounds: Tyrosol, 2(p-hydroxyphenyl) ethanol and tryptophol, (-ind olyl ethyl alcohol) are respectively produced by decomposition of tyrosine or tryptophan. The first is abundant, easily observed and assayed, but the peak of the second lies in a confusing part of the chromatogram. It could have a taxonomic interest, but is difficult to assay precisely.

Trans-resveratrol recently took on increasing importance for many researchers. The growing interest for that molecule results from its supposed role in wine's protective action against coronary heart diseases. We had for several years detected in wine two compounds of retention time 104 and 119 min having very close uv spectra, but we never were able to identify them until Siemann and Creasy (6) reported the presence of *trans*-resveratrol in wine and showed its uv spectrum. Thus, resveratrol was quickly identified in our chromatograms, and on the basis of its retention time and uv spectrum, we postulated that the other compound may be a resveratrol-glycoside. That hypothesis was recently confirmed by the discovery of piceid (resveratrol 3-glucoside) in wine by Waterhouse, Lamuela-Raventos and co-workers (7,8).

The only difference between trans-resveratrol and trans-resveratrol-glycoside spectra lies in the 200-230 region and the use of a solvent constituted with phosphoric acid instead of acetic acid is necessary to observe that difference.

Many authors have indicated the presence of *cis*-resveratrol in wine. In our research we proved that gentle uv illumination of *trans*-resveratrol induces the formation of the *cis* isomer. Intense irradiation leads to the formation of an unknown compound, a derivative of which is present in wine. These two compounds of max absorbance at 260 nm are highly fluorescent at 372 nm when excited at 270 nm and then easily detected using a fluorescence detector (9). *Cis*-resveratrol is also present in wine, but not in the grape berry skins of many varieties; it may be formed during fermentation. It should be noted that the greater part of the resveratrol in the skins is in piceid state.

Assay of the components

For the phenolics, which may be purchased in pure state from various commercial companies, the external standard mode is used without any difficulty. In most cases, the peak area gives a linear plot versus concentration, but when large variations are observed, as for gallic acid which is very abundant in some wines, Beer's law may be not followed, and the assay requires using of a calibration curve.

In other cases, we tentatively used a uv response identical to that of a closely related compound. So, we consider that caftaric acid may be assayed using the molar calibration factor of caffeic acid at 328 nm, and coutaric acid by using the molar calibration factor of p-coumaric acid at 310 nm. These assumptions allow an element of comparison between the different samples.

For *cis*-resveratrol, which is practically impossible to obtain in pure state, we used a partial light induced isomerization of the *trans* isomer and we measured the peak areas of both forms. The calculated absorbency of 12,000 at 286 nm is in line with that of cis-stilbene which is 13,500 at 280 nm.

Conclusions

Despite its apparent heaviness, the present method holds many advantages over prior extraction methods. As detection and assay are done by less handling of the sample, its main interest is to give, qualitatively and quantitatively, the actual content of the wine, because problems involved by extraction are avoided. Another advantage of the method is to show most of the phenolic constituents in a single analysis. However, many peaks remain unidentified at the present time.

Naturally, the analysis requires a diode array detector, an efficient column and a thermostatic device. The one we use consists of a cryogenic coil immersed in an ordinary thermostatic bath. The time for analysis is 2-1/2 hours and hence is similar to that required for extraction and cleanup of a sample.

The main difficulty, which is not inherent to this method of analysis, was the presence of acetic acid in the mobile phase. That solvent permits use of a ternary gradient, but results in a cut-off at 240 nm and then does not permit recording uv spectra at lower wavelengths. In several cases this limitation may cause doubtful identification of phenolics. For this reason, we are now working on the use of phosphoric acid.

Literature cited

1 Roggero, J-P., Archier, P. Mise au point d'une méthode de dosage des phénols simples des vins. Application à des vins d'origines et d'ages différents. *Connaiss. Vigne Vin*, **1989**, *23,* 25-37.
2 Roggero, J-P., Coen, S., Archier, P. Wine phenolics : Optimization of HPLC Analysis. *J. Liquid. Chromatogr.* **1990**, *13,* 2593-2603.
3 Roggero, J-P., Archier, P., Coen, S. Wine Phenolics Analysis via Direct Injection : Enhancement of the Method. *J. Liquid. Chromatogr.* **1991**, *14,* 533-538.
4 Roggero, J-P., Archier, P., Coen, S. Etude par CLHP des compositions phénolique et anthocyanique d'un moût de raisin en fermentation. *Sci Aliments*, **1992**, *12,* 37-46.
5 Roggero, J-P., Archier, P. Dosage du resvératrol et de l'un de ses glycosides dans les vins. *Sci Aliments*, **1994**, *14,* 99-107.
6 Siemann, E. H., Creasy, L. L. Concentration of the phytoalexin resveratrol in wine. *Am J Enol.Vit*, **1992**, *43,* 49-52.
7 Waterhouse, A. L. The occurence of piceid, a stilbene glucoside, in grape berries. In: Compositions phénolique et anthocyanique d'un moût de raisin en Lamuela-Raventos, R. M., ed.; *Phytochemistry,* **1994**, *37,* 571-573.
8 Lamuela-Raventos, R. M., Romero-Perez, A.I., Waterhouse, A.L., de La Torre, C. Direct HPLC analysis of *cis-* and *trans-* resveratrol and piceid isomers in spanish red *Vitis vinifera* wines. *J Agric Food Chem.* **1995**, *43,* 281-283.
9 Roggero, J-P., Garcia-Parilla, C. Effects of ultraviolet irradiation on resveratrol and changes in resveratrol and various of its derivatives in the skins of ripening grapes. *Sci Aliments*, **1995**, *15*

Chapter 3

Levels of Phenolics in California Varietal Wines

Andrew L. Waterhouse and Pierre-Louis Teissedre[1]

Department of Viticulture and Enology, University of California, Davis, CA 95616-8749

California wines are abundant sources of phenolic compounds, with some flavonoid classes having average concentrations of 250 mg/L in some wine varieties. Total phenol levels ranged from 1850-2200 mg/L for reds and 220-250 mg/L for white wines. The variability in the levels of individual components is striking, and thus it is essential to analyze wines for their content of individual phenolic components to ensure that the composition of a particular wine is known. This is of specific importance to ensure that nutritional and health-related studies are reproducible. Since phenolic compounds have both antioxidant activity and platelet inhibitory activity, they may be the wine components responsible for the decreased rate of cardiac heart disease mortality observed in wine drinkers, but further studies are needed to ascertain the validity of this hypothesis.

The interest in wine's potential to improve health is based on numerous epidemiological studies, both ecological and prospective, which have shown strong correlations between increased wine consumption and reduced cardiac heart disease. Cross cultural (or ecological epidemiology) studies, which compare average attributes of specific populations, show that when whole populations increase their average consumption of wine, average cardiac heart disease (CHD) mortality rates drop. In the first such study, St. Leger *et al* showed that there was an association between reduced cardiac disease mortality and increased wine consumption (*1*). More recently, Renaud and de Lorgeril used World Health Organization data to demonstrate that dairy fat consumption is highly correlated with CHD mortality. People in a few French (and other) cities however, had very high dairy fat consumption and high serum lipid levels, but CHD

---
[1]Current address: Université de Montpellier I, Faculté de Pharmacie, 15 Avenue Charles Flahault, 34060 Montpellier, France

© 1997 American Chemical Society

mortality rates that were far too low to fit the correlation—thus the "French Paradox". When the authors included wine consumption in the correlation as a factor that reduced CHD mortality, these cities were no longer outliers and overall a much better correlation was obtained (2). The authors could not explain the low rate of disease in these populations solely by the alcohol content of the diet. Criqui and Ringel have subsequently investigated similar data but compared intake of many different dietary components with mortality from many different causes and came to a similar conclusion—wine was one of the few dietary factors that correlated significantly with reduced CHD mortality, although it was not related to total mortality (3). However, one other result was even more intriguing—they also showed that one other dietary component was significantly correlated with reduced CHD mortality, fruit consumption. This is of particular interest because common components may be responsible for the two associations, a likely supposition because wine is made from fruit.

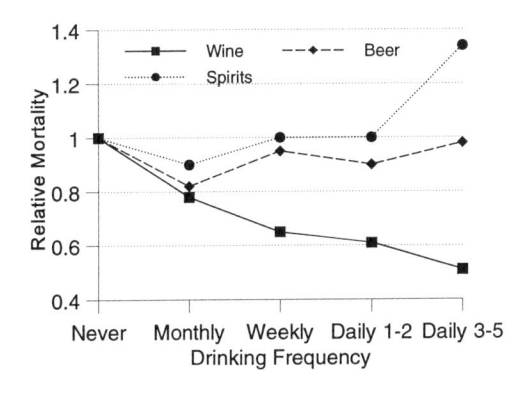

Figure 1 Relative Mortality Rates at Varying Consumption Rates for Specific Beverages. Adapted from (5).

In addition, prospective epidemiology studies have shown that wine consumption is correlated with a greater reduction in CHD mortality than other alcoholic beverages. Klatsky and Armstrong showed that drinkers who consume predominantly wine have mortality rates 50-70% of spirits drinkers (4). Nonetheless, they were unwilling to attribute this significant reduction in mortality to wine constituents, saying that U.S. wine consumers typically had lifestyle factors predisposing them to lower mortality, in particular, higher incomes and different exercise and eating habits. However, a recent prospective study from Denmark concludes that the reduction in CHD mortality attributed to alcohol is in fact solely due to wine (5) (Figure 1). At different levels of consumption, wine drinkers had total mortality rates 78-55% of non drinkers. The reduction was due primarily to lower CHD mortality rates. The authors did not suspect that in their population that lifestyle factors could explain this striking difference in mortality. These data strongly suggest that wine contains components absent in other alcoholic beverages, and it is these unique components which favorably affect CHD mortality.

A study relating increased flavonoid intake with reduced CHD mortality (6) definitely points to this class of substances, and perhaps by extension, to all phenolic substances, as the components responsible for the correlations seen with wine (7). The best correlation between reduced CHD mortality and specific dietary components was with tea, onions and apples (6). Two of these foods, tea and apples, are very rich sources of catechins, while onions are significant sources of quercetin glycosides (see

Figure 2) (8). So, the evidence appears to be quite compelling that flavonoid phenols are a very significant dietary factor in reducing CHD mortality. And wine, especially red wine, is a very rich dietary source of flavonoids compared to many other potential sources. A serving of wine provides an amount of flavonoids that is comparable to a similar serving of many fruits. Thus the flavonoid or other phenolic compounds in wine may be the critical dietary component that causes the observed reduction in CHD mortality in wine drinkers.

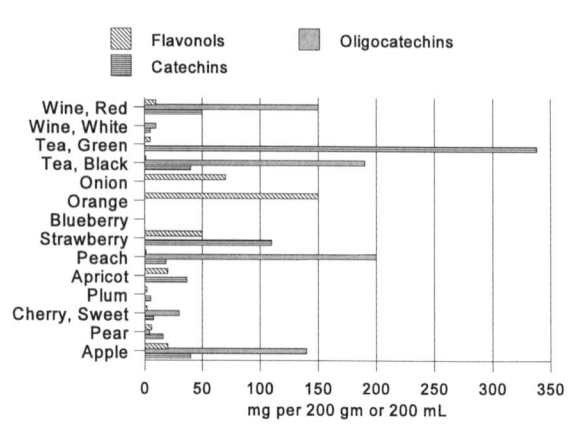

Figure 2 Levels of flavanol and flavonol phenolics in wine tea, and selected fruits.

Phenolic Compounds Found in Wine. The phenolic compounds which are found in wine are a class of phytochemicals widely distributed in plants, and ubiquitous in the

A flavan-3-ol, Catechin

An anthocyanin, Malvidin-3-glucoside

A flavan-3-ol oligomer, Procyanidin-B1

A flavonol, Quercetin

Figure 3 A representative selection of flavonoid compounds found in wine.

diet (9). There are several chemical classes of phenolic compounds found in food, broadly separated into two classes, the flavonoids and the non-flavonoids.

In grapes, the most significant sub-classes of the flavonoids are the flavan-3-ols (the monomers are also called the catechins), their oligomers (the proanthocyanidins) and polymers (the condensed tannins). In addition, there are the flavonols, and the anthocyanins, (Figure 3). There are numerous other classes of flavonoids, however, the quantities of these other classes in wine are generally low; as these other classes generally occur as biosynthetic intermediates in the production of the major classes.

The classes of flavonoids are distinguished by differences in the central oxygen-containing "C" ring (Figure 3). The "A" ring rarely has a different substitution pattern, typically having hydroxyl groups at positions 5 and 7. In most cases, class members are distinguished by differences in substitution on the "B" ring. On the B ring, two or three hydroxy or methoxy substituents at the 3', 4', and 5' positions are most common.

Nearly 5000 individual flavonoids have been characterized, (10). However, differences in the flavonoid nucleus account for only a few of these. In most cases, the different compounds arise by glycosylation or other substitution, and very large number of different sugars have been found to substitute flavonoids, in particular the flavonol class (9). The presence of specific flavonoids, based largely on the presence of specific glycosides can be used to verify the identity of the fruit species or occasionally the variety used to make a processed product such as juice or wine (11,12).

There are also several classes of non-flavonoids, dominated by a few groups including the benzoic acids and the hydroxycinnamates. There are other classes, such as the stilbene derivatives, but again the levels of these other components is low (Figure 4).

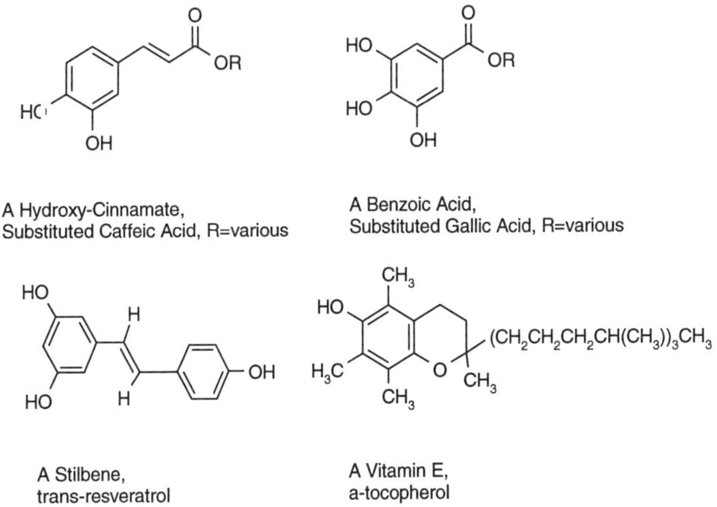

A Hydroxy-Cinnamate,
Substituted Caffeic Acid, R=various

A Benzoic Acid,
Substituted Gallic Acid, R=various

A Stilbene,
trans-resveratrol

A Vitamin E,
a-tocopherol

Figure 4 A selection of the non-flavonoid phenolics found in wine, fruit and tea.

Mechanisms of Action. Much current research focuses on deriving a mechanistic explanation by which wine consumption could reduce cardiac heart disease. One explanation for the effect of phenolics and or flavonoids arises from the oxidation theory of atherosclerosis (13,14). In this theory, arterial plaque develops from a series of steps that is initiated by the oxidation of blood lipid particles, in particular LDL. The oxidation occurs due to uncontrolled free radical reactions. When this occurs to LDL particles that are under the endothelial lining of the arterial wall, they are attacked by macrophages which cannot digest the entire particle as they contain cholesterol. This leaves a residue, which after several stages of development becomes arterial plaque. The potential benefits of antioxidants in retarding this process has been shown in animal models of the disease where synthetic antioxidants have had a significant effect (15).

Thus the question arises, could wine phenolics affect atherogenesis? In many situations, but not all, these phenolic compounds are antioxidants. A key study of wine by Frankel et al (16) showed that wine contained antioxidants towards the oxidation of LDL *in vitro*, and thus may slow the development of arterial plaque. Based on this interpretation, these authors hypothesized that the phenolic compounds (generally known to be antioxidants) found in wine were responsible for the French Paradox. A follow-up investigation on three wine phenolics showed that all were antioxidants towards LDL—the most potent were epicatechin and quercetin, while resveratrol was less potent, and the control, α-tocopherol (vitamin E), not found in wine, was least so (17). These results have engendered a large number of investigations into the antioxidant properties of these compounds as it is possible that these substances inhibit LDL oxidation *in vivo*.

In addition, wine phenolics are known platelet activity inhibitors (18) and thus may inhibit the formation of thrombotic clots. Wine and grape juice consumption has been shown to reduce the formation of blood clots in Folts' animal model (19). The fact that grape juice had an effect further supports the hypothesis that the phenolic compounds are the active component in wine. In addition, a study of quercetin, one of the flavonoid phenolics in wine also showed inhibition of aggregation (20). Grape extracts have also been shown to have vasorelaxing activity (21).

Absorption Studies. An important factor in determining the significance of phenolic compounds is the issue of absorption, but progress in understanding of these potential effects is severely limited by the lack of absorption data (22). The few previous studies on phenolic absorption and metabolism have shown, on a few flavonoids, that they are absorbed at widely different rates. Catechin has been shown to be one of the more efficiently absorbed materials, about half being absorbed (23). On the other hand, no absorption was observed for quercetin (24).

Analysis of California Wine Samples

Many flavonoids and non-flavonoids are found in wine and all originate from the grape. However, they can be modified by the wine production process and as a wine ages, its phenolic constitution changes. We analyzed a selection of California wines for the concentration of a some of the major phenolic constituents.

Wines Samples. Red—Cabernet Sauvignon, Pinot noir, Syrah, Zinfandel, Merlot, Cabernet Franc, others; and white—Chardonnay and Sauvignon blanc, were obtained by a solicitation to 200 California wineries in all viticultural regions. For individual varieties, the numbers varied and Cabernet Sauvignon had the highest sample numbers. Syrah had a total of 7 wines, Chardonnay 14, and Sauvignon blanc, 7. See Table I for the number of wines in individual vintages where there were many wines.

Table I. Red Wine Sample Set

Vintage	Cabernet Sauvignon	Pinot Noir	Zinfandel	Merlot
	Number of Wines			
1986	4			
1987	12			
1988	14	3	1	1
1989	19	4	2	5
1990	13	4	5	4
1991	6	4	7	2

Phenolic Compounds. Gallic acid, caffeic acid, catechin, epicatechin, sinapic acid, malvidin-3-glucoside, rutin, and quercitin were purchased from Aldrich (Milwaukee, WI, USA) and Sigma (St. Louis, MO, USA). Malvidin-3-glucoside was purchased from Extrasynthese, (Genay, France). Cyanidin-3-glucoside was provided by Vernon L. Singleton.

HPLC Analysis. A Hewlett-Packard (Palo Alto, CA, U.S.A.), Model 1090 with three low pressure pumps and a diode-array UV-visible detector coupled to an HP Chem Station was used for solvent delivery and detection. A Novapack C18 column, 3.9 x 150mm, 4 µm particle size, (Waters, Milford, MA, USA) thermostatted at 40° C was used for the stationary phase with a flow of 0.5 mL/min. The solvents used for the separation were: Solvent A = 30 mM dichloroacetic acid adjusted to pH 1.5 with sulfuric acid; Solvent B = Methanol (Fisher-HPLC grade). The solvent gradient consisted of linearly increasing the percent of MeOH in the solvent mixture from 0% at the start to 10 at 7 min, 12.3 at 19 min, 25 at 27.5 min, 39.5 at 42 min, 50.5 at 48 min, 70 at 53 min, 80 at 55 min with a 3 min hold. Detection was at 280 nm, 313 nm, 520 nm, 620 nm, and UV-Vis spectra were acquired of peaks higher than 1 mAU.

Resveratrol Analysis. Wine, 4 mL, was placed in a test tube and 4 mL water was added. Then, 2-naphthol, internal standard (100 µL of a solution in ethyl acetate-to achieve 10 ppb), was added, and 50-100 µL samples of resveratrol standard in ethyl acetate solution was added when desired for spiking purposes. These solutions are then added to "10 mL" diatomaceous earth cartridges (Extrelut, EM Merck). After 5 minutes exactly, 12 mL ethyl acetate is added to the cartridges. After another 5 minutes, another 12 mL ethyl acetate is added, and solvent then elutes from the cartridges, approximately 12 mL volume over 2 min. This solution is dried with sodium sulfate (approx 8 g). This solution (5 mL) was then transferred by syringe to 20 mL scintillation vials for evaporation in a centrifugal vacuum evaporator (Savant). After 40 minutes, the vials were removed with approximately 200 µL solvent remaining. The solution was transferred to 300 µL vials for GC analysis, 50 µL BSTFA (bis-trimethylsilyl-trifluoroacetamide) added, the vials capped and heated at 70° C for 15 min. Then the samples were analyzed by GC/MS on a HP 5890/5970 system using a 30 m, 0.25 mm capillary column DB-5 (J&W Scientific), monitoring at mass 216 for 2-naphthol and 444 for cis and trans resveratrol—TMS derivatives. The resveratrol results express total cis and trans as trans-resveratrol equivalent levels (the cis isomer is assumed to have the same response as trans).

Total Phenol Content. The "total" phenol levels were determined using the Folin-Ciocalteu reagent to develop a blue color quantitated spectrophotometrically at 765 nm (25). The analysis is calibrated with gallic acid, and results are reported in Gallic Acid Equivalents (GAE).

Results of Analysis. Catechin, Figure 5, is known as the most abundant monomeric phenolic compound in wine (26,27). It is also an important monomeric unit that is a constituent of the many procyanidins dimers, trimers, etc, and condensed tannins, along with epicatechin and its gallate ester. This flavan-3-ol appears to be highest in Pinot noir wines, averaging 250mg/L. This result is comparable to previous studies (27) which found that both Pinot noir grapes and wine had high levels of catechin compared to other *vinfera* grapes and wines made from other grapes. In order of decreasing levels, the red wines are Merlot, Syrah, Zinfandel, Cabernet Franc and Cabernet Sauvignon in the range (220-150 mg/L). The white varieties contain lower concentrations, averaging 40 mg/L of this compound, averaging six times less for Sauvignon blanc and Chardonnay compared to the average level of the red varieties.

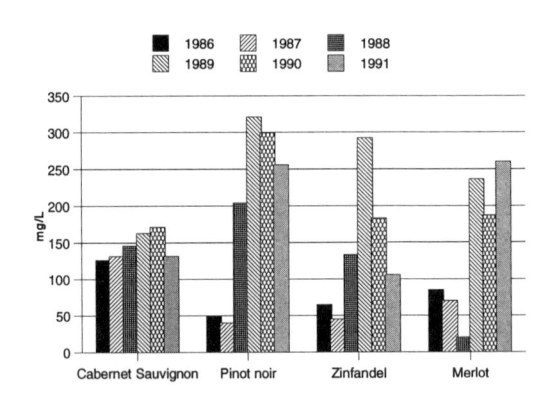

Figure 5 Average catechin levels in selected red wines, by vintage

In the histogram shown in Figure 6 only 15% of the red wines are in the class 0-50 mg/L but, not shown, 90% of the white wines are in this class. Most (59%) of the red wines are between 50 and 200 mg/L, 25% are between 200-400 mg/L and just a few outliers are found at concentrations higher than 400 mg/L. Such a distribution illustrates the

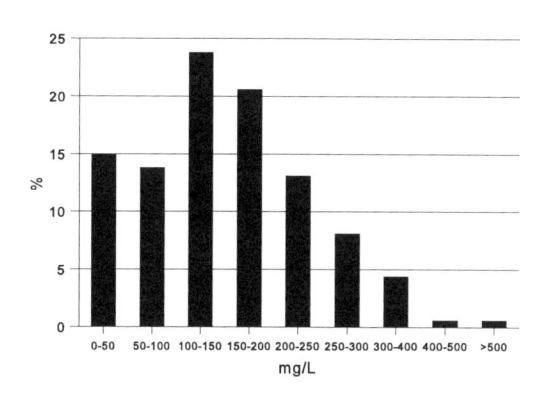

Figure 6 Histogram of catechin levels in all red wines.

very wide range of levels that can be expected for phenolic compounds. Here, there are significant number of wines below 50 mg/L and above 250 mg/L, a range of 500%. Thus a single wine could have a level of this compound, the most abundant single phenolic in wine, that could be very different from the average wine. This large variation illustrates the importance of analyzing the levels of these substances in any wine used for health-related studies.

Epicatechin an isomer of catechin which comprises much of the procyanidins and condensed tannins is typically found at a lower concentration than catechin in grapes, as noted by others (28). The varieties which have high concentrations are Merlot, Zinfandel, Cabernet Sauvignon, and Pinot noir, averaging around 80mg/L, a level one third than of catechin. We found the average levels in Syrah and Cabernet Franc varieties only about half as much (40-50mg/L), and in white varieties like Sauvignon blanc and Chardonnay levels were only a quarter as much, averaging 20 mg/L. The order of the epicatechin levels by variety is the same order as for catechin. Also, 47% of the white wines are between 0 and 20 mg/L and 42% in the group 20-40 mg/L. In the red wines, about half fall into these categories-only 19% and 20% are in the classes 0-20 mg/L and 20-40 mg/L respectively. Around 50% of the red wines are between the levels of 40-100 mg/L and nearly 10% of the reds have more than 100 mg/L.

One of the most common flavonols, quercetin, was observed at the highest average level in Cabernet Franc, at 13 mg/L, while the other red varieties had levels in a range from 6 to 11 mg/L. The levels varied depending on vintage, but only in Pinot noir was the variation very large (Figure 7). In the white varieties this flavonol was not detected. Over 35% of the red wines had less than 5 mg/L, 30% had between 5 and 10 mg/L, 15% had 10-15, and 8% 15-20 with 11% over 20 mg/L. Price has noted that in Pinot noir, the level of quercetin in controlled almost exclusively by sun exposure of the grape (29).

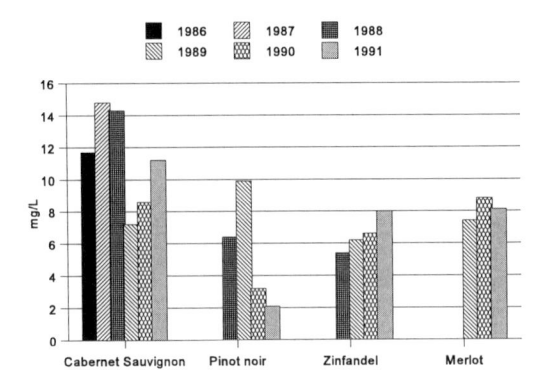

Figure 7 Average levels of quercetin in selected red wines, by vintage

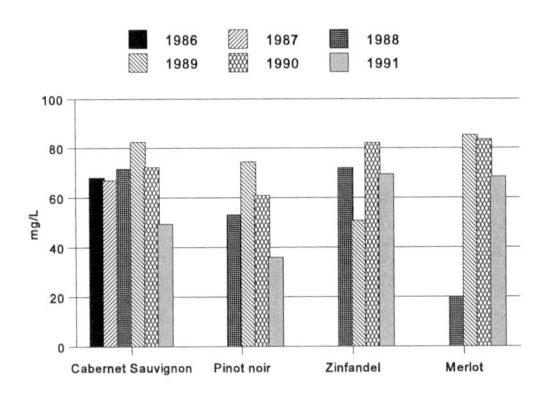

Figure 8 Average levels of gallic acid in selected red wines, by vintage

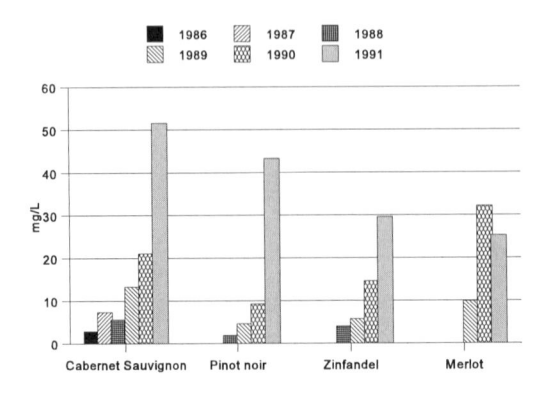

Figure 9 Average levels of malvidin-3-glucoside in selected red wines, by vintage

The cinnamate sinapic acid was not detected in the white varieties Sauvignon blanc or Chardonnay and ranged from 0.3 to 2 mg/L in the red wines. Syrah had the highest concentration for this minor component. The majority of the red wines (60%) are between 0 and 1 mg/L and 24% between 1 and 2mg/L.

Another cinnamate, caffeic acid had levels that were very similar in Pinot noir, Cabernet Sauvignon, Merlot, Zinfandel and Cabernet Sauvignon wines, being between 7 and 9 mg/L. On average it is three times higher in Syrah (26 mg/L), but lower in Sauvignon blanc and Chardonnay (6mg/L). For both white and red wines we observed approximately the same percentage of wines (70-80%) between 3 and 9 mg/L. We observed that 23% of the reds were at a concentration higher than 9mg/L but only 5% for the white wines.

Gallic acid has been described as increasing during aging, but in this set of wine, there is no clear trend in that direction (Figure 8) *(30)*. The levels observed here were between 65 and 85 mg/L for the red varieties, with the higher concentrations observed in Cabernet Franc, Syrah and Zinfandel. In the white varieties Sauvignon blanc and Chardonnay, the levels averaged about one tenth (7 and 10 mg/L) of the reds. Of the whites, 74% are in the class 0-10 mg/L but only 5% of the red wines. The levels of the red wines range from 0 to 100 mg/L with nearly two thirds between 40 and 90 mg/L.

Myrecitin was detected and identified in wine by Alonso *(31)*. In our work this aglycon was not detected in white wines and average levels varied between 5 and 13 mg/L for the red varieties. Syrah was found to have the highest average concentration. In reds overall, there was a regular decrease number of wines in the classes, 35% being between 0 and 5 mg/L, 30% in the class 5 to 10 mg/L, and down to 6% of the wines with a concentration above 20 mg/L.

Cyanidin-3-glucoside was not found in the white wines. It appeared in trace amounts (0.3 to 2 mg/L) in the Pinot noir, Cabernet Sauvignon, Merlot, Zinfandel, and Cabernet Franc wines. Only Syrah contains high amounts (18 mg/L) of this anthocyanin, a level which is ten to sixty times more than the other red varieties. Looking at the population of level classes, 63% of the red wines are between 0 and 0.5 mg/L. The other classes shows percentages around 0 to 5. Only 9% of the red wines have a level above 5 mg/L.

Malvidin-3-glucoside was not detected in the white wines, but, as the major anthocyanin in most red wines, significant quantities were found in the reds. Syrah had an average concentration near 50 mg/L and Cabernet Franc near 35 mg/L, the highest levels by variety. Merlot had half that of the Syrah, and Pinot noir, Cabernet Sauvignon and Zinfandel had only about a third as much (around 15mg/L). Separating the levels into three classes, of all the reds, 55% are between 0 and 10 mg/L, 25% are between 10 and 30 mg/L; and 16% have more than 35 mg/L. By vintage the decrease in levels as the wines age is quite striking as seen in Figure 9. The older wines have only a small fraction of the malvidin-3-glucoside observed in the younger wines. This observation corroborates many other studies which have made the observation that the monomeric anthocyanins decrease on aging.

By the Folin-Ciocalteau procedure, the white varieties had average levels close to 220-250 mg/L GAE which about one tenth of the red varieties. The Syrah was the variety with the highest average total phenol level (2220 mg/L GAE). The other varieties clustered in two groups, Zinfandel and Pinot noir around 1850 mg/L GAE and Cabernet Sauvignon, Cabernet Franc, Merlot 2000 mg GAE/L.

The wine variety which contained the highest average concentration of resveratrol was Pinot noir (500 µg/L) corroborating the results many studies (*32,33*). This is 2½ times more than for Cabernet Sauvignon and Merlot, four times more than Syrah, seven and 18 times more than Zinfandel and Cabernet Franc respectively. The white varieties appear to have very low average levels compared to the red varieties, 50 and 80 µg/L for the Sauvignon blanc and Chardonnay respectively, approximately 65 to 100 times less than the Pinot noir average level. All the white wines all had levels between 0 and 0.5 mg/L. In the red wines, 42% had levels between 0 and 1 mg/L, 26% between 1 and 2 mg/L, 22% between 2-5 mg/L and 10% over 5 mg/L.

Conclusions

Wine phenolics appear to have the properties that could reduce the heart disease mortality rates observed in wine drinkers-they are antioxidants and antiaggregatory. It appears that absorption of some phenols is significant, although the levels must still be established. The variability of the levels of these substances in red wine demands that health studies be carried out with well described wines to ensure their reproducibility. These data may be useful in understanding the typical sensory properties of different wine varieties, and perhaps their effects on human physiology. Many more studies are needed to prove whether or not dietary phenolic compounds have any health effects.

Literature Cited

1. St. Leger, A.S.; Cochrane, A.L.; Moore, F. *Lancet* **1979**, i, 1017-1020.
2. Renaud, S.; de Lorgeril, M. *Lancet* **1992**, 339, 1523-1526.
3. Criqui, M.H.; Ringel, B.L. *Lancet* **1994**, 344, 1719-1723.
4. Klatsky, A.L.; Armstrong, M.A. *Am. J. Card.* **1993**, 71 (5), 467-469.
5. Gronbæk, M.; Deis, A.; Sorensen, T.I.A.; Becker, U.; Schnohr, P.; Jensen, G. *BMJ* **1995**, 310, 1165-1169.
6. Hertog, M.G.L.; Feskens, E.J.M.; Hollman, P.C.H.; Katan, J.B.; Kromhout, D. *Lancet* **1993**, 342, 1007-1011.
7. Hertog, M.G.L.; Hollman, P.C.H.; Katan, M.B. *J. Agric. Food Chem.* **1992**, 40, 2379-2383.
8. Waterhouse, A.L.; German, J.B.; Frankel, E.N.; Walzem, R.L.; Teissedre, P.L.; Folts, J., In *Hypernutritous Foods*; Finley, J.W.; Roussef, R.; Nagy, S.; Robinson, S.F. Eds.; Agscience Inc, Auburndale, 1996; in press.
9. Kühnau, J. *Wld Rev. Nutr. Diet* **1976**, 24, 117-191.
10. Harborne, J.B., Ed. *The flavonoids: Advances in research since 1986*; Chapman and Hall: London, 1993.
11. Albach, R.F.; Kepner, R.E.; Webb, A.D. *Am. J. Enol. Vitic.* **1959**, 10, 164-172.
12. Fernández de Simon, B.; Pérez-Ilzarbe, J.; Hernández, T.; Gómez-Cordovés, C.; Estrella, I. *J. Agric. Food Chem.* **1992**, 40, 1531-1535.

13. Steinberg, D.; Parthasarathy, S.; Carew, T.E.; Khoo, J.C.; Witztum, J.L. *New Eng. J. Med.* **1989**, 320, 915-924.
14. Esterbauer, H.; Gebicki, J.; Puhl, H.; Jürgens, G. *Free Radical Res. Commun.* **1992**, 13, 341-390.
15. Xiu, R.J.; Freyschuss, A.; Ying, X.; Berglund, L.; Henriksson, P.; Bjorkhem, I. *J. Clin. Invest.* **1994**, 93, 2732-2737.
16. Frankel, E.N.; Kanner, J.; German, J.B.; Parks, E.; Kinsella, J.E. *Lancet* **1993**, 341, 454-457.
17. Frankel, E.N.; Waterhouse, A.L.; Kinsella, J.E. *Lancet* **1993**, 341, 1103-1104.
18. Casenave, J.P.; Beretz, A.; Anton, R., In *Flavonoids and Bioflavonoids*; Studies in Organic Chemistry 23; Farkas, L.; Gábor, M.; Kállay, F., Eds.; Elsevier: Amsterdam, 1985; pp. 373-380.
19. Demrow, H.S.; Slane, P.R.; Folts, J.D. *Circulation* **1995**, 91, 1182-1188.
20. Slane, P.R.; Folts, J.D. *Clin. Res.* **1994**, 42, 394.
21. Fitzpatrick, D.F.; Hirschfield, S.L.; Coffey, R.G. *Am. J. Physiol.* **1993**, 265, H774-H778.
22. Halliwell, B. *Biochemist* **1995** (Feb/Mar), 3-6.
23. Hackett, A.M.; Griffiths, L.A.; Broillet, A.; Wermeille, M. *Xenobiotica* **1983**, 13, 279-283.
24. Gugler, R.; Leschik, M.; Dengler, H.J. *Eur. J. Clin. Pharmacol.* **1975**, 9, 229-234.
25. Singleton, V.L.; Rossi, J.A. *Am. J. Enol. Vitic.* **1965**, 16, 144-158.
26. Singleton, V.L. *Proc. Symposium Univ. Calif. Davis, Grape & Wine Centennial, 1980* **1982**, 215-227.
27. Bourzeix, M.; Weyland, D.; Heredia, N.; Desfeux, C. *Bull. O.I.V.* **1986**, 59 (669-670), 1171-1254.
28. Bourzeix, M.; Dubernet, M.O. *Ind. Aliment. Agricol.* **1975**, 1057-1064.
29. Price, S.F.; Breen, P.J.; Valladao, M.; Watson, B.T. *Am. J. Enol. Vitic.* **1995**, 46, 187-194.
30. Archier, P. Doctorate Dissertation, Université de Droit, 1992.
31. Alonso, E.; Estrella, M.I.; Revilla, E. *Chromatogr.* **1986**, 22, 268-270.
32. Lamuela-Raventos, R.M.; Waterhouse, A.L. *J. Agric. Food Chem.* **1993**, 41, 521-523.
33. Goldberg, D.M.; Yan, J.; Ng, E.; Diamandis, E.P.; Karumanchiri, A.; Soleas, G.; Waterhouse, A.L. *Am. J. Enol. Vitic.* **1995**, 46, 159-165.

Chapter 4

Identification and Assay of Trihydroxystilbenes in Wine and Their Biological Properties

David M. Goldberg[1], G. J. Soleas[2], S. E. Hahn[1,4], E. P. Diamandis[1], and A. Karumanchiri[3]

[1]Department of Clinical Biochemistry, University of Toronto, 100 College Street, Toronto, Ontario M5G 1L5, Canada
[2]Andres Wines Limited, 697 South Service Road, Grimsby, Ontario L8E 5S3, Canada
[3]Quality Assurance, Liquor Control Board of Ontario, 55 Lake Shore Boulevard East, Toronto, Ontario M5E 1A4, Canada

> We have developed a series of methods to assay the isomers and glucosides of resveratrol including GC-MS techniques by direct-injection and derivatisation procedures, and HPLC techniques using normal phase isocratic elution with UV detection and reverse phase gradient elution with diode array detection. Their application to commercial wines has revealed major differences in resveratrol isomer and glucoside concentrations showing specific influences of cultivar and climate. Prospective studies performed during fermentation and subsequently have defined the kinetics of release of resveratrol isomers and demonstrated the varying roles of duration of skin contact, oak ageing and filtration. Resveratrol alters the synthesis and secretion of lipids and lipoproteins by a human liver cell line; blocks human platelet aggregation *in vitro*; and inhibits the synthesis of pro-aggregatory and pro-inflammatory eicosanoids by platelets and neutrophils respectively. This spectrum of effects places it among the most powerful anti-atherosclerotic phenolics yet identified as a constituent of wines.

Current interest in the potential health benefits of the phenolic constituents of wine stimulated an explosion of research activities focused upon these compounds. The most significant results to emerge from this research have been well described by earlier contributors to this Symposium, and no further elaboration is required in the present report. Indeed, an adequate introductory account of the trihydroxystilbene resveratrol and its glucoside polydatin has already been provided. Further information relevant to resveratrol and its biological activities is recorded in two recent review publications by our group which also present the rationale underlying

---
[4]Current address: Allelix Biopharmaceuticals, 6850 Goreway Drive, Mississauga, Ontario L4W 1Y7, Canada

© 1997 American Chemical Society

our current research program (1, 2). This is targeted towards the following objectives:
1. Identification of the biologically active components of wine that are particularly relevant to the prevention of coronary heart disease (CHD) and cancer.
2. Development of assays to allow their quantitation in wine and other beverages.
3. To survey their concentrations in wines from different regions and countries with a view to defining the enological factors that can lead to their enrichment.
4. Testing the biological potency of these compounds in laboratory experiments involving cultured cells.
5. Performance of clinical studies validating their effectiveness in human subjects.

In this paper, we will review the progress that has been accomplished in the past three years with particular reference to resveratrol and related trihydroxystilbenes. Much of this work has already been published, and other findings have been presented at scientific meetings such as the present, but we will also describe some very recent results which are being reported for the first time.

Assay of Resveratrol

Direct-Injection GC-MS Procedure. At the time we started this work, the reference method for *trans*-resveratrol was that of Siemann and Creasy (3). This was time-consuming and called for considerable technical expertise, since it required multiple solvent extractions followed by two sequential HPLC procedures culminating in differential spectrophotometry after UV-irradiation. Our first approach was based upon direct injection of an ethyl acetate eluate, derived from a 1 mL sample of wine that had been extracted on a C-18 column, into a gas-chromatograph fitted with a highly thermostable capillary column, DB-5 and subsequently DB-17 (4). Detection and quantitation was by mass-spectrometry with selective ion monitoring using the molecular ion at mass 228; ions at mass 229 (carbon isotope) and 227 (M-H) were employed as qualifiers, and pure *trans*-resveratrol as standard, initially prepared by organic synthesis and subsequently obtained commercially. The method was linear over a wide range (0.05 - 10 mg/L) with recovery averaging 100% and precision varying from 5.3 - 7.4% depending on concentration. The same principles permitted the determination of *cis*-resveratrol which generated an identical mass spectrum but eluted several minutes earlier than *trans*-resveratrol (5). Both isomers could be analyzed simultaneously in 1 mL of wine at a rate of 20 min per sample. A disadvantage of the method is the high cost of the column which needs to be replaced after 150-300 assays due to increased baseline and some degradation of peak contours occasioned by the very high temperatures (290-350°C) at which the chromatography is performed, causing more rapid 'bleeding' than occurs when conventional temperatures are used.

Derivatisation GC-MS Procedure. Simultaneously, we developed a GC-MS method in which 1 mL of wine was subjected to solid phase extraction and the dried residue was derivatised with BSTFA before chromatography on a DB-5 HT column (6). The target ion at mass 444 was used for quantitation with ions at mass 445 and

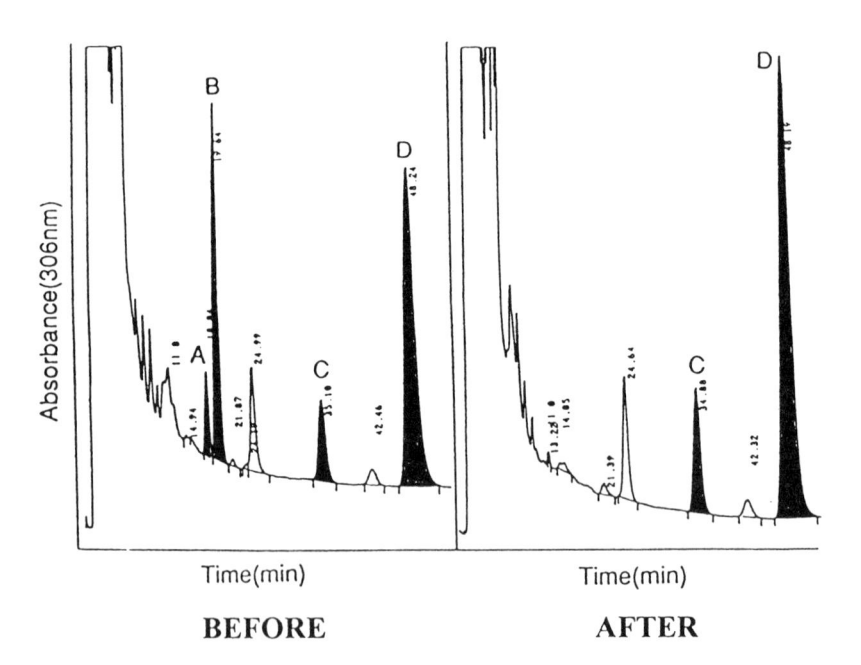

Figure 1. HPLC separation of *cis*-polydatin (A), *trans*-polydatin (B), *cis*-resveratrol (C) and *trans*-resveratrol (D) before and after treatment of a red wine sample for 12 hours at room temperature. Adapted from ref. 8.

443 employed as qualifiers. Identical mass ion spectra were yielded by *trans* and *cis*-resveratrol which eluted approximately 3-min apart. The method was linear from 10-3,000 µg/L, gave recoveries in the range 91-98%, with precision varying from 2.6 - 9.9% depending upon the concentration. Although it is more time-consuming than the direct method, since evaporisation and derivatisation are required, the method is very versatile and has been further elaborated into a multi-residue method capable of simultaneously analyzing up to 15 biologically active phenolics by on-line selective ion monitoring. These include *trans* and *cis*-polydatin, quercetin, catechin, epicatechin, morin, and p- and m- coumaric acid (Soleas *et al*, In Preparation).

Assay of Resveratrol Glucosides

The next phase of our work was devoted to the development of methods to assay the β-glucosides of resveratrol, *cis* and *trans*-polydatin (piceid). These have been shown to share at least one major biological property with the free isomers, namely, inhibition of protein kinase activities (7). Their solubility and susceptibility to enzymatic hydrolysis by intestinal glucosidases suggest that they may have higher bioavailability than the hydrophobic free isomers, and they hold further interest as possible sources of the latter during fermentation.

Normal-Phase HPLC. Our first approach involved normal-phase HPLC with isocratic elution of the polyphenols in 20 µL of wine directly injected onto a LiChrospher 100-CN column by a mobile phase of water-acetonitrile-methanol (8). In this system, the glucosides eluted between 16 and 18 min while the isomers of resveratrol appeared much later: around 35 min for *cis* and 45 min for *trans* (Fig 1). All four were well resolved from each other and from neighbouring peaks and could therefore be quantitated simultaneously in the same sample over a 50-min run. Detection was at 306 nm, corresponding to the peak absorbance of *trans*-resveratrol and although the peak of *cis*-resveratrol was around 280 nm, the former wavelength could be successfully used for all four compounds. The spectra of the glucosides were almost identical to those of the free isomers, with a minor shift to the left approximating 2.5 nm. Thus, pure *trans*-resveratrol could be used to standardize both the free isomer and the glucoside, while *cis*-resveratrol prepared by UV-irradiation of *trans*-resveratrol was the only other standard required. The polydatins were quantitatively converted to the corresponding isomers on treatment with β-glucosidase (Figure 1). GC-MS criteria were also used to identify and validate the 4 peaks. Excellent linearity, recovery and precision were obtained for all constituents.

Reverse-Phase HPLC. More recently, we have developed a reverse-phase HPLC method utilizing diode array detection to measure a wide array of wine phenolics (9). ODS-Hypersil serves as the stationary phase, and gradient elution is accomplished in 40 min with a mobile phase of water-methanol-acetic acid. 20 µL of sample is applied directly through a guard column of LiChrospher 100 RP-18. The isomers of resveratrol and polydatin are well-resolved in this system which allows their determination with excellent analytical characteristics. Virtually all other wine phenolics for which standards are available can be adequately resolved and quantitated. A powerful feature of the software developed for these assays, which routinely records the absorbance at 5 wavelengths (265, 280, 306, 317 and 369 nm), is the ability to utilize purity checks and match-factor analysis to authenticate each peak and eliminate interference. Although HPLC analyses of wine phenolics with diode array detection have been described earlier, the authors have not stressed the importance of validating the purity and authenticity of each peak. In our experience, 5% of all peaks obtained during the analysis of commercial wines which match the retention times of the relevant standards demonstrate unacceptable spectral properties due to impurities and should not be reported (Goldberg *et al*, In Preparation).

Method Comparison. The availability of several methods for the analysis of trihydroxystilbenes raises the issue of which ought to be adopted for general use. Unfortunately, there is no easy answer to this question. While all methods provide results which demonstrate good inter-method correlation, similar relative differences between wines, and virtually identical conclusions of a general nature, the absolute values obtained reveal systematic variations which are method-dependent and cannot be attributed to the use of different standards or standardization procedures (10). Higher results for *trans*-resveratrol with direct injection GC-MS may be due to fragmentation of *trans*-polydatin which will release the same ion spectrum. The two-hour evaporation and derivatization steps in our second GC-MS procedure may allow some *trans:cis* isomerization, with underestimation of the first and overestimation of the second. The normal-phase HPLC method with single wavelength monitoring is susceptible to significant peak contamination which defies visual inspection but can be identified by diode array detection and use of appropriate software for purity checks and spectral comparisons. It has already been shown that liquid phase extractions as used in several methods (3,11,12) are associated with poor recovery and losses due to oxidation (13). The choice of method will therefore be governed by considerations of capital and running costs and whether the method selected can also measure other compounds of interest.

Regional Differences in Trihydroxy Stilbene Content

***Trans*-Resveratrol Concentrations.** Our first survey, involving approximately 1,000 wines, was restricted to *trans*-resveratrol (14). There were striking differences based on cultivar and region. The salient findings were the following:

a) Highest concentrations were encountered in wines from Pinot Noir grapes. These included the wines of Burgundy, Oregon and Switzerland whose most prominent red wine, Dole, is vinted from a clone of Pinot Noir. Wines made from this cultivar in other regions of France (Alsace and Loire Valley) or in other countries (California, Australia, Italy, Central Europe) invariably had much higher concentrations than wines made in the same regions by the same producers from different cultivars. There were no apparent temperature-dependent influences upon the *trans*-resveratrol content of Pinot Noir wines.

b)   Wines vinted from Cabernet Sauvignon grapes had much lower *trans*-resveratrol concentrations with the exception of red Bordeaux and Canadian wines. Especially low values were found in Cabernet Sauvignon wines from countries noted for warmer drier climates such as California, Australia, South America, South Africa, Italy and Spain, but similar wines from Central Europe and the Midi region of France had moderately high concentrations. Thus, in general, this cultivar generated wines of higher *trans*-resveratrol content when grown under unfavorable climatic conditions.

c)   Whether as the predominant cultivar (e.g., St. Emilion), or the exclusive cultivar as in many Italian and New World wines, Merlot generated wines that tended to span a narrower range than those of Cabernet Sauvignon and showed a less profound impact of climatic conditions. In all countries and regions (including the Northern Rhone Valley), those wines vinted from Shiraz grapes had low *trans*-resveratrol concentrations and climate seemed to exercise no effect.

d)   Wines from the Southern Rhone Valley, Midi and Provence had moderately high concentrations of *trans*-resveratrol. The predominant cultivars contributing to the cepage in these regions include Carignan, Cinsault, Mourvedre and Grenache which appear to be quite high in trihydroxystilbenes (15). It is important to emphasize, as will become apparent subsequently, that these relatively simple wines do not receive the length of oak ageing accorded the more prestigious wines of the Northern Rhone, or those of the Rioja region of Spain which utilize some of these cultivars as well as the indigenous Tempranillo grape.

e)   The lowest *trans*-resveratrol concentrations of any of the commercial wines tested were found in Italian wines. It mattered little whether these were from Piemonte where the Nebbiolo grape predominates, Tuscany which is the home of Sangiovese, or Veneto where a wide range of cultivars are used in red wine production. The red wines of Spain and Portugal also had relatively low *trans*-resveratrol concentrations. The data collected at that time did not define the predominant influence as due to climate, wine-making techniques such as fining and oak-ageing, or the intrinsic genetic properties of the cultivars from which the wines were produced.

f)   In confirmation of many reports that white wines are almost invariably low in *trans*-resveratrol, few if any such wines had concentrations within 10% of those found in the lowest range of red wines. Rose wines were almost as low, and so were fortified red wines such as Ports and Madeiras. Among white wines, only the occasional German Riesling or Swiss (e.g. Neuchatel or Fendant) had modest concentrations which overlapped the lower range of concentrations for red wines.

Cis-Resveratrol Concentrations. Once the methods for *cis*-resveratrol assay had been developed (5), we were able to measure the concentrations of both isomers in commercial wines, and we have recently described our findings in considerable depth (Goldberg, D.M.; Ng, E.; Yan, J.; Karumanchiri, A.; Soleas, G.J.; Diamandis, E.P. *J. Wine Res*, in press). The same generalizations that applied to *trans*-resveratrol were largely true of the *cis*-isomer. Thus, Pinot Noir wines (Burgundy,Oregon), those of Switzerland, and red Bordeaux had highest concentrations, with wines from Canada, the Southern Rhone Valley, Beaujolais and the Midi next in line. Wines from warm New World regions and the Mediterranean basin had very low concentrations, with Cabernet Sauvignon wines showing a definite temperature-dependence.

A few unexpected findings are worth emphasizing. Although the *cis*-resveratrol concentrations generally averaged 50-60% those of the *trans*-isomer, there were some notable exceptions. The ratio of *cis:trans* averaged 0.34 in South African and 0.46 in South American wines. By contrast, very high ratios characterized Pinot Noir wines from Burgundy (0.87) and Oregon (0.95) as well as those of Beaujolais (0.92). These trends were reflected in the wines from individual cultivars. For example, among wines from Cabernet Sauvignon, the lowest ratios occurred in those from South Africa (0.33) and South America (0.36). Variations were seen among the different regions of Italy with the ratio averaging 0.35 in Tuscan wines, 0.40 in those from Piemonte, rising to 0.62 in the Veneto and 0.81 in wines grouped together from areas including Umbria, Campagna, Sardegna and Puglia, i.e., further South than the first three regions listed.

Resveratrol Glucoside Concentrations. The most striking and unexpected results were uncovered by our analyses of commercial wines in which their concentrations of resveratrol isomers and glucosides were compared (16). To summarize briefly:

a) Those countries whose wines were especially high in *trans* and *cis*-resveratrol (e.g. Burgundy, Bordeaux, Oregon) had low concentrations of both *trans* and *cis*-polydatin, whereas many wines with low concentrations of the free isomers (South America, South Africa, Italy, Spain and Portugal) had very high concentrations of both glucosides. However, some countries such as Australia and California whose wines were low in free resveratrol isomers also had low concentrations of both glucosides. Canadian wines and those from the Rhone Valley were unique in having very high glucoside concentrations as well as above average concentrations of the free isomers.

b) With most wines, *trans*-polydatin was present in higher concentrations than the *cis*-isomer, but in Canadian wines in particular, and to a lesser extent in red Burgundy, Australian and South American wines, higher concentrations of *cis*-polydatin were present.

c) Fortified wines such as Ports, Madeiras and Sherries that were virtually devoid of free resveratrol had significant concentrations of the glucosides, often exceeding those present in regular table wines.

d) The ratio of total glucoside to total isomer concentrations was absolutely characteristic for several wines. This ratio averaged 4.0 in wines from Spain and Portugal, 3.0 in wines from Italy, and <1 in wines from California, Bordeaux, Burgundy and Australia (Fig 2).

e) The results are consistent with the notion that the overall content of resveratrol isomers and glucosides in wine is a function of genetic factors (e.g., cultivar) and acquired factors (e.g., climate, soil, vinification techniques), and that to a certain extent there is a reciprocal relationship between the glucoside and free isomer content of wines, possibly due to the fact that the latter originate (at least in part) from the former, and this conversion is influenced by viticultural and enological practices characterictic of each wine-producing region.

Influence of Enological Procedures

We have been able to conduct a very detailed investigation of the enological factors that influence the resveratrol isomer concentrations of wines produced in the Niagara region of Southern Ontario (17) and we believe that the conclusions drawn from this study are generally applicable to the production of wines elsewhere. These include the following observations:

a) During fermentation there is negligible isomerization of *trans* to *cis*-resveratrol, presumably due to absence of light and oxygen.

b) The extraction of resveratrol isomers during skin fermentation follows one of two patterns which seem to be characteristic of the cultivar concerned. With Cabernet Franc, Villard Noir and Chambourcin, a rapid increase in *trans*-resveratrol occurred within 24 hours of fermentation reaching a maximum over the next 2 days and followed by a plateau and, in some cases, by a slight fall in concentration (Fig 3a). Simultaneously or one day later, the *cis*-resveratrol concentration started to increase, but much more slowly and throughout the period of observation, over which time neither a plateau or a decrease was observed. The second pattern seen with De Chaunac, Pinot Noir, Cabernet Sauvignon and Merlot (Fig 3b) was characterized by a more gradual and parallel increase in the concentrations of both isomers, accelerating after day 3 of fermentation, reaching a peak around day 6 and declining thereafter.

c) Striking differences in resveratrol content were noted in wines from different vintages. For example, the *cis*-resveratrol concentrations of Pinot Noir wines of the 1992 vintage were one-quarter those of the 1993 vintage; the *trans*-resveratrol concentrations of 1993 Niagara Pinot Noir wines were only about 50% higher than those of the 1992 vintage. In contrast to Pinot Noir wines which were higher in

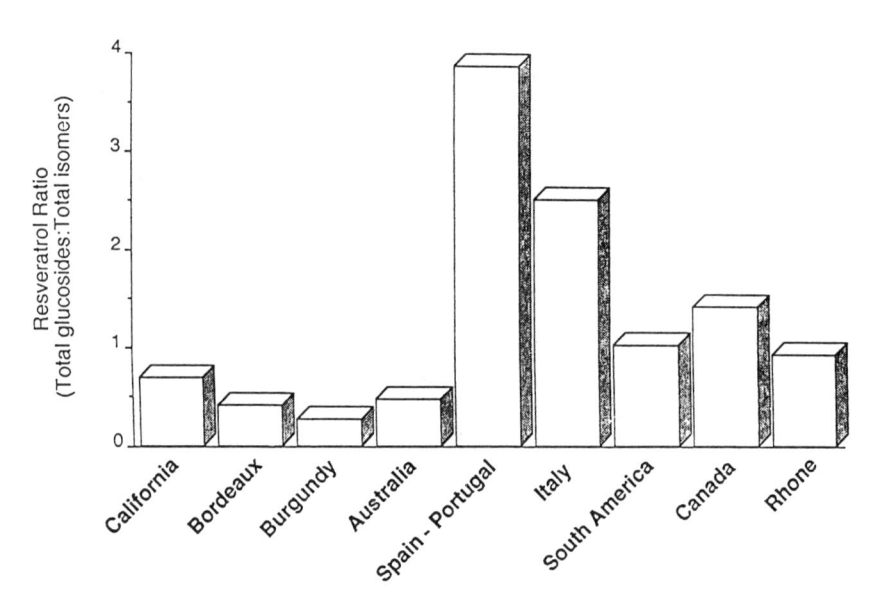

Figure 2. Mean ratio of total resveratrol glucosides to total resveratrol free isomers in red wines from different regions.

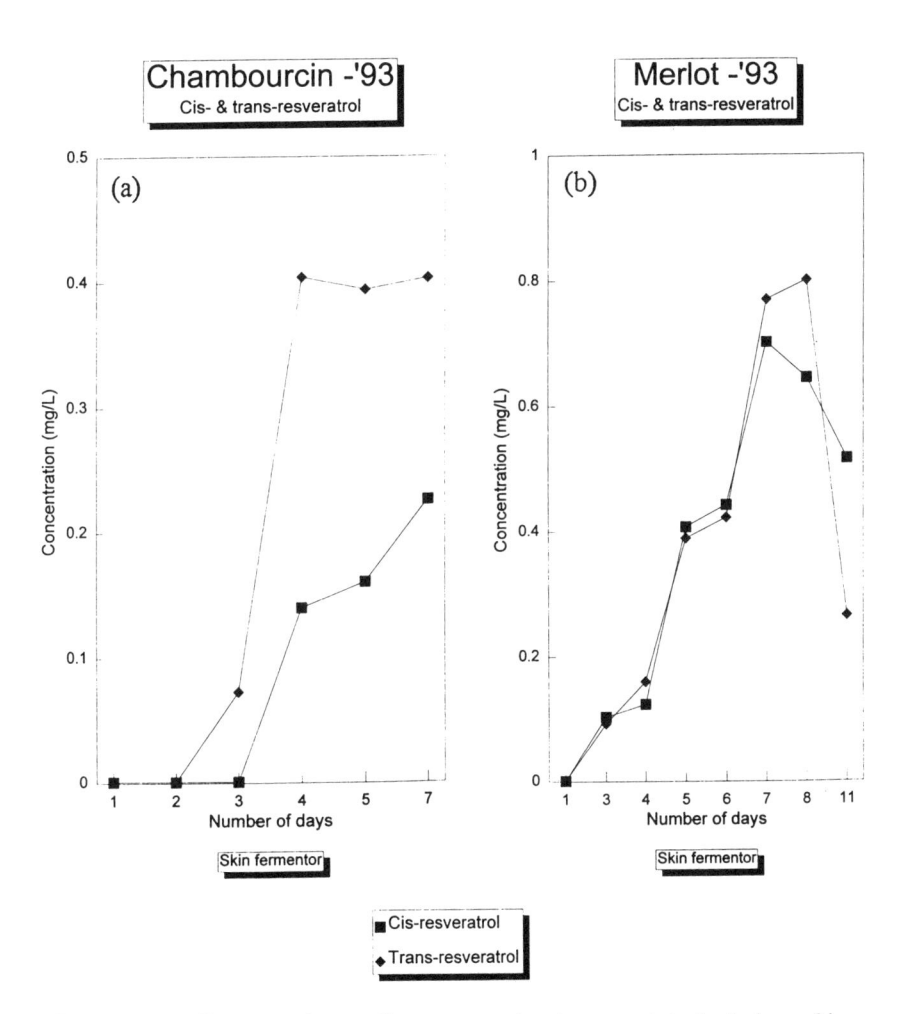

Figure 3. Concentrations of *trans-* and *cis-* resveratrol during skin fermentation of (a) Chambourcin and (b) Merlot grapes. Reproduced with permission from ref. 17. Copyright 1995, Carfax Publishing.

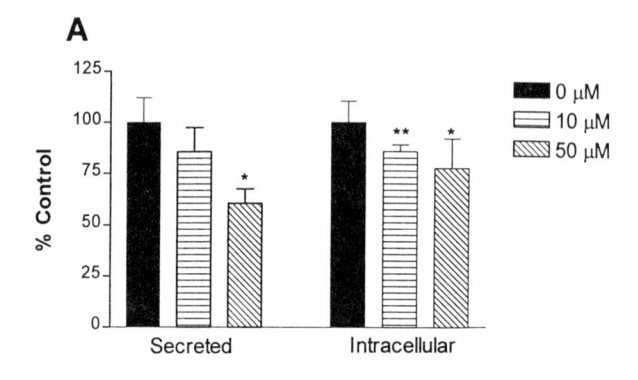

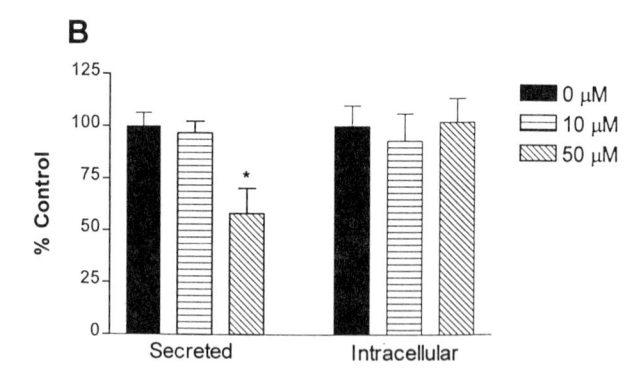

Figure 4. Effect of *trans*-resveratrol on the secretion and intracellular concentrations of cholesteryl esters (A) and triglycerides (B). Confluent Hep G2 cells were incubated for 24 hours at the stated concentrations. Results are mean ± SD of 4 plates assayed in duplicate and expressed as a percentage of control cultures (no resveratrol). *$P < 0.05$; ** $P < 0.01$.

1993 than in 1992, Niagara wines from Merlot and Cabernet Sauvignon cultivars were slightly lower in resveratrol free isomer concentrations in 1993.

d)   We were unable to detect *cis*-resveratrol in the skins of any wine-producing cultivars. Surprisingly, the *trans*-resveratrol concentrations of white grape skins were in the range of those from most red grapes. Clearly, the very low resveratrol concentrations that we observed in white wine and which have been consistently noted by ourselves and others (3,6,12,14) are due to the absence of skin contact during fermentation. It should also be emphasized that for most grapes, the *trans*-resveratrol concentrations of the finished wines were less than those of the corresponding skins, indicating either incomplete extraction or loss during vinification and processing. Length of skin contact was an important variable. Doubling of the skin fermentation time increased *trans*-resveratrol nearly 3-fold, and *cis*-resveratrol by about 150%.

e)   Wide variations occurred in the *trans*-resveratrol content of skins from the same cultivar harvested at the same time but grown in regions of Niagara up to 20 miles apart at different elevations and degrees of exposure.

f)   Certain materials used in clarification, but not others, caused reduced concentrations of resveratrol isomers. Losses tended to be greater with *trans* than with *cis*-resveratrol. Bentonite and gelatin had little effect. Silica caused minor losses and charcoal major losses in both isomers. Interestingly, cellulose filter pads retained *trans* but not *cis*-resveratrol to the extent that the two isomers could be separated by replicate passage. Oak ageing led to major reduction in both isomers even though the wines were kept cool and free of light.

In Vitro Studies

Our objectives in these investigations were to examine the effect of resveratrol on: a) lipid and lipoprotein metabolism; b) platelet aggregation; c) eicosanoid metabolism. The first objective was accomplished by utilizing the human hepatocarcinoma cell line, Hep G2, which has preserved the major functions of human liver parenchymal cells (18). The third involved the impact of resveratrol upon thromboxane and hepoxillin synthesis by platelets, and the 5- and 15-lipoxygenase pathways in leukocytes.

Lipid Metabolism. A slight but significant reduction of apolipoprotein B content and secretion takes place when Hep G2 cells are grown in the presence of *trans*-resveratrol in the 1-50 µM concentration range, although a true dose-dependent response was not demonstrated (2). The intracellular content and the rate of secretion of cholesteryl esters as well as the rate of secretion of triglycerides were reduced by resveratrol in a dose-dependent manner (Fig 4), but the intracellular triglyceride content was unaffected. Overall, these changes would tend to diminish the rate of secretion of VLDL which are converted to atherogenic LDL in the circulation, and are therefore consistent with an anti-atherogenic role of resveratrol.

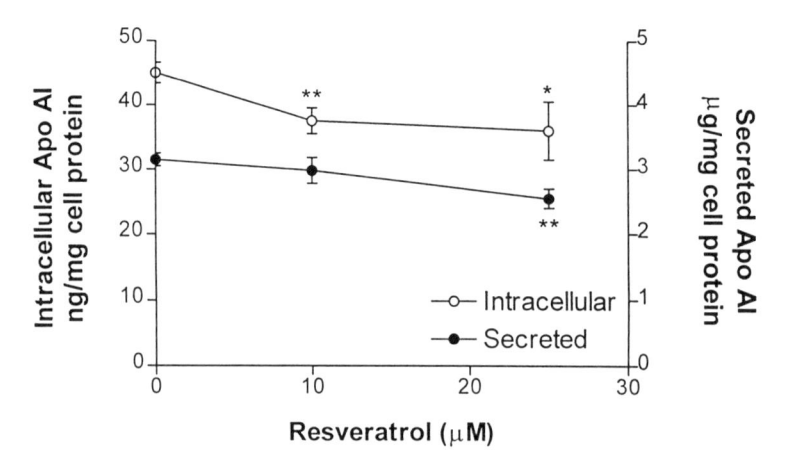

Figure 5. Effect of *trans*-resveratrol on the secretion and intracellular concentration of apolipoprotein AI. Confluent Hep G2 cells were incubated for 24 hours at the stated concentrations. Results are mean ± SD of 4 plates assayed in duplicate * $P < 0.05$; ** $P < 0.01$.

The effects of *trans*-resveratrol on apo-AI metabolism of Hep G2 cells were not entirely reproducible, and seemed to depend upon the duration of exposure, but in general there was reduced intracellular content and secretory rate of this apolipoprotein when the cells were grown in its presence, the results of a typical experiment being exhibited in Fig 5. We were unable to demonstrate a clear dose-response relationship in 4 independent experiments over the range of 5-50 µM, and, paradoxically, greater inhibition was encountered when cells were incubated for 24 h than for 72 h. Since apo-AI is the dominant apolipoprotein of HDL and is essential for initiating reverse cholesterol transport as well as esterification of free cholesterol (19), our results suggest that *trans*-resveratrol may lead to some inhibition of these processes and in this regard it could have deleterious consequences from the standpoint of protection against atherosclerosis.

For this reason, it was instructive to examine the effects of another phenolic constituent of wine, quercetin, upon these processes. In 4 independent experiments, there was a consistent reduction of the intracellular concentration and rate of secretion of apoB which was more pronounced than the comparable effects of *trans*-resveratrol, but which did not show a clear dose-response relationship or time-dependence. Whereas the rates of secretion of cholesteryl esters and triglycerides were decreased by quercetin, their intracellular concentrations were increased (Fig 6). Finally, the synthesis and secretion of apoAI by Hep G2 cells were reduced to a greater extent by this polyphenol than by resveratrol (Fig 7). Whereas *trans*-resveratrol over the concentrations used in these experiments had no effect upon protein synthesis as judged by incorporation of ^{14}C-leucine into TCA-precipitable protein, concentrations of quercetin >20 µM strongly inhibited this process, a finding that makes it difficult to interpret our results. It does appear, however, that the effects of quercetin upon hepatic lipoprotein metabolism are less beneficial than those of resveratrol in protecting against atherosclerosis.

Platelet Aggregation. The significance of this process in the initiation of vascular endothelial damage in atherosclerosis and in precipitating lumenal occlusion leading to acute CHD has been described by earlier contributors to this Symposium. Our experiments were designed to examine the ability of *trans*-resveratrol to inhibit this aggregation and to ascertain its contribution to the overall anti-aggregatory potential of red wine (20).

Using ADP and thrombin as agonists, we demonstrated a dose-dependent inhibition by both *trans*-resveratrol and quercetin of aggregation by human platelets provoked by these agents which was more powerful than that caused by the total phenolics derived from dealcoholized wine on a molar basis . The IC_{50} for resveratrol was a little higher than that for quercetin with both agonists, but the IC_{50} for ethanol was three orders - of - magnitude higher for thrombin-induced aggregation whereas it had no inhibitory effect upon ADP-induced aggregation in the millimolar range. None of the other wine phenolics (catechin and epicatechin) or antioxidants (α-tocopherol, hydroquinone, butylated hydroxytoluene) tested had any effect on this process. The anti-aggregatory properties of red wine are thus in

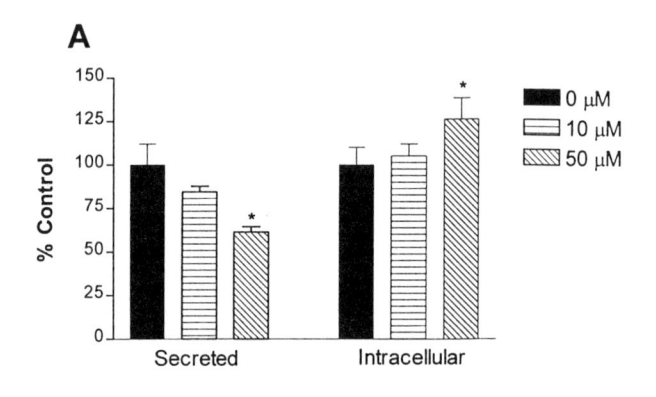

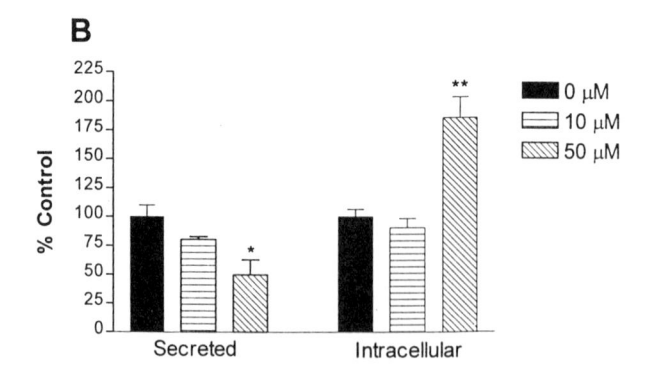

Figure 6. Effect of quercetin on the secretion and intracellular concentrations of cholesteryl esters (A) and triglycerides (B). Details as for Figure 4.

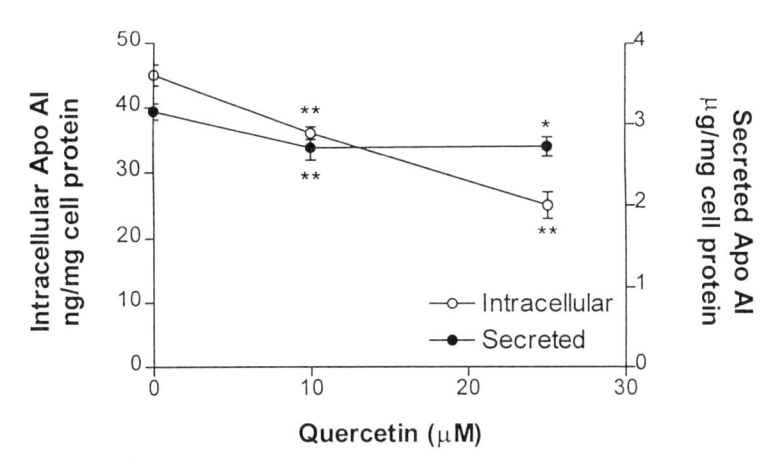

Figure 7. Effect of quercetin on the secretion and intracellular concentration of apolipoprotein AI. Details as for Figure 5.

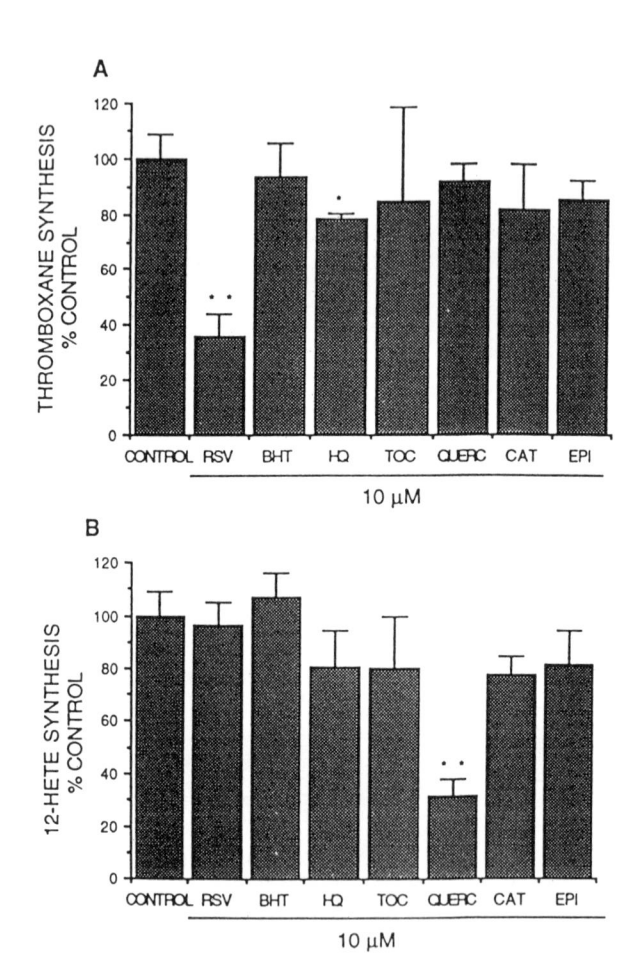

Figure 8. Effect of *trans*-resveratrol, antioxidants and other wine phenolics on the synthesis of thromboxane B_2 (A, top) and 12-HETE (B, bottom) from labelled arachidonate by washed human platelets at a fixed concentration of 10 µmol/L as a percentage of the control (DMSO) in which they were dissolved. Data are mean ± SD of 4 experiments. RSV, *trans*-resveratrol; BHT, butylated hydroxytoluene; HQ, hydroquinone; TOC, alpha-tocopherol; QUERC, quercetin; CAT, catechin; EPI, epicatechin. * $P< 0.05$; ** $P< 0.001$. Reproduced with permission from ref. 20. Copyright 1995, with kind permission from Elsevier Science - NL.

considerable measure due to these two polyphenols. Varying their content in red wine or in a de-alcoholized extracts of red wine caused marked changes in anti-aggregatory potential suggesting that the other phenolics had little or no effect, or were present in grossly sub-optimal concentrations. Indeed, applying information obtained from dose-response curves, we could compute the anti-aggregatory effect of a particular wine to approximate that expected from the sum of its concentrations of resveratrol and quercetin.

Eicosanoid Metabolism

Platelets. The effects of *trans*-resveratrol and quercetin were tested on two pathways of eicosanoid synthesis from arachidonic acid. The first was the cyclo-oxygenase pathway leading to the production of thromboxane A_2, a powerful pro-aggregatory eicosanoid which is synthesized by stimulated platelets and plays a crucial role in the propagation of aggregation once this process is initiated. Because of its very short half-life this component cannot be assayed with meaningful results, but the overall activity of the pathway and its rate of synthesis can be assessed by measuring the production from labeled arachidonate of thromboxane B_2 and HHT, two stable products of the pathway dowstream from thromboxane A_2. By these criteria, *trans*-resveratrol exercised a profound inhibitory effect upon thromboxane A_2 production, approximating 60% at a concentration of 10 µM (Fig 8a   ). Neither quercetin or any of the other wine phenolics or antioxidants tested had any effect at this concentration, with the exception of hydroquinone which caused a slight inhibition of 15-20%.

The other major eicosanoids produced from arachidonic acid by human platelets include the hepoxillins which are mediators of calcium mobilization, vascular permeability and neutrophil activation (21). This pathway involves the enzyme 12-lipoxygenase and one of its active and stable products is 12-HETE which has been postulated to be pro-atherogenic by virtue of impairing endothelial function and prostacyclin production (22). At a concentration of 10 µM, quercetin reduced the formation of 12-HETE by 70% (Fig 8b) but none of the other compounds tested were effective at this concentration, although at higher concentrations *trans*-resveratrol caused moderate inhibition.

Neutrophil Leukotriene Production. The production of leukotrienes by neutrophils through the lipoxygenase pathway represents the most important aspect of arachidonic acid metabolism in these cells (23). These compounds are powerful mediators of inflammatory reactions and are likely to play a role in at least some of the cellular processes that lead to the development of atherosclerosis (24,25). The two principal lipoxygenase enzymes in neutrophils are those of the 5- and 15- series, and their intracellular activity can be assessed by measuring the production from arachidonic acid of their stable products 5-HETE and 15-HETE, respectively.

In preliminary experiments, neither catechin, epicatechin, or the various antioxidants tested (hydroquinone, butylated hydroxytoluene or α-tocopherol) altered the rates of production of 5-HETE or 15-HETE from arachidonic acid by human neutrophil homogenates. On the other hand the synthesis of both products was profoundly inhibited by both resveratrol and quercetin. Dose-response studies provided IC_{50} estimates of 22.4 µM (resveratrol) and 2.8 µM (quercetin) for inhibition of 5-HETE synthesis, and 8.7 µM (resveratrol) and 0.75 µM (quercetin) for inhibition of 15-HETE synthesis. These effects must be independent of free-radical scavenging activity since they do not occur in the presence of more powerful anti-oxidants than resveratrol, such as catechin and epicatechin.

Conclusion

Taking into account its actions on apolipoprotein B and lipid secretion by liver cells, its inhibition of platelet aggregation and of the synthesis of thromboxane A_2 and leukotrienes as delineated by the studies reported herein, as well as its moderately high antioxidant activity as reported by others (26), resveratrol, together with quercetin, ranks as the most potent wine phenolic as defined by an array of biological properties likely to prevent the development of atherosclerosis.

Acknowledgement

We thank the National Research Council of Canada (IRAP) for their support of this work, and Mrs. Patricia Machado for preparation of the manuscript.

Literature Cited

1. Goldberg, D.M. *Clin. Chem.* **1995**, *41*, 14-16.
2. Goldberg, D.M.; Hahn, S.E.; Parkes, J.G. *Clin. Chim. Acta* **1995**, *237*, 155-187.
3. Siemann, E.H.; Creasy, L.L. *Am. J. Enol. Vitic.* **1992**, *43*, 49-52.
4. Goldberg, D.M.; Yan, J.; Ng, E.; Diamandis, E.P.; Karumanchiri, A.; Soleas, G.; Waterhouse, A.L. *Anal. Chem.* **1994**, *66*, 3959-3963
5. Goldberg, D.M., Karumanchiri, A.; Ng, E.; Yan, J.; Diamandis, E.P.; Soleas, G.J. *J. Agric. Food Chem.* **1995**, *43*, 1245-1250.
6. Soleas, G.J.; Goldberg, D.M.; Diamandis, E.P.; Karumanchiri, A.; Yan, J.; Ng, E. *Am. J. Enol. Vitic.* **1995**, *46*, 342-352.
7. Jayatilake, G.S.; Jayasuriya, H.; Lee, E.-S.; Koonchanok, N.M.; Geahlen, R.L.; Ashendel, C.L.; McLaughlin, J.L.; Chang, C.-J. *J. Nat. Prod.* **1993**, *56*, 1805-1810.
8. Goldberg, D.M.; Ng, E.; Karumanchiri, A.; Yan, J.; Diamandis, E.P.; Soleas, G.J. *J. Chromatogr. A* **1995**, *708*, 89-98.
9. Karumanchiri, A.; Tsang, E.; Ng, E.; Goldberg, D.M.; Soleas, G.J.; Diamandis, E.P.; *Am. J. Enol. Vitic.* **1995**, *46*,409.
10. Soleas, G.J.; Ng, E.; Yan, J.; Karumanchiri, A.; Diamandis, E.P.; Goldberg, D.M. *Am. J. Enol. Vitic.* **1995**, *46*, 409-410.
11. Jeandet, P.; Bessis, R.; Maume, B.F.; Sbaghi, M. *J. Wine Res.* **1993**, *4*, 79-85.

12. Lamuela-Raventos, R.M.; Waterhouse, A.L. *J. Agric. Food Chem.* **1993**, *41*, 521-523.
13. Pezet, R.; Pont, V.; Cuenat, P. *J. Chromatogr. A.* **1994**, *663*, 191-197.
14. Goldberg, D.M.; Yan, J.; Ng, E.; Diamandis, E.P.; Karumanchiri, A.; Soleas, G.J.; Waterhouse, A.L. *Am. J. Enol. Vitic.* **1995**, *46*, 159-165.
15. Roggero, J-P.; Archier, P. *Sci. Aliments* **1994**, *14*, 99-107.
16. Goldberg, D.M.; Ng, E.; Karumanchiri, A.; Diamandis, E.P.; Soleas, G.J. *Am. J. Enol. Vitic.* **1995**, *46*, 400.
17. Soleas, G.J.; Goldberg, D.M.; Karumanchiri, A.; Diamandis, E.P.; Ng, E. *J. Wine Res.* **1995**, *6*, 107-121.
18. Zannis, V.I.; Breslow, J.L.; San Giacomo, T.R.; Aden, D.P.; Knowles, B.B. *Biochemistry*, **1981**, *20*, 7089-7096.
19. Dolphin, P.J. *Can. J. Biochem. Cell Biol.* **1985**, *63*, 850-869.
20. Pace-Asciak, C.R.; Hahn, S.; Diamandis, E.P.; Soleas, G.J.; Goldberg, D.M. *Clin. Chim. Acta* **1995**, *235*, 207-219.
21. Pace-Asciak, C.R. *Gen Pharmacol.* **1993**, *24*, 805-810.
22. Spector, A.A.; Moore, S.A.; Gordon, E.E.L.; Gordon, J.A.; Kaduce, T.L. In *Proceedings of the Ninth International Symposium on Atherosclerosis*; Stein, O.; Eisenberg, S.; Stein, Y., Eds.; Creative Communications: Tel-Aviv, Israel, **1992;** pp 367-370.
23. Samuelsson, B. *Science* **1983**, *220*, 568-575.
24. Parsatharathy, S.; Wieland, E.; Steinberg, D. *Proc. Nat. Acad. Sci. USA.* **1989**, *86*, 1046-1050.
25. Ross, R. *Nature* **1993**, *362*, 801-809.
26. Frankel, E.N.; Waterhouse, A.L.; Kinsella, J.E. *Lancet* **1993**, *341*, 1103-1104.

Chapter 5

Resveratrol in Wine

Kenneth D. McMurtrey

Department of Chemistry and Biochemistry, University of Southern Mississippi, Hattiesburg, MS 39406–5043

ABSTRACT

Levels of *trans*-resveratrol in commercial red and white *Vitis vinifera* wines from several regions in Europe, South America, California, and Australia, which were purchased as individual bottles from vendors in this region, were determined using HPLC with electrochemical detection. In addition some white wines prepared in Mississippi from muscadine grapes, *Vitis rotundafolia*, were also analyzed. HPLC conditions suitable for simultaneous analysis of both *trans*-resveratrol and free quercetin were developed. Concentration of free quercetin is also reported for many of the wines analyzed.

Unlike white *V. vinifera* wines, white *V. rotundafolia* wines contain appreciable levels of resveratrol. Measured values ranged from about 0.3 to 1.2 mg/L (ppm), which is similar to resveratrol levels in some red California wines. We are not aware of other analyses of muscadine wines for resveratrol.

Highest resveratrol levels were found in a California Barbera (9.2 ppm), California Pinot noir (8.7 ppm), and a French Bordeaux (Merlot/Cabernet Sauvignon blend, 8.3 ppm). Bottles of the same type of wine from different vintners contained widely varying amounts of resveratrol. We also found that levels of resveratrol in multiple bottles of the same wine also varied considerably. Fourteen bottles of a California non vintage blended red wine contained resveratrol levels from 2.74 to 5.77 ppm while eight bottles of a California 1993 Cabernet Sauvignon had levels from 0.46 to 0.74 ppm, nearly the same degree of variation.

INTRODUCTION

It is now reasonably well accepted that red wine has potentially positive effects on human cardiovascular health. Resveratrol (*trans*-3, 4', 5-trihydroxy-stilbene, produced by certain plants as an antifungal agent) has been suggested as one of the components which may provide some of these health benefits. In addition, wine components such as the flavanol, quercetin have also been nominated as potentially positive dietary components. Others papers in this volume will provide details on potential health benefits of wine and wine components. The primary focus of this paper will be to discuss application of HPLC with electrochemical detection to measurement of resveratrol levels in wines at the point of consumption. Levels of free quercetin have also been measured for some wines. While quercetin analysis is still preliminary, available data will be presented.

© 1997 American Chemical Society

Analysis of wines for resveratrol began with an account published in 1992 by Siemann and Creasy, the seminal paper of this area. These researchers used an analytical technique which involved a complicated multistep process requiring extraction with ethyl acetate, freezing overnight to remove water, rotary evaporation, normal phase preparative HPLC, irradiation with UV light to convert *trans*-resveratrol to the *cis*-isomer and finally analysis by reversed-phase HPLC with UV detection.

Jeandet, *et al.* (1993) analyzed wines using a process involving multistep extraction followed by derivitization to give trimethylsilyl ethers followed by analysis on gas chromatography.

Lamuela-Raventós and Waterhouse (1993) shortened the extraction procedure required somewhat and analyzed the resulting extracts using HPLC with diode-array UV detection. Both of the above reports found relatively low levels of resveratrol.

Analysis of resveratrol was simplified further by Mattivi (1993), who used disposable extraction cartridges follow by analysis of extracts using HPLC with UV detection. This report found somewhat higher levels of resveratrol than had previously been reported.

Pezet, *et al.* (1994) reported analysis of *trans*-resveratrol and related pterostilbenes in grape berries and wines using HPLC with fluorescence detection. Because of the greater sensitivity of fluorescence to *trans*-resveratrol, wines were analyzed by direct injection without the sample treatments which had previously been used. These authors found levels of resveratrol consistent with those reported by Mattivi and higher than those given in earlier reports. Pezet, *et al.*, reported that *trans*-resveratrol was unstable to conditions used during rotary evaporation in earlier accounts.

We employed direct injection of 10 μL samples of wine on liquid chromatographs with electrochemical detectors operated in an oxidative mode (McMurtrey, *et al.*, 1994). We examined eleven wines and found low levels of *trans*-resveratrol ($\leq$ 0.02 mg/L) in four white wines and levels of from 1 to 5 mg/L in the seven red wines studied. These levels were consistent with those reported by Mattivi and Pezet, *et al.*

Goldberg *et al.* (1994) has reported details of a method for determining *trans*-resveratrol using octadecylsilyl extraction cartridges eluted with ethyl acetate followed by analysis using combined gas chromatography/mass spectrometry. These authors report finding resveratrol levels in red wines from 0.1 to 12 mg/L. They indicate that resveratrol concentrations follow geographical distribution with relatively low levels in wines from California, Australia, and Italy, and relatively high levels in wines from Oregon, Canada, and France.

Lamuela-Raventós and co-workers (1995) have extended analysis of wines to include determination of both *cis*- and *trans*-resveratrol and their glycoside conjugates, the piceids, in wine using direct injection (after filtration) and diode array UV detection. In this account these researchers found combined *cis*-, and *trans*-resveratrol and the *cis*-, and *trans*-piceid levels of up to 13.8 mg/L in a Spanish Merlot with high levels also in Pinot noir wines from that country. The *cis*-resveratrol and piceid and *trans*-piceid compounds could apparently be converted in the body to *trans*-resveratrol by combined isomerization and hydrolysis reactions.

Further details of the analytical procedures used by the research groups of Drs. Lamuela-Raventós and Goldberg, as well as results from application of these procedures, are to be found in papers in this collection.

RESULTS AND DISCUSSION

We were initially interested in the analysis of wine for the *trans*-isomer of resveratrol and have not performed analyses specifically for the *cis* analog.

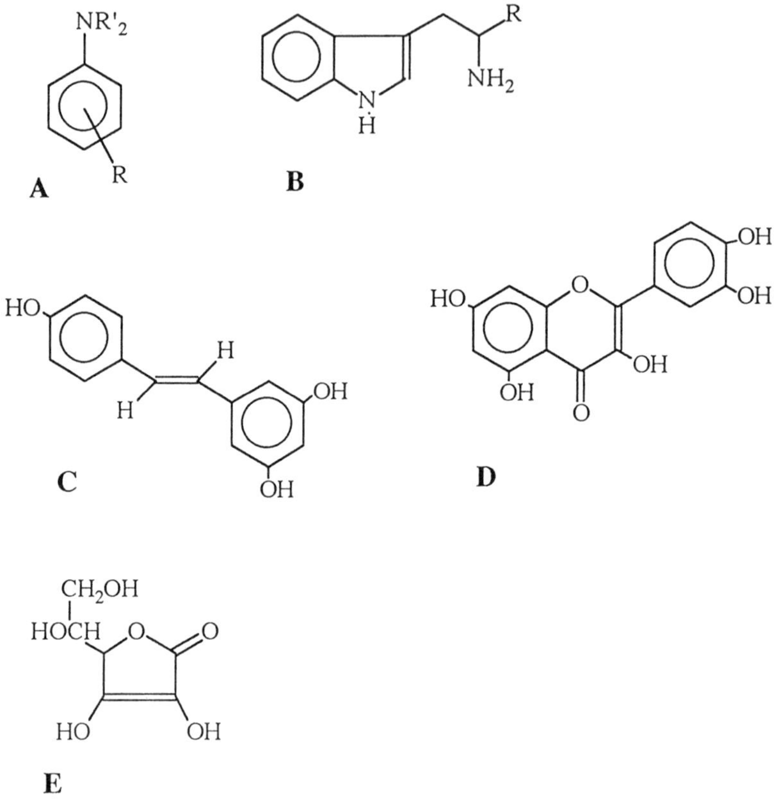

Figure 1. Substances readily detected using HPLC with electrochemical detection in the oxidative mode. A. aniline derviatives, B. tryptamine, tryptophan and other indoles; phenols such as C. *trans*-resveratrol, D. quercetin; and enols such as E. ascorbic acid.

Resveratrol levels quoted below are for *trans*-resveratrol only, and unless specified the use of the term resveratrol is meant to indicate the *trans*-isomer only.

Analytical Conditions: Analysis of substances such as resveratrol by chromatography or other analytical techniques is dependent on a balance of selectivity and sensitivity. In this regard, for a successful analytical method based on HPLC the column must be capable of separating the components of interest from interfering substances while the detector must be capable of detecting and quantitating the analyte at the levels available. The chromatography column can affect sensitivity primarily through peak sharpness, while the detector may also contribute to selectivity if it is insensitive to materials in the matrix.

We chose an electrochemical detection as the method for monitoring resveratrol in wines primarily because of its excellent sensitivity to phenolic substances. When used under the conditions which were employed (glassy carbon working electrode, silver/silver chloride reference electrode, stainless steel auxiliary electrode, oxidative mode), the detector responds very well to two groups of organic compounds: aromatic amines and phenols, Figure 1. Aromatic amines including substituted analines and biologically important substances such as tryptamine and tryptophane are readily detected as are phenols including resveratrol, quercetin, and any of the other many phenolic substances contained in wine. Some enolic materials such as ascorbic acid are also detected. Thus, the electrochemical detector would also respond well to *cis*-resveratrol, the piceid derivatives of the two isomers of resveratrol, and to various sugar conjugates of flavonoids such as quercetin, assuming that at least one phenolic hydroxyl group remains unconjugated.

Sensitivity levels obtained with the electrochemical detector are more than sufficient for quantitation of resveratrol or quercetin at the parts-per-million or parts-per-billion levels. We have not tested the ultimate limit of sensitivity but they appear to be at least in the mid ppt (ng/L) range for resveratrol, well below the levels currently of interest.

Initial conditions for resveratrol analysis are those used in Figure 2. A mobile phase of 25% acetonitrile afforded separation of resveratrol from other components with a retention time of about 16 minutes. Although resveratrol was easily quantitated, quercetin eluted partially overlapping an interfering peak, ca. 25 and 26 min, respectively. We have modified the original conditions of analysis with the goal of being able to quantitate both trans-resveratrol and free quercetin during the same chromatographic analysis.

The mobile phase was changed from acetonitrile-ammonium phosphate buffer to one composed of methanol and formic acid. To keep the analysis time within the same interval (approximately 30 min, or less) the percent of organic modifier was increased to 45% and the counterion used was formic acid, which also decreased the pH of the mobile phase from a value of about 4.5 to 2.5. An example of analysis of a red wine with these conditions is given if Figure 3. In this case while separation of quercetin in near optimum, the resveratrol peak elutes early in the chromatogram and may provide less than ideal conditions for quantitation.

We next employed a mixture of acetonitrile and methanol as the organic modifier of the mobile phase. In addition, it appeared that formic acid may lead to early failure of the reference electrodes. Ammonium phosphate (0.05 M, pH adjusted to 3.0) was used instead. We desired a blend of methanol and acetonitrile which would provide good conditions for analysis of both *trans*-resveratrol and quercetin and have an analysis time of approximately 25 minutes. A simple graph was constructed, see Figure 4. Boundary mobile phases of 25% CH_3CN with 0.05 M ammonium phosphate, pH 3.0, and 47% methanol with the same buffer were used as graph end points. These two mobile phases provided equal retention time for quercetin although resveratrol is eluted more rapidly in the methanolic phase. This graph allow rapid selection of percent acetonitrile and methanol which should give approximately equal total analysis time for quercetin. Thus, a mixture of 20%

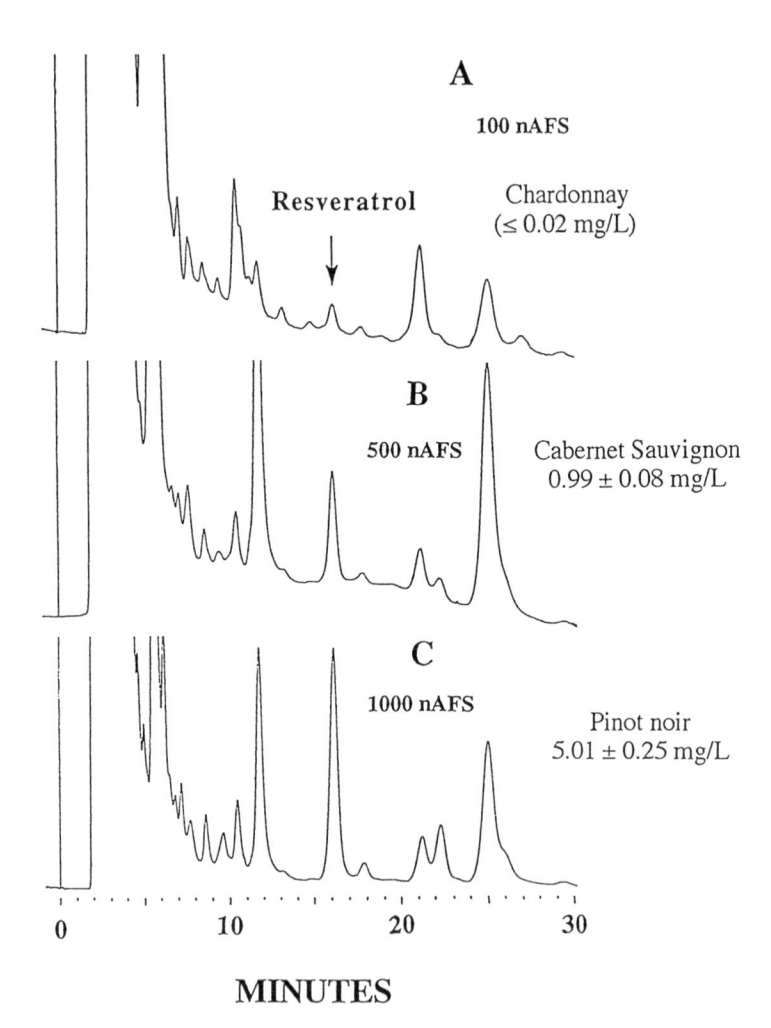

Figure 2. Analysis of three wines by HPLC with electrochemical detection. Chromatographic conditions were: Nucleosil C18, 5 μm, 4.6 X 150 mm, mobile phase 25 % (v/v) acetonitrile 75 % 0.05 M $NH_4H_2PO_4$, 1.0 mL/min. Resveratrol elutes at ca. 16 min. Sensitivity in trace A is 5 times that in trace B and 10 times that of trace C. Quercetin elutes at about 25 min with an unresolved unknown substance (trailing edge). The electrochemical detector was operated at 0.5 V vs. the Ag/AgCl reference electrode.

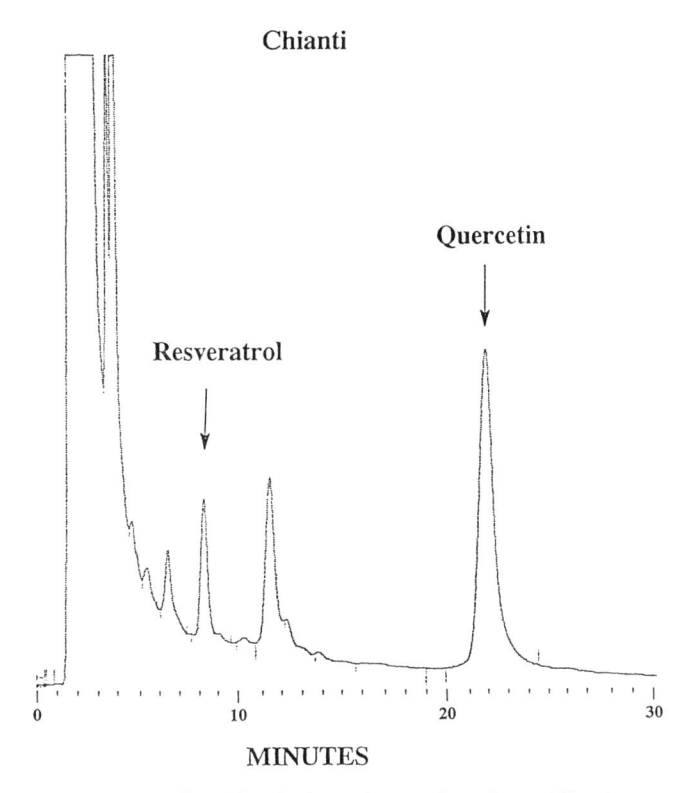

Figure 3. Analysis of a Chianti wine using methanolic mobile phase. Chromatography conditions similar to those employed in Figure 2 were used except that the mobile phase was 45% (v/v) methanol in 0.5% formic acid.

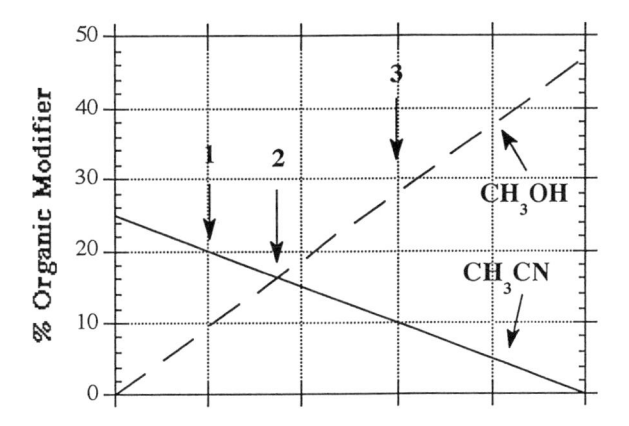

Figure 4. Graph for selecting acetonitrile–methanol mixtures. Methanol (– – –), acetonitrile (——).

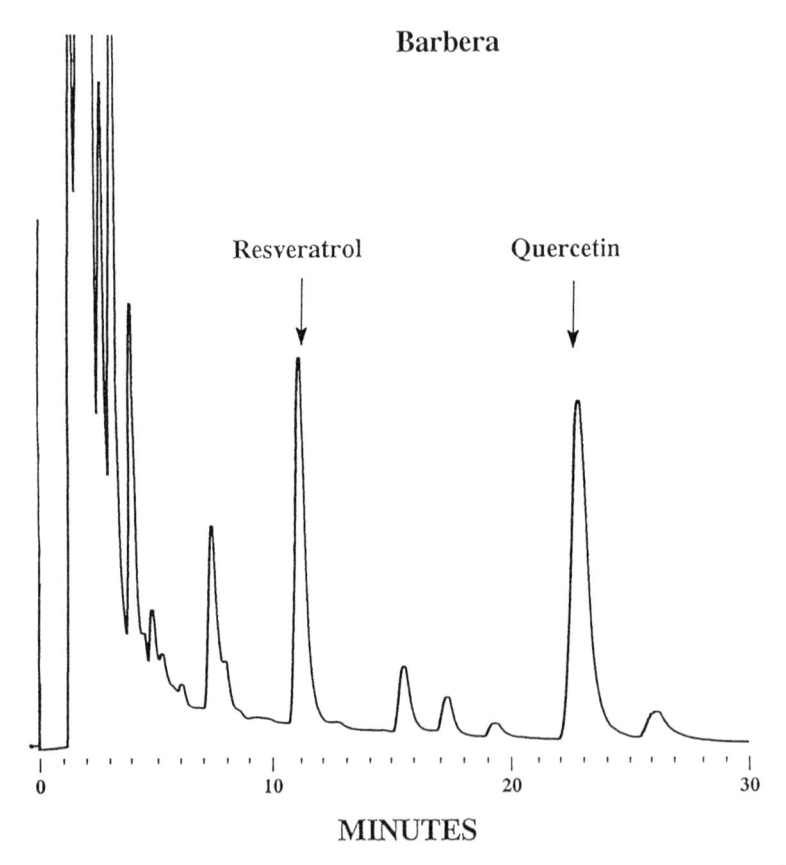

Figure 5. Analysis of Barbera wine under conditions that allow quantitation of both *trans*-resveratrol and quercetin in a single chromatographic analysis. Nucleosil C18 column, 4.6 X 150 mm, 16% each CH_3CN and MeOH + 68% 0.05 M $NH_4H_2PO_4$, pH 3.0, 1.0 mL/min. EC detector 0.700 V vs. Ag/AgCl, 1000 nAFS

acetonitrile and 9% methanol + 71% ammonium phosphate buffer (1, Figure 4), a mixture of 16% of each organic solvent + 68% ammonium phosphate (2, Figure 4), or 10% acetonitile and 28% methanol + 62% ammonium phosphate (3, Figure 4) should give approximately equivalent quercetin retention with respective decreasing resveratrol retention time. It was found that a 16% mixture of the two solvents provided a mobile phase which separated the two analytes well, see Figure 5. These conditions are now used in the analysis of wines in our laboratory.

Results of Wine Analyses: A number of commercial wines were analyzed for resveratrol, with some analyses also quantitating free quercetin. As others have found, white wines from *vinifera* grapes contain little resveratrol, see Table 1. Even wines from grapes grown in England (with its relatively moist climate) contain little.

Table 1

Resveratrol and Free Quercetin Levels in Commercial White *Vitis vinifera* Wine

Variety (Vintner)	Vintage	Origin	Resveratrol	Quercetin
Chardonnay (Marcus James)	NA	Brazil	≤ 0.02*	----
Chardonnay (Blossom Hill)	NV	Calif.	≤ 0.02	0.20 ± 0.02
White blend (Deer Valley)	NV	"	≤ 0.02*	0.54 ± 0.17
Sauvignon blanc (Gallo)	1991	"	≤ 0.02*	0.06 ± 0.01
Dry Sherry (Gallo)	NV	"	≤ 0.01*	nil
White Zinfandel (Beringer)	1993	Calif.	≤ 0.02	----
Gewürtztraminer (Fetzer)	1992	"	≤ 0.02	----
Schönburger (Battle)	NV	England	≤ 0.02	----
Wurzer	NV	"	≤ 0.02	----

*data from McMurtrey, *et al*., 1994.

We have found one group of white wines which do have relatively high levels of resveratrol. These wines are prepared from muscadine grapes, *Vitis rotundifolia*, rather than *V. vinifera*, see Table 2. All of the muscadine wines have more than ten times as much resveratrol as any of the white *vinifera* wines which we have tested. Indeed, resveratrol levels in these muscadine wines are equivalent to or greater than those in some California red wines. With one exception, these muscadine wines are produced in laboratories at Mississippi State University as part of a program to increase use of muscadine grapes. The single exception is produced at a commercial winery in Mississippi. We are unaware of previous analyses of resveratrol in muscadine wines.

It is not completely surprising that wines prepared from *V. rotundifolia* contain relatively high levels of *trans*-resveratrol. This grape species grow well in the very high humidity areas of the Gulf Coast where conditions are excellent for development of fungal infections. Accordingly, the plants require as much protection from these infections as possible.

Table 2

Resveratrol Levels in White *Vitis rotundifolia* Wines

Variety (Vintner)	Vintage	Origin	Resveratrol
Noble	1992	Mississippi	0.73 ± 0.04
Noble	1993	"	0.46 ± 0.03
Noble Rosé	1993	"	0.66 ± 0.03
Cowart	1993	"	0.58 ± 0.04
Carlos (Old South)	NV*	"	0.65 ± 0.05
Carlos	1993	"	0.66 ± 0.07
Carlos	1992	"	0.62 ± 0.07
Doreen	1993	"	1.18 ± 0.06
Magnolia	1993	"	0.29 ± 0.05

*commercial wine

Resveratrol and quercetin content of red wines appear to be extremely variable, Table 3. Our earlier observation, and the observation of others, that Pinot noir wines from California appear to have high levels of resveratrol relative to wines of other varieties grown in that state still appears to be valid, however, this generalization does not appear to be as striking as it seemed when fewer results were available. For example, the single Barbera wine analyzed had the highest resveratrol level of any wine that we have tested. The most striking aspect of our data appears to be the considerable variability in resveratrol (and quercetin) concentrations even in wines produced from the same variety of grape. Resveratrol concentration in a wine is expected to vary with a number of factors. Genetics of the variety of grape, growing conditions, conditions of preparation and storage all should affect resveratrol content of the wines.

We next examined resveratrol variation in multiple samples of two California wines, Table 4. The wines selected were a blended non vintage wine prepared from Barbera, Pinot noir, Zinfandel, and Ruby Cabernet grapes and a Cabernet Sauvignon wine, vintage 1993. Single bottles of these wines were purchased from several merchants in the area as individual purchases. The blended wine was purchased over about 30 months while the Cabernet Sauvignon was obtained over about six months. This selection pattern was chosen to mimic purchase of wines by consumers. Not surprisingly the blended wine showed considerable variation in resveratrol content, which ranged from approximately 2.7 to about 5.8 ppm. This might be expected because the different grapes (Barbera, Pinot noir, Zinfandel, and Ruby Cabernet) are different genetically, may have been grown in different vineyards, and may even be from different years. Furthermore, the percentages of each grape variety making up the blend may have changed from one bottle to the next. Results of the analyses of the Cabernet Sauvignon selected, however, were unexpected. Although the resveratrol levels were considerably less than those in the blended wine, nearly the same variation was apparent: the greatest concentration of resveratrol was about 1.6 times that of the lowest level.

Table 3

Resveratrol and Free Quercetin Levels in Red Wines

Wine (Vintner)	Vintage	Origin	Resveratrol	Quercetin
Merlot/ Cabernet Sauvignon	1990	France	8.26 ± 0.24	3.57 ± 0.06
"Burgundy"	NV	CA	0.50*	3.33 ± 0.37
75% Cab. Sauv./ 25% Mer.	1991	Chile	1.56 ± 0.08*	1.46 ± 0.07
Barbera, Pinot noir, Zinfandel, Ruby Cab.	NV	CA	2.74 ± 0.08*	----
Barbera (Sebastiani)	1991	CA	9.20 ± 0.40	13.40 ± 0.60
Beaujolais (Jadot)	1992	France	3.55 ± 0.06*	0.15 ± 0.02
" (St. Louis)	1992	France	3.27 ± 0.0.14*	0.19 ± 0.02
Cabernet Sauvig.(Gallo)	1986	CA	0.99 ± 0.08*	----
" (Gallo)	1992	CA	2.78 ± 0.16	3.06 ± 0.28
" (Avia)	1989	Slovenia	0.95 ± 0.01	3.33 ± 0.37
" (Kendall-Jackson)	1991	CA	4.33 ± 0.54	----
" (Vendange)	1993	CA	0.53 ± 0.02	5.03 ± 0.48
Chianti (Ruffino)	1993	Italy	4.80 ± 0.10	----
" (Placido)	1993	Italy	2.76 ± 0.10	7.34 ± 0.08
Citra (Montapulcitano)	1993	Italy	2.60 ± 0.15	3.37 ± 0.21
Gamay Beaujolais	1994	CA	2.09 ± 0.17	----
Merlot (Marcus James)	1991	Brazil	3.30 ± 0.10	4.00 ± 0.27
" (Walnut Creek)	1992	CA	5.42 ± 0.23	3.04 ± 0.00
" (Rosemount Estate)	1993	Australia	5.78 ± 0.09	9.62 ± 0.13
" (Deer Valley)	1992	CA	3.57 ± 0.33	----
Petit Sarah (Mirassou)	1991	CA	1.76 ± 0.11	----
Pinot noir (Sebastiani)	1990	CA	5.01 ± 0.25*	1.82 ± 0.16
" (Mt. View)	1991	CA	7.99± 0.09	3.32 ± 0.06
" (Beaulieu)	1991	CA	3.72 ± 0.10	0.90 ± 0.12
" (Mirassou)	1992	CA	8.70 ± 0.10	----
Zinfandel (Sutter Home)	1991	CA	1.38 ± 0.18*	0.90 ± 0.10
" (Sebastiani)	1991	CA	4.90 ± 0.50	4.96 ± 0.58

*data from McMurtrey, et al., 1994.

Table 4

Resveratrol and Free Quercetin Levels in Replicate Samples of Two California Red Wines

Variety(Vintner)	Resveratrol	Quercetin
blended (Deer Valley)	2.74 ± 0.08*	----
"	3.42 ± 0.13	----
"	3.50 ± 0.42	----
"	3.51 ± 0.18	----
"	3.61 ± 0.08	----
"	3.85 ± 0.25	----
"	4.43 ± 0.03	----
"	4.76 ± 0.14	----
"	4.81 ± 0.05	----
"	4.90 ± 0.21	----
"	5.14 ± 0.44	----
"	5.34 ± 0.32	----
"	5.35 ± 0.26	----
"	5.49 ± 0.27	----
"	5.77 ± 0.05	----
Cabernet Sauvignon, 1993 (Vendange)	0.46 ± 0.01	3.62 ± 0.25
"	0.49 ± 0.02	3.87 ± 0.10
"	0.51 ± 0.02	3.60 ± 0.15
"	0.53 ± 0.01*	4.83 ± 0.18
"	0.53 ± 0.02	5.03 ± 0.48
"	0.63 ± 0.03	5.28 ± 0.17
"	0.66 ± 0.04	5.46 ± 0.08
"	0.74 ± 0.03	5.35 ± 0.03

blended: Barbera, Pinot noir, Zinfandel, and Ruby Cabernet
*data from McMurtrey, et al., 1994

Comparison of resveratrol and quercetin content of the Cabernet Sauvignon detailed in Table 4 might suggest some sort of relationship between the levels of these two compounds. However, consideration of the data in all Tables indicates that if there is a relationship it is not a simple one, particularly if different varities of wines are compared.

From the standpoint of a consumer, the data in Table 4 indicate that it would be very difficult or impossible to predict with great precision the amount of resveratrol being ingested in the diet from consumption of a particular wine. Even if analyses are available for a particular vintage and brand of wine the actual resveratrol level in a particular bottle of that wine may be no closer than a factor of two to the presumed value. If it becomes established that resveratrol does confer significant health benefits it may be important that analysis of wine for the substance be performed on a routine basis. Because of its sensitivity, lack of sample treatment and low cost HPLC with electrochemical detection is certainly a valuable technique which compares favorably to other methods of analysis.

ACKNOWLEDGMENT

We would like to thank Dr. Betty Ector, Department of Home Economics, Mississippi State University, for providing samples of wines prepared from *Vitis rotundafolia* grapes.

LITERATURE CITED

Goldberg, D.M.; Yan, J.; Ng, E.; Diamandis, E.P.; Karumanchiri, A.; Soleas, G.; Waterhouse, A.L. Direct injection gas chromatographic mass spectrometric assay for *trans*-resveratrol, *Anal. Chem.*, **1994**, *66*, 3959-3963.

Jeandet, P.; Bessis, R.; Maume, B.F.; Sbaghi, M. Analysis of resveratrol in burgundy wine, *J. Wine Res.*, **1993**, *4*, 79-85.

Lamuela-Raventós, R.M.; Waterhouse, A.L. Occurrence of resveratrol in selected California wines by a new HPLC method, *J. Agric. Food Chem.*, **1993**, *41*, 521-523.

Lamuela-Raventós, R.M; Romero-Pérez, A.I.; Waterhouse, A.L.; de la Torre-Boronat, M.C. Direct HPLC analysis of *cis*- and *trans*-resveratrol and piceid isomers in Spanish red *Vitis vinifera* wines, *J. Agric. Food Chem.*, **1995**, *43*, 281-283.

Mattivi, F. Solid-phase ectraction of *trans*-resveratrol from wines for HPLC analysis, *Z. Lebensm. Unters. Forsch.*, **1993**, *196*, 522-525.

McMurtrey, K.D.; Minn, J.; Pobanz, K.; Schultz, T.P. Analysis of wines for resveratrol using direct injection high-pressure liquid chromatography with electrochemical detection, *J. Agric. Food Chem.*, **1994**, *42*, 2077-2080.

Pezet, R.; Pont, V.; Cuenat, P. Method to determine resveratrol and pterostilbene in grape berries and wines using high-performance liquid chromatography with highly sensitive fluorometric detection, *J. Chromatogr. A* **1994**, *663*, 191-197.

Siemann, E.H.; Creasy, L.L. Concentration of the phytoalexin resveratrol in wine. *Am. J. Enol. Vitic.*, **1992**, *43*, 49-52.

Chapter 6

Resveratrol and Piceid Levels in Wine Production and in Finished Wines

Rosa M. Lamuela-Raventós[1], A. I. Romero-Pérez[1],
Andrew L. Waterhouse[2], M. Lloret[1], and M. C. de la Torre-Boronat[1]

[1]Nutrició i Bromatologia, Facultat de Farmàcia, Universidad de Barcelona, Avinguda Joan XXIII s/n, 08028-Barcelona, Spain
[2]Department of Viticulture and Enology, University of California, Davis, CA 95616–8749

A direct HPLC method has been developed for the quantification of four resveratrol derivatives, the *cis* and *trans* isomers of resveratrol and their glucosides, the piceids. The concentration of these compounds was determined in 60 samples of red, rosé and white wine. Analysis of the low levels in the white wines required an additional sample concentration step. This method was also applied to following the levels of these four compounds during the fermentation and maceration, at a winery scale, of one Merlot and two Cabernet Sauvignon wines. The presence or absence of glycosylation affected the extraction rate while a comparison of the three fermentations showed that each compound had a characteristic extraction behavior.

Heart disease is the first leading cause of death in developed countries. A healthy diet is one of the factors that can contribute to reduce cardiac disease mortality. The traditional Mediterranean diet is accepted as a relatively healthy diet and it has been promoted by the Harvard School of Public Health, United Nations World Health Organization/Food and Agriculture Organization (WHO/FAO), and Oldways Preservation & Exchange Trust. One of the components included in this diet is wine, in moderation, normally with meals. Epidemiological studies show that wine consumption is related to a decrease in cardiovascular disease (1) (2); however, these beneficial effects are not observed among beer and spirits drinkers (2). It has been hypothesized that the compounds responsible for this positive effect are the phenols present in wine (3). The presence of the phenols, *trans*-resveratrol and its glucoside, piceid, (see Figure 1) in wines has been of much interest for their physiological properties. *trans*-Resveratrol is one of the compounds present in wines that could be responsible for the decrease in coronary heart disease observed among wine drinkers, since it

© 1997 American Chemical Society

inhibits LDL oxidation (4), it blocks platelet aggregation (5); (6) and eicosanoid synthesis (6, 7). Piceid, the 3-β-glucoside of *trans*-resveratrol, also shows antiplatelet aggregation properties (6, 7), and it may release *trans*-resveratrol by the β-glucosidase hydrolysis, after ingestion (8). However, the levels of these compounds required to inhibit platelet aggregation are not very clear, since big differences are found among the antiaggregation reports. Pace-Asciak et al. (1995) (6) reported that 129.9±64.4 μmol/L of *trans*-resveratrol can inhibit platelet aggregation by 50%, when ADP is used as inducer, or 164.7±67.3 μmol/L, when thrombin is the inducer; while Bertelli et al (1995) (5) found that 0.016 μmol/L inhibited platelet aggregation by 50.3%, when collagen was the inducer. Similar disparities are reported with the inhibition of eicosanoid synthesis; the levels which have physiological effects by Pace-Asciak et al (1995) (6) are 10 times higher than those reported by Kimura et al (1985) (7).

The activity of the *cis* isomers in LDL oxidation. The *cis* isomers show that they also have, as the *trans* isomers, potential anticancer activity by inhibiting protein-tyrosine kinase (9).

In grape berries, resveratrol synthesis is primarily located at the skin cells and it is absent or low, in the fruit flesh. In red vinification, maceration with skins and seeds, during fermentation, contribute to the extraction of the phenols present in the firmer tissue. Resveratrol requires relatively long maceration time on the skins to be extracted (10-13). The extraction of resveratrol in fermentation is controlled by the increase in ethanol concentration, the enzymatic activity (14) and presumably phenols are affected by absorptive interaction with yeast (15, 16), which settle out after fermentation, and by the fermentation temperature.

Red wines have the highest *trans*-resveratrol content, since they are macerated with skins for a longer time (13, 17-20). In the only study done in rosé wines (20), *trans*-resveratrol levels were between 0.005 to 1.19 mg/L, with higher amounts in the wine related to longer maceration.White wine is reported to have much lower resveratrol content than the red wine (19, 21, 22), presumably due to minimal skin contact associated with white wine production. Jeandet et al. (1995) (19) noted that white wines macerated with skins had a higher resveratrol content, than non-macerated ones. Goldberg et al. (1993) (23) describe the minimum and a maximum levels for white wines, and they note that one Sauvignon blanc had the highest level, 1.3 mg/L, while the levels in other white wines were so low that they could not be quantified.

Since 1992, when Siemann and Creasy (17) described the presence of the phytoalexin *trans*-resveratrol in wines, many different methods have been described to determine this compound in wines, including these based on HPLC with UV detection (18, 22, 24, 25), and by GC/MS (19, 23, 26, 27), these method required prior sample treatment, before injection. In 1994, McMurtrey et al,. (21) and Pezet et al (22) developed a direct HPLC analysis using electrochemical and fluorimetric detectors, respectively. These methods were very sensitive and rapid. However, they only analyzed *trans*-resveratrol.

The HPLC method developed by Lamuela-Raventós et al (28) allowed the determination of the four resveratrol derivatives in red, rosé and white wines; however, in white wines a concentration step was necessary to quantify the four resveratrol isomers. Since two reports have claimed that *trans*-resveratrol is unstable to rotary

evaporation (22, 24), and this technique is used in the analysis of white wines, the stability of these compounds in the rotovap was confirmed.
We report the levels of the four resveratrol derivatives in red, rosé and white Spanish wines and we also follow the evolution pattern of the four compounds during fermentation to establish the extraction kinetics of these compounds during fermentation.

Material and Methods

Samples. Red wines. Wines from different harvests and appellations were analyzed. The varieties tested were Cabernet Sauvignon, Merlot, Pinot noir, Tempranillo, and Grenache.
Rosé wines. Three different varieties were tested Cabernet Sauvignon, Pinot noir, and Grenache, being the only varietal rosé wines in the Barcelona market.
White wines. The white wine grape varieties analyzed were Albariño, Chardonnay, Macabeo, Parellada, White Riesling, Sauvignon blanc, Verdejo and Xarel.lo.
Fermentation curves in red vinification. Cabernet Sauvignon (40,000 Kg) and Merlot (20,000 Kg) were destemmed, crushed, and fermented in the presence of the skins and seeds. Three different tanks of approximately 12,000 L were vinified separately, two of Cabernet Sauvignon and one of Merlot. Samples were collected every two days until the fermentation had finished. Samples of the musts were treated with 1 g/L of NaF to stop the fermentation, and frozen at - 21 °C. Samples were centrifuged (1800g x 20 min.). Absorbance at 280 nm for total phenols and 320 nm for hydroxycinnamates were determined in these samples, in 1 mm and 10 mm cells, respectively, in a Hewlett-Packard 8452A diode array spectrophotometer, according to the method described by Somers and Ziemelis (1985) (29). Total anthocyanins were measured following Somers and Evans (1977) (30).

Stilbenes determination. Red and rosé wine samples were analyzed by direct HPLC injection, after filtration through Whatman inorganic Anopore membrane filters (Anodisc. 0.2 μm).Quantitation of the low levels of the *cis* forms in some white wines required an additional sample concentration step; 10 mL was concentrated to 1 mL by rotary evaporation (30°C, in vacuo) and the concentrate was filtered through a Whatman inorganic Anopore membrane filter, with a prefilter of glass microfiber to avoid plugging the membrane filter (Anotop 10 PlusTM, 0.2μm). The precision, recovery and reproducibility, of the method were established following The U. S. Pharmacopoeia (USP XXII) (31).
All the samples were protected from light to avoid light-induced isomerization.

HPLC analysis. A Hewlett-Packard (HP) 1050 instrument equipped with a Rheodyne injection valve (Model 7125), (100 μL fixed loop) and a diode-array UV-vis detector HP 1040 M coupled to a Chem Station HP 79995A. The column used was a Tracer Nucleosil, C18 120 (25 cm x 0.4 cm), 5 μm particle size, with a precolumn of the same material, maintained at 40 °C.
Results of the analyses are expresses in equivalents of *trans*-resveratrol, based on absorbance of the *trans* and *cis* isomers at 306 and 285 nm, respectively.

Results and Discussion

The validation of the HPLC method was described previously (28).

Red wines. Pinot noir wines have the highest levels of *trans*-resveratrol, as was observed previously in California (18, 21) and in French wines (25). However, the total amount of resveratrol derivatives were very similar in Merlot and in Pinot noir (see Figure 2).
trans-Resveratrol was the major compound followed by *trans*-piceid. So the *trans* forms predominate compared to the *cis* ones. The compound present at lowest concentration was *cis*-resveratrol.

Rosé wines. The levels of resveratrol monomers are between the levels of white and red wines. *trans*-Resveratrol levels were similar to those described in the only previous study done on rosé wines (20). On these rosé wines, the content of resveratrol does not depend on variety (see Figure 3), presumably because the time of maceration with the skins depends on the technology applied by each winery. In average, the levels of *trans*-resveratrol were very similar to *trans*-piceid. Rosé wines are made with short maceration time with skins, so *trans*-resveratrol, because of its polarity, is not totally extracted from the skins. Again, *cis*-resveratrol is the compound present at the lowest concentration.

White wines. The degradation of resveratrol during rotary evaporation, as described by Pezet et al. (22) was not observed, and the amounts of the four compounds were the same before and after concentration.
White wines had the lowest resveratrol content (see Figure 4). The variety affected the amount of resveratrol isomers present. The traditional Spanish varieties, Xarel.lo, Parellada, Albariño, Verdejo, and Macabeo, had higher amounts of these compounds than the varieties more recently introduced to Spain, Sauvignon blanc, white Riesling, and Chardonnay, ($p<0.01$).
trans-Piceid was the compound present on average at the highest level, however the concentrations were 10 times lower than the levels described in Spanish red wines.
trans- Resveratrol was the second most abundant compound, however the levels of *trans*-resveratrol were 20 times lower than in red wine.
cis-Resveratrol, as in the cases of red and rosé wines, was the compound present at the lowest concentrations.

Evolution of Resveratrol during Fermentation. During the Merlot fermentations, the aglycons were always at lower concentrations than their respective glucosides (see Figure 5). However, in the two Cabernet Sauvignon fermentations, the glucosides predominated at the beginning of the fermentation, but at the end, the aglycons were higher (see Figure 6). This same pattern was observed by Mattivi with the Lambrusco a foglia frastagliata variety (14).
The total amount of resveratrol (*cis* and *trans* resveratrol plus *cis* and *trans* piceid) had its maximum in all cases on the eighth day of fermentation, and levels then

Figure 1. Structures of the *Trans* Isomers and the *Cis* Isomers of Resveratrol and Piceid.

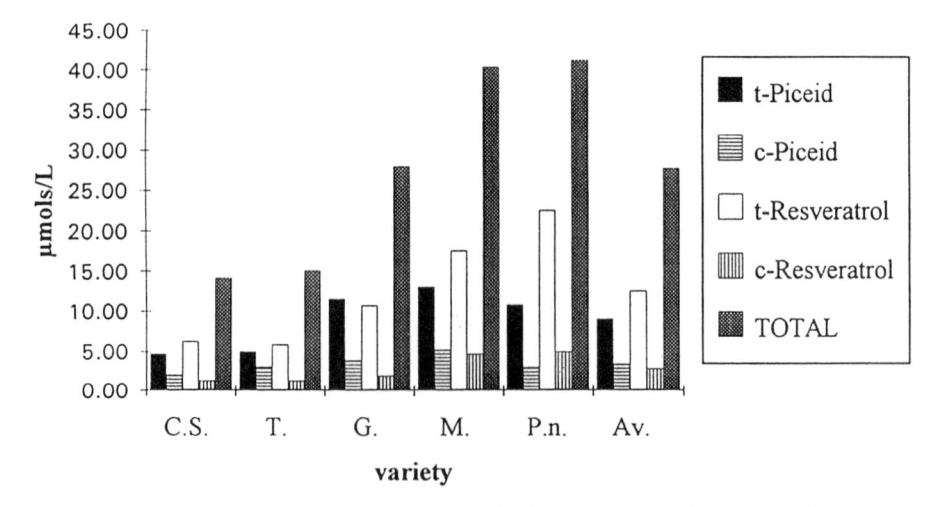

Figure 2. Levels of Resveratrol Monomers in Spanish Red Wines. C.S., Cabernet Sauvignon; T., Tempranillo; G., Grenache; M., Merlot; P.n., Pinot noir; Av., average.

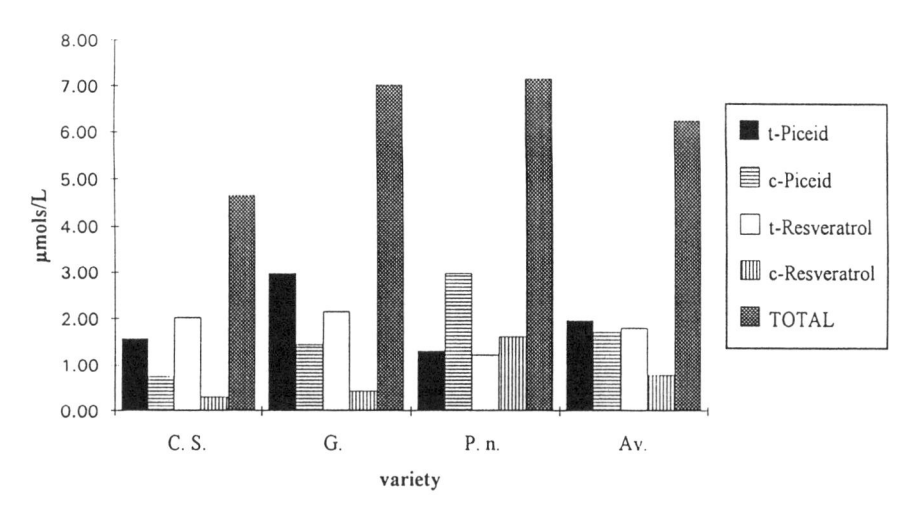

Figure 3. Levels of Resveratrol Monomers in Spanish Rosé Wines. C.S., Cabernet Sauvignon; G., Grenache; P.n., Pinot noir; Av., average.

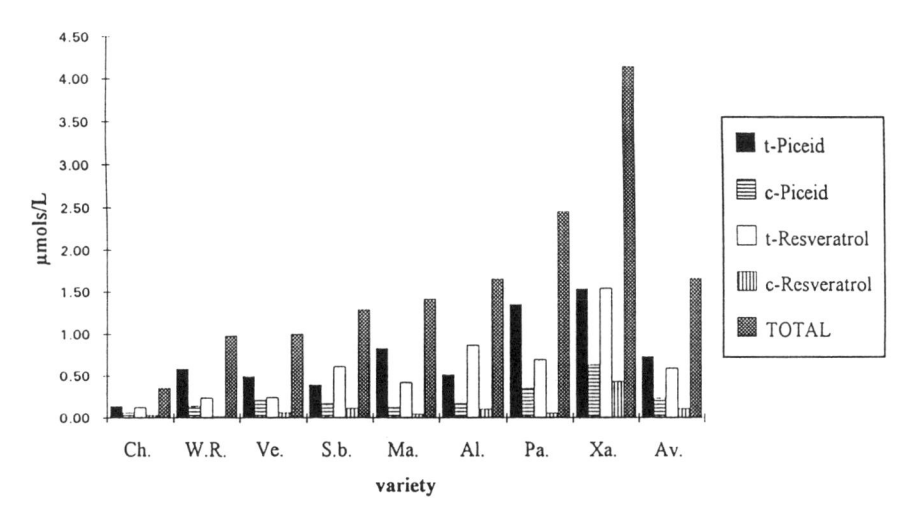

Figure 4. Levels of Resveratrol Monomers in Spanish White Wines. Al. Albariño; Ch., Chardonnay; Ma., Macabeo; Pa., Parellada; W.R., white Riesling; S.B., Sauvignon blanc; Ve., Verdejo; Xa., Xarel.lo; Av., average.

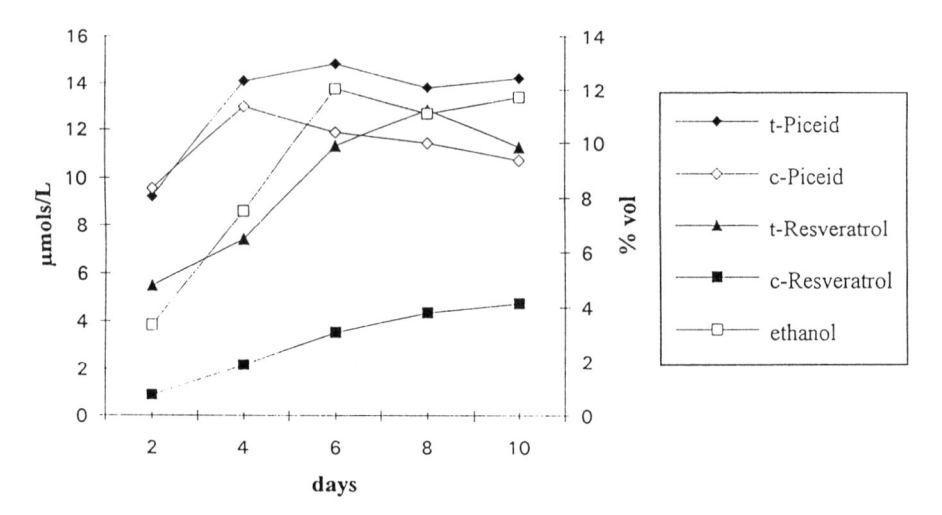

Figure 5. Evolution of Resveratrol during Merlot Fermentation.

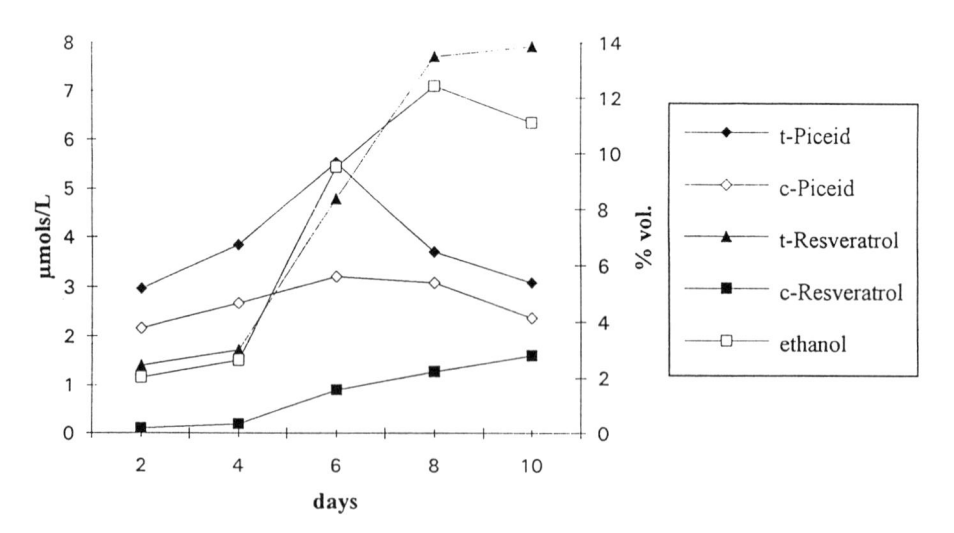

Figure 6. Evolution of Resveratrol during Cabernet Sauvignon Fermentation.

decreased. It would appear that once the maximum had been extracted from the skins, these compounds were adsorbed by the yeast and/or oxidized. However, total phenols (absorbance at 280 nm), hydroxycinnamates (absorbance at 320) and anthocyanins (see Figures 7, 8 and 9) continued increasing, so the other phenols, including hydroxycinnamates and anthocyanins, were still being extracted from the skins, while resveratrol decreased.

The glucosides (*trans* and *cis*) evolution patterns were very similar in the three fermentations, and the aglycons also had similar extraction kinetics.The glucosides were extracted more quickly, appearing at the beginning of the fermentation, the aglycons, being less polar, seemed to be more influenced by the ethanol concentration. These results were similar to those obtained by Mattivi et al (1995) (14). For this reason, white wines, which are obtained from free run juice, had higher amounts of the glucosides than aglycons (See Figure 4).

trans-Piceid was the major compound in the three musts at the beginning of the fermentation. However, in the Cabernet Sauvignon, *trans*-resveratrol was the major component at the end. The extraction curve for *trans*-resveratrol was very similar to the ethanol evolution, so when the ethanol increased, as between the fourth and the sixth day and also between the sixth and eighth day of fermentation, there was also a significant increase in *trans*-resveratrol along with significant yeast activity.

The fermentation curve for *cis* piceid was the same in the two Cabernet Sauvignon wine fermentation tanks, and it increased through the eighth day of fermentation, while in the Merlot it decreased after day four. The decrease in the concentration of the glucosides is probably related to the yeast glucosidase activity. Mattivi et al (1995) (14) show that it decreases during the fermentation, however, in their assay, yeast activity (ethanol increase) is very high from the beginning of the fermentation.

cis-Resveratrol increased during fermentation, probably due to isomerization of the *trans* forms and hydrolysis of its glycoside. This hydrolysis seems to be the main source of this compound, because *cis*-piceid decreases, while *cis* resveratrol increases, as is noted by Mattivi et al (14) and, moreover, *cis*-resveratrol is not reported in *Vitis vinifera* grapevines (13, 32); however, in a recent study, Jeandet et al (1995) detected it, in small amounts, in Pinot noir grape skins (12).

Conclusions

The quantification of the four resveratrol monomers changes the potentially-available amount of resveratrol for a physiological effect. Consumption of red wine will provide the highest levels of these compounds, followed by rosé and, finally white wines. If consumers of wine absorbed a significant portion of the resveratrol, their serum levels could reach those at which enzymatic activities are observed. However, studies of the absorption and metabolism of these compounds in humans are necessary to ascertain whether or not this could happen. Resveratrol synthesis seems to be in part genetically controlled, because grape variety plays an important role in the amount present in wine. Consequently, the amount ingested will depend also on the wine varietal consumed. The evolution curves of these compounds during fermentation in red vinification depend on their polarity, except for *cis*-resveratrol which seems to be formed during fermentation. The concentration of the stilbene compounds in must reaches a maximum

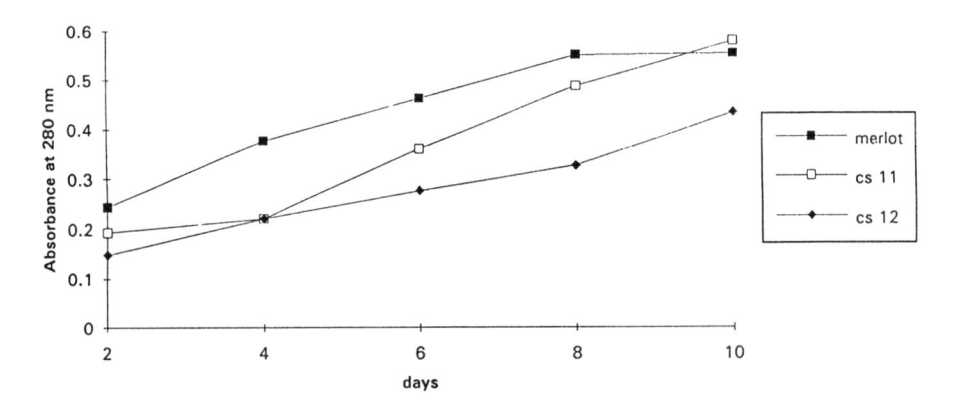

Figure 7. Evolution of Absorbance at 280 nm.

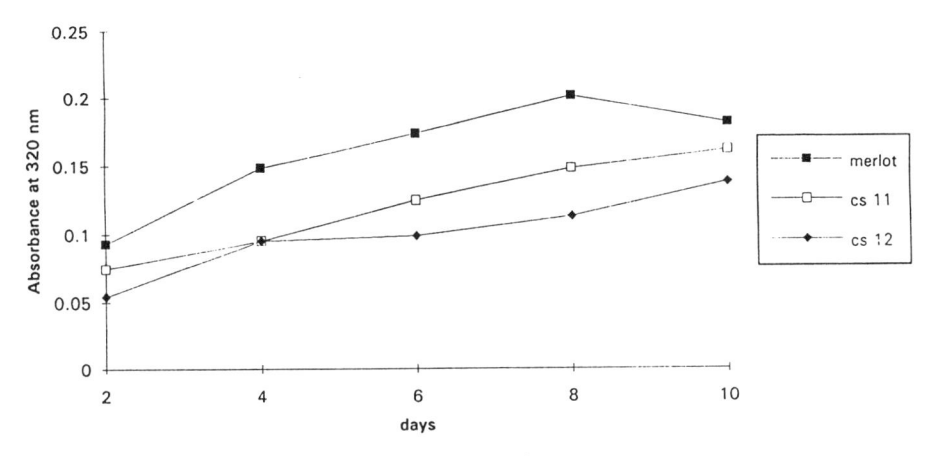

Figure 8. Evolution of Absorbance at 320 nm.

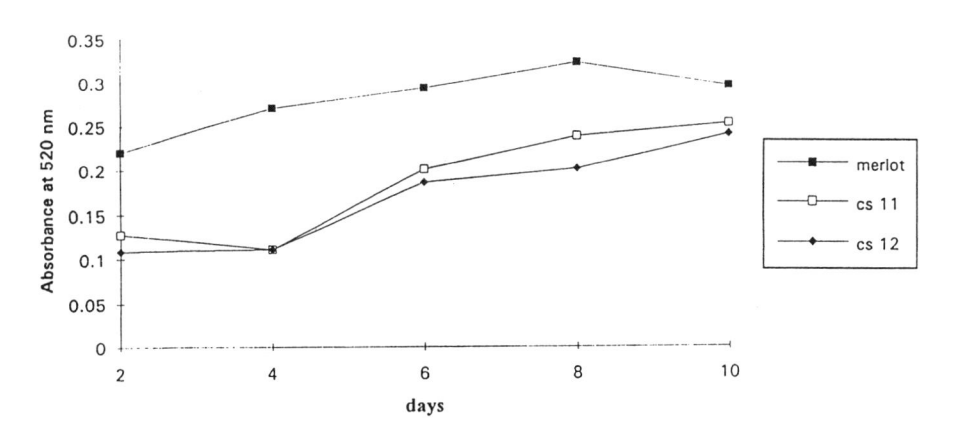

Figure 9. Evolution of Absorbance at 520 nm.

after one week and does not follow the same evolution curve as the other phenols, which continue to increase with maceration time.

Acknowledgment

The authors would like to thank Fundación para la Investigación del Vino (FIVIN) for financial support.

References

1. St. Leger, A.S.; Cochrane, A.L.; Moore, F. Factors associated with cardiac mortality in developed countries with particular reference to the consumption of wine, *Lancet* **1979**, *i*, 1017-1020.
2. Gronbæk, M.; Deis, A.; Sorensen, T.I.A.; Becker, U.; Schnohr, P.; Jensen, G. Mortality associated with moderate intakes of wine, beer and spirits, *BMJ* **1995**, *310*, 1165-1169.
3. Frankel, E.N.; Waterhouse, A.L.; Teissedre, P.L. Principal phenolic phytochemicals in selected California wines and their antioxidant activity in inhibiting oxidation of human low density lipoprotein, *J. Agric. Food Chem.* **1995**, *43*, 890-894.
4. Frankel, E.N.; Waterhouse, A.L.; Kinsella, J.E. Inhibition of human LDL oxidation by resveratrol, *Lancet* **1993**, *341*, 1103-1104.
5. Bertelli, A.A.E.; Giovannini, L.; Giannessi, D.; Migliori, M.; Bernini, W.; Fregoni, M.; Bertelli, A. Antiplatelet activity of synthetic and natural resveratrol in red wine, *Office International de la Vigne et du Vin* **1995**.
6. Pace-Asciak, C.R.; Hahn, S.E.; Diamandis, E.P.; Soleas, G.; Goldberg, D.M. The red wine phenolics trans-resveratrol and quercetin block human platelet aggregation and eicosanoid synthesis: Implications for protection against coronary heart disease, *Clin. Chimica Acta* **1995**, *235*, 207-219.
7. Kimura, Y.; Okuda, H.; Arichi, S. Effects of stilbenes on arachidonate metabolism in leukocytes, *Biochim. Biophys. Acta* **1985**, *834*, 275-278.
8. Hackett, A.M. The metabolism of flavonoid compounds in mammals, In *Plant Flavonoids in Biology and Medicine: Biochemical Pharmacologocal and Structure-Activity Relationships*; Progress in clinical and biological research 213; Cody, V.; Middleton, E.J.; Harborne, J.B., Eds.; Liss: New York, 1986; pp. 177-194.
9. Jayatilake, G.S.; Jayasuriya, H.; Lee, E.S.; Koonchanok, N.M.; Geahlen, R.L.; Ashendel, C.L.; McLaughlin, J.L.; Chang, C.J. Kinase inhibitors from Polygonum cuspidatum, *J. Nat. Prod.* **1993**, *56*, 1805-1810.
10. Creasy, L.L.; Coffee, M. Phytoalexin Production Potential of Grape Berries, *J. Amer. Soc. Hort. Sci.* **1988**, *113*, 230-234.
11. Jeandet, P.; Bessis, R.; Gautheron, B. The Production of Resveratrol (3,5,4")-trihydroxystilbene by Grape Berries in Different Development Stages, *Am. J. Enol. Vitic.* **1991**, *42*, 41-46.

12. Jeandet, P.; Bessis, R.; Maume, B.F.; Meunier, P.; Peyron, D.; Trollat, P. Effect of Enological Practices on the Resveratrol Isomer Content of Wine, *J. Agric. Food Chem.* **1995**, *43*, 316-319.
13. Soleas, G.J.; Goldberg, D.M.; Diamandis, E.P.; Karumanchiri, A.; Yan, J.; Ng, E. A derivatized gas chromatographic-mass spectrometric method for the analysis of both isomers of resveratrol in juiece and wine, *Am. J. Enol. Vitic.* **1995**, *46*, 346-351.
14. Mattivi, F.; Reniero, F.; Korhammer, S. Isolation, chracterization, and evolution in red wine vinification of resveratrol monomers, *J. Agric. Food Chem.* **1995**, *43*, 1820-1823.
15. Nagel, C.W.; Wulf, L.W. Changes in the anthocyanins, flavonoids and hydroxycinnamic acid esters during fermentation and aging of Merlot and Cabernet Sauvignon, *Am. J. Enol. Vitic.* **1979**, *30*, 111-116.
16. Somers, T.C.; Vérette, E.; Pocock, K.F. Hydroxycinnamate esters of *V. vinifera*: changes during white vinification and effects of exogenous enzyme hydrolysis, *J. Sci. Food Agric.* **1987**, *40*, 67-78.
17. Siemann, E.H.; Creasy, L.L. Concentration of the phytoalexin resveratrol in Wine, *Am. J. Enol. Vitic.* **1992**, *43*, 49-52.
18. Lamuela-Raventos, R.M.; Waterhouse, A.L. Occurence of resveratrol in Selected California Wines by a New HPLC Method, *J. Agric. Food Chem.* **1993**, *41*, 521-523.
19. Jeandet, P.; Bessis, R.; Maume, B.F.; Sbachi, M. Analysis of resveratrol in burgundy wines, *J. Wine Res.* **1993**, *4*, 79-85.
20. Mattivi, F. Resveratrol content in red and rosé wines prodeuced in Trentino (Italy) and currently available on the market, *Riv. Vitic. Enol.* **1993** (1), 37.
21. McMurtrey, K.D.; Minn, J.; Pobanz, K.; Schultz, T.P. Analysis of wines for reseveratrol using direct injection High-Pressure Liquid Chromatography with electrochemical detection, *J. Agric. Food Chem.* **1994**, *42*, 2077-2080.
22. Pezet, R.; Pont, V.; Cuenat, P. Method to determine resveratrol and pterostilbene in grape berries and wines using high-performance liquid chromatography and highly sensitive fluorimetric detection, *J. Chromatogr.* **1994**, *A 663*, 191-197; 673, 303 (1994) erratum.
23. Goldberg, D.M.; Karumanchiri, A.; Eng, E.; Diamandis, E.P.; Yan, Y.; Soleas, G.J.; Waterhouse, A.L. Resveratrol content of wines assayed by a direct gas chromatographic-mass spectrometric technique, *Am. J. Enol. Vitic.* **1993**, *44*, 344.
24. Mattivi, F. Solid phase extraction of trans-resveratrol from wines for hplc analysis, *Z. Lebensm. Unters. Forsch.* **1993**, *196*, 522-525.
25. Roggero, J.-P.; Archier, P. Quantitative determination of resveratrol and one of its glycosides in wines, *Sci. Aliments* **1994**, *14*, 99-107.
26. Goldberg, D.M.; Van, J.; Ng, E.; Diamandis, E.P.; Karumanchiri, A.; Soleas, G.; Waterhouse, A.L. A Direct Injection Gas Chromatographic Mass Spectrometric Assay for Resveratrol, *Analyt. Chem.* **1994**, *66*, 3959-3963.
27. Soleas, G.J.; Goldberg, D.M.; Diamandis, E.P.; Karumanchiri, A.; Ng, E.; Yan, J. A gas chromatographic-mass spectrometric method for the analysis of resveratrol in juice and wine samples, *Am. J. Enol. Vitic.* **1993**, *44*, 344.

28. Lamuela-Raventós, R.M.; Romero-Pérez, A.I.; Waterhouse, A.L.; de la Torre-Boronat, M.C. Direct HPLC analysis of *cis*- and *trans*-resveratrol and piceid isomers in Spanish Red *Vitis vinifera* wines, *J. Agric. Food Chem.* **1995**, *42*, 281-283.
29. Somers, T.C.; Ziemelis, G. Spectral Evaluation of Total Phenolic Components in *Vitis vinifera*: Grapes and Wine, *J. Sci. Food Agric.* **1985**, *36*, 1275-1284.
30. Somers, T.C.; Evans, M.E. Spectral evaluation of young red wines: anthocyanin equilibria, total phenolics, free and molecular SO2, "chemical age", *J. Sci. Food Agric.* **1977**, *28*, 279-287.
31. Validation of comendial methods The United States Pharmacopoeia (USP XXII), **1989**, *1225*, 1710-1711.
32. Langcake, P.; Pryce, R.J. The production of resveratrol by *Vitis vinifera* and other members of the Vitaceae as a response to infection or injury, *Physiol. Plant Pathol.* **1976**, *9*, 77-86.

Chapter 7

The Content of Catechins and Procyanidins in Grapes and Wines as Affected by Agroecological Factors and Technological Practices

Eugenio Revilla[1], E. Alonso[1], and V. Kovac[2]

[1]Departamento de Quimica Agricola, Geologia y Geoquimica, Universidad Autónoma de Madrid, 28049 Madrid, Spain
[2]Tehnoloski Fakultet, 21000 Novi Sad, Yugoslavia

Within the past several years, the content of catechins and procyanidins in several grape cultivars, grown under different agroecological conditions, and in red wines, made using different technological practices, has been studied. Grape seeds contain a higher amount of catechins and procyanidins than cluster stems and grape skins, and the relative amount of these molecules in the different parts of the grape cluster is closely related to the year of production, the site of production and the degree of maturation. The content of catechins and procyanidins in red wines is affected by the length of maceration of grape pomace, by the destemming of grape clusters and by adding supplementary quantities of seeds during fermentation. The amount of catechins and procyanidins in young red wines decreases after the treatment with several fining agents.

Experiments carried out by Flanzy and Causeret in 1951 (*1*) first pointed out that wine intake by rats does not produce the same toxic effects as those caused by the intake of spirits or ethanol. These researchers suggested that wine should contain some ethanol antidote, which is absent in the spirit of wine.

Several epidemiological inquiries on coronary heart disease, CHD, have shown that, in most developed countries, high intake of saturated fat is positively related to high mortality from CHD (*2-5*). However, France had a lower-than-expected CHD mortality rate, in spite of high intake of saturated fat (similar to that in Germany, UK, and other central and northern European countries). This fact has been known as the 'French paradox', and may be partially attributed to high wine consumption (*3, 5*).

© 1997 American Chemical Society

Grapes and red wines contain a relatively high amount of different phenolic compounds (6) that act as antioxidants (7-9) or have effects on thrombosis (10). Among the major phenolic compounds present in grapes and red wines, catechins and procyanidins are considered to be responsible for the protective effect of red wine with regard to atherosclerosis (7). Other studies have shown that these molecules exhibit a wide variety of biological activities, like free radical scavenging ability (11), and the inhibition of eicosanoid synthesis (12) and platelet aggregation (13). In addition, it was demonstrated that some minor wine polyphenols (resveratrol and derivatives) possess similar biological properties (14-16); however, their concentration in red wines is very low compared to that of catechins and procyanidins (17-18).

On the other hand, catechins and procyanidins are molecules of great interest in enology. They are involved in a drying and puckering sensation called astringency (19), due to the ability of catechins and procyanidins to bond to salivary glycoproteins, and are involved in complex condensation reactions with flavilium salts which lead to polymeric wine pigments (20), which are the major contributors to color in aged red wines.

Thousands of grape cultivars are grown all over the world, and may be classified according to their use (table grapes, winemaking grapes and raisins), their color (white, red, rosé, roux, teinturier, etc.), the presence or absence of seeds (seeded grapes, Sultanina type seedless grapes, and Corinthe type seedless grapes), their precocity, etc. (21). In most cases, grapes are grown in temperate regions, the harvest takes place in September and October, and their quality is affected by weather conditions during the growing season (21). This relation of quality and weather conditions is specially evident in the case of grape cultivars used for making red wines, hence the French concept of "millésime".

Once in the cellars, a number of different technologies may be used in the production of wines (22). Thus, wines which clearly differ in their chemical composition and in their sensory characteristics may be made with the grapes harvested a day in a vineyard, using different technological practices. If a shipment of grapes is divided into three parts, and each part is processed in a different way (e.g., a conventional French type red winemaking, carbonic maceration and thermovinification), it will be possible to obtain three different young wines with a different capacity of ageing (22).

For several years, we have focused our research on the effect of several agroecological factors on the content of catechins and procyanidins in grapes, and the influence of different technological practices on the levels of catechins and procyanidins of red wines made with the same grapes (23-30). For these purposes, analytical methods for the fractionation and the quantitation of catechins and procyanidins present in grapes and wines described in the literature (31) and other developed in our laboratories (24, 32) were used. Some results of our research are presented in this paper.

Agroecological Factors

The literature indicates that several agroecological factors may affect the phenolic composition of grapes when harvested (33-35). Among them, four have been selected for their influence on the content of catechins and procyanidins of grapes: cultivar, year of production, site of production and degree of maturity.

The Content of Catechins and Procyanidins in Different Grape Cultivars. In 1987, the content of catechins and procyanidins in 19 different grape cultivars used for winemaking grown in the Ampelographic Collection located at Sremski Karlovci, Yugoslavia, was determined. Samples were harvested with a similar degree of maturity, including 11 *Vitis vinifera* cultivars used for winemaking (seven white, one grey and three red), and eight hybrid white cultivars obtained by crossing *V. vinifera* and *V. amurensis* cultivars: two of them were selected in Hungary, and contained a 25% of theoretical genetic charge of *V. amurensis*; the other six were selected at Sremski Karlovci by crossing the Hungarian hybrids above mentioned with several *V. vinifera* cultivars, and their theoretical genetic content of *V. amurensis* was 12.5%. These hybrids were selected due to their high cold hardiness (*36*).

Table I shows the total content of catechins and procyanidins (sum of (+)-catechin, (-)-epicatechin, dimeric procyanidins B1, B2, B3 and B4, and trimeric procyanidin C1) in the skins, the seeds and the cluster stems of those 19 cultivars,

Table I. Total content of catechins and procyanidins (mg/kg grapes) in seeds, skins, cluster stems and entire clusters of 19 grape cultivars sampled at Sremski Sremski Karlovci in 1987

Group of cultivars	Grape cultivar	Seeds	Skins	Cluster stems	Entire clusters
V. vinifera	Italian Riesling	415	27	113	555
	Rhin Riesling	415	27	41	483
	Sauvignon	402	20	62	484
	Pinot blanc	558	24	112	694
	Chardonnay	463	60	96	619
	Gewürztraminer	1178	100	51	1329
	Neoplanta	617	58	146	821
	Pinot gris	2400	121	72	2593
	Pinot noir	1922	181	53	2156
	Cabernet-Sauvignon	874	185	72	1131
	Merlot	625	63	86	774
Hungarian hybrids	Kunleany	455	59	308	822
	Kunbarat	685	2	88	775
Yugoslavian hybrids	Zlata	456	75	80	611
	Petra	1339	19	48	1406
	Lela	797	16	146	959
	Rani Rizling	564	189	180	933
	Lisa	732	49	122	903
	Mila	250	41	123	414

SOURCE: Adapted from ref. 26

expressed as milligrams per kilogram of grapes. The content of catechins and procyanidins is very different depending on the cultivar. The total content of catechins and procyanidins in seeds varied from 250 mg/kg grapes (cv. Mila) to 2400 mg/kg grapes (cv. Pinot gris). Skins and cluster stems often contain less than 100 and 150 mg of catechins and procyanidins per kg of grapes, respectively. Also, the content of catechins and procyanidins in white cultivars may be as high as in red cultivars. Thus, cvs. Gewürztraminer and Petra contained more catechins and procyanidins than cv. Cabernet-Sauvignon, and cvs. Neoplanta, Kunleany, Kunbarat, Lela, Rani Rizling and Lisa are richer in catechins and procyanidins than cv. Merlot. These results are close to other previously reported in the literature for several grape cultivars grown in France (*37*). From the data displayed in Table I, it may be noted that the contribution of seeds to the total content of catechins and procyanidins of grapes is more important than the contribution of cluster stems and skins. In most cases, catechins and procyanidins contained in seeds represented more than 60% of the total content of these molecules in grape clusters. The most remarkable exception is cv. Kunleany, which contained a relatively high amount of catechins and procyanidins in cluster stems.

The situation is quite similar in table grapes. In 1992, the content of catechins and procyanidins in skins and seeds of 11 white and nine red table grape cultivars sampled with a similar degree of maturity in the Ampelographic Collection located at El Encín, Spain, was measured. Table II summarizes the results obtained for those cultivars. Once again, the content of catechins and procyanidins was quite different depending on the cultivar considered, ranging from 243 mg/kg grapes (cv. Dominga) to 1108 mg/kg grapes (cv. Muscat of Hambourg). These values are quite similar to those reported for grape cultivars used for winemaking (*23, 26, 31*), and reinforce the finding that the content of catechins and procyanidins in white cultivars may be as high as in red cultivar (e.g., cv. Chelva cointained more catechins and procyanidins than seven red cultivars, and cv. Napoleón contained less catechins and procyanidins than eight white cultivars). Seeds contained more than 89% of catechins and procyanidins present in grapes, except in cv. Dominga, that contained a remarkable amount of these compounds in skins (23.9% of catechins and procyanidins were located in the skins).

Year of Production. Data displayed in Table III show the effect of the year of production on the content of catechins and procyanidins in seeds of cv. Muscat of Hambourg grown at El Encin in 1992 and 1993. Of course, grapes presented a similar degree of maturity both years. As can be noted, the different climatic conditions from year to year clearly affect the total amount of catechins and procyanidins in grape seeds, and also the relative amount of each one of these molecules. The results obtained for other cultivars (Chelva, Dominga, Mantúo, Ohanes, Alphonse Lavallée, Moscatel Tinto, Napoleón and Valencí Tinto) were quite similar (*30*). These data agree with other previously reported for several white cultivars used for winemaking (Gewürztraminer, Italian Riesling, Sauvignon and Neoplanta), sampled at Sremski Karlovci in 1986, 1987 and 1988 (*23*).

Table II. Total content of catechins and procyanidins (mg/kg grapes) in seeds, skins and entire berries of 20 table grape cultivars sampled at El Encín in 1992

Group of cultivars	Cultivar	Seeds	Skins	Entire berries
White cultivars	Albillo	451	9	460
	Aledo	368	14	382
	Aledo Real	303	14	317
	Chelva	924	30	954
	Dominga	185	58	243
	Malvasía	376	7	383
	Malvasía de Sitges	452	28	480
	Mantuo	647	11	658
	Moscatel de Málaga	509	31	540
	Ohanes	225	4	229
	Valencí Blanco	647	34	681
Red cultivars	Alphonse Lavallée	922	61	983
	Barlinka	352	42	394
	Gros Colman	728	18	746
	Moscatel Tinto	588	17	605
	Muscat of Hambourg	1074	34	1108
	Napoleón	295	32	327
	Negra Tardía	773	46	819
	Planta Mula	534	44	578
	Valencí Tinto	555	14	569

SOURCE: Adapted from ref. 29
Copyright 1995 with kind permission from Elsevier Science - NL.

Table III. Total content of catechins and procyanidins, C+P, (mg/kg grapes) and percentages (%) of the different catechins and procyanidins in seeds of cv. Muscat of Hambourg sampled at El Encín in 1992 and 1993

Year	C+P	CAT[a]	EPI[b]	DIM[c]	C1[d]
1992	1074	49.8	24.3	19.6	6.3
1993	877	50.4	35.6	12.3	2.7

[a](+)-catechin. [b](-)-epicatechin. [c]dimeric procyanidins B1, B2, B3 and B4.
[d]procyanidin C1
SOURCE: Adapted from ref. 29
Copyright 1995 with kind permission from Elsevier Science - NL.

Site of Production. The characteristic varietal chemical composition of grapes may be affected by the growing area, despite a similar degree of maturity. This fact has been demonstrated for monoterpenes (38). The effect of this factor on the content of catechins and procyanidins in grapes is not well known. Table IV show some results obtained for Tempranillo grapes grown in different sites around Madrid, sampled by September 20th 1994, with a similar degree of maturity. As can be noted, the content of catechins and procyanidins is quite different, in seeds and in skins, depending on the geographic origin of grapes, despite their similar degree of maturity. Also, the ratio between the contents of catechins and procyanidins in seeds and in skins is considerably different.

Table IV. Total content of catechins and procyanidins (mg/kg grapes) in seeds, skins and entire berries of Tempranillo grapes sampled in different sites around Madrid in 1994

Site	Seeds	Skins	Entire berries
Aranjuez	163	58	221
Escalona del Alberche	122	27	149
Madrid-Moncloa	108	9	117
Valdilecha	225	17	242

Degree of Maturity. Some authors have studied the changes in the content of catechins and procyanidins during growth and development of grapes (*39-40*). These collegues have shown that the highest concentrations of these molecules are found in the early stages of development. The level then decreases quickly, and becomes virtually stabilized by the beginning of September. Unfortunately, the behaviour of these molecules during September is not well known. During the summer, the climate in Central Spain is very warm, and the temperature easily rises up to 35 C (95 F) or even more. Thus, the biosynthesis of anthocyanins virtually stops (*41*), and red grapes usually are harvested after the 15th of September to obtain a well colored product for making red wines. For these reasons, the changes in the content of catechins and procyanidins in skins and seeds of three cultivars (Cabernet-Sauvignon, Garnacha and Tempranillo) have been studied from the end of September to the beginning of October 1994 in Escalona del Alberche, near Madrid. The level of anthocyanins in the skins of cultivars above mentioned dramatically rose. At the same time, the content of catechins and procyanidins decreased, specially in the seeds, and the levels by the end of September were dramatically low. Table V shows the results obtained for Tempranillo grapes: the total content of catechins and procyanidins in seeds decreased dramatically during September. Thus, the amount of these molecules in seeds by the end of August was nearly five-fold more than by the beginning of October. A similar situation has been observed in Garnacha and Cabernet-Sauvignon grapes. Of course, the different catechins and procyanidins behaved in a similar way.

Technological Practices

Dozens of different technological practices are used to make red wines, that may modify their phenolic composition. We have selected four to elucidate their effect on the content of catechins and procyanidins of wines: length of maceration, destemming of grape clusters, and clarification or fining, that clearly modify the phenolic composition of wines according to the literature; and the addition of supplementary quantities of seeds during maceration, which is a new technological practice assayed to obtained wines "enriched" in catechins and procyanidins (*25, 27, 28*).

Table V. Total content of catechins and procyanidins, C+P, (mg/kg grapes) in seeds, skins and entire berries, and content of free anthocyanins (mg/kg grapes) in Tempranillo grapes sampled at Escalona del Alberche from August to October 1994

Date	C+P, seeds	C+P, skins	C+P, entire berries	Free anthocyanins
8/31	240	25	265	613
9/10	230	31	251	519
9/20	122	27	149	733
10/4	48	20	68	801

Length of Maceration. The length of maceration affects the extraction of phenolics contained in skins, seeds and cluster stems. Usually, the maceration does not exceed ten days, because the level of anthocyanins in wine decreases after this time (*33-34*). In 1989, several experimental microvinifications with entire clusters of Vranac grapes were conducted to understand the effect of the length of maceration on the content of catechins and procyanidins in wines. As may be observed in Table VI, the extraction of catechins and procyanidins from grape pomace was higher as the maceration was longer. The effect was quite similar for (+)-catechin, (-)-epicatechin and dimeric procyanidins.

Destemming of Grape Clusters. In many cellars, the destemming of grape clusters is a current enological practice. The effect of this technology on the content of catechins and procyanidins in red wines was studied in 1987 by conducting four experiments with Vranac grapes: two experiments were carried out with entire clusters, the maceration lasting 7 and 14 days, and two other with destemmed grapes, the maceration lasting 7 and 14 days. Table VII shows the results obtained for wines whose maceration lasted 7 days. As may be noted, the destemming of grape clusters leads to wines with a lower amount of catechins and procyanidins than wines made with entire clusters. Similar results were obtained for wines whose maceration lasted 14 days (*27*).

Table VI. Effect of the length of maceration on the content of catechins and procyanidins in Vranac wines

Length of maceration (days)	(+)-catechin (mg/L)	(-)-epicatechin (mg/L)	Dimeric procyanidins (mg/L)
2	55	25	111
3	78	36	130
4	80	38	146
5	84	46	166
6	88	56	190
7	130	65	241
14	137	76	291

SOURCE: Adapted from ref. 27

Table VII. Effect of destemming on the content of catechins and procyanidins of Vranac wines. Maceration lasted seven days

Experiment	(+)-catechin (mg/L)	(-)-epicatechin (mg/L)	Dimeric procyanidins (mg/L)
Entire clusters	130	65	241
Destemmed clusters	99	63	175

SOURCE: Adapted from ref. 27

Fining of Wines. The fining or clarification of wines is a technological practice used to eliminate colloidal materials of proteic or phenolic nature to avoid undesirable turbidity and precipitates during the ageing and/or the storage of wines (42-44). Several substances commonly used as fining agents were assayed, at a laboratory level, to understand their effect on the phenolic composition of red wines. Table VIII shows the effect of sodic bentonite, gelatine and PVPP, at enological doses, on the content of catechins and procyanidins of a Garnacha wine. As may be observed, gelatine and PVPP affect dramatically the content of catechins and procyanidins in this wine. On the other hand, the effect of sodic bentonite is not so intense. Anyway, the relative loss of catechins and procyanidins depends on their level in wine before clarification; thus, the effect of clarification in wines relatively rich in phenolics may be not so intense like in wines with a relatively low level of phenolic compounds (30, 45).

Table VIII. Effect of different fining agents on the content of catechins and procyanidins of a Garnacha wine

Experiment	(+)-catechin (mg/L)	(-)-epicatechin (mg/L)	Dimeric procyanidins (mg/L)
Control	43	37	37
Sodic bentonite (0.5 g/L)	35	29	23
Gelatine (0.05 g/L)	27	17	22
PVPP (0.5 g/L)	14	12	14

Addition of supplementary quantities of seeds during fermentation. Grape seeds contain a very large amount of catechins and procyanidins if compared with skins and cluster stems. Thus, it would be possible to obtain wines with relatively high amounts of catechins and procyanidins by adding a supplementary quantity of seeds during fermentation. Several microvinification experiments have been conducted, from 1988 to 1994, with seven different red cultivars in order to understand the effect of this new practice on the content of phenolic compounds in wines. As a general rule, the addition of a supplementary quantity of seeds during fermentation leads to wines with a higher content of catechins and procyanidins than in a control wine made with the same grape shipment.

Table IX summarizes the results obtained for experiments carried out in 1989 to evaluate the effect of adding supplementary seeds in Vranac wines. Three sets of Vranac grapes were destemmed and crushed. In the first experiment (control wine), a conventional red-type vinification was carried out. In the other two experiments, the fermentation was carried out by doubling and tripling the quantity of seeds present in pomace ("double" and "triple" wines). The maceration lasted seven days in every case. As can be observed, when the quantity of seeds was doubled, the amount of catechins and procyanidins was slightly higher than double in relation to the control wine, and when tripled, it was slightly higher than triple. The effect was quite similar for (+)-catechin, (-)-epicatechin and dimeric procyanidins.

Table IX. Effect of adding supplementary quantities of seeds on the content of catechins and procyanidins in Vranac wines

Experiment	(+)-catechin (mg/L)	(-)-epicatechin (mg/L)	Dimeric procyanidins (mg/L)
Control wine	99	63	175
"Double" wine	235	155	483
"Triple" wine	334	212	724

SOURCE: Adapted from ref. 27

Table X displays the results obtained with Cabernet-Sauvignon wines in 1994. Three wines were made at Novi Sad, Yugoslavia: control (0), double quantity of seeds (+100) and triple quantity of seeds (+200). Like in the experiments previously carried out, when doubling or tripling the quantity of seeds in contact with the must, the amount of catechins and procyanidins in wines was sligthly higher than the double or the triple in relation to control wine. Three other wines were made at Madrid, Spain (wines 0, +30 and +60). In this case, the suplementary quantities of seeds were relatively low: 30% and 60%. Even with this relatively low supplementation, wines became enriched in catechins and procyanidins in relation to control wine. As can be observed, the levels of catechins and procyanidins were quite different in both control wines. These data also point out that the quality of grapes may be dramatically important in relation to the levels of catechins and procyanidins in wines.

The addition of supplementary quantities of seeds also affects the levels of anthocyanins in wines, as well as other physico-chemical parameters related to the phenolic content of wines, like color intensity, Folin-Ciocalteu index and the UV absorbance at 280 nm (25, 27-28). Table XI displays the content of catechins, dimeric procyanidins and free anthocyanins in three Tempranillo wines made in 1993: control (0), double quantity of seeds (+100) and triple quantity of seeds (+200). As may be noted, the amount of free anthocyanins in the wine made doubling the quantity of seeds was higher than in control wine. This may be explained by the fact that the phenolic compounds extracted from supplementary seeds caused the stabilization of wine color. Nevertheless, when the quantity of seeds was tripled, the content of free anthocyanins was quite similar to that of control wine. In this case, it seems that the retention of coloring matter by pomace is more intense than color stabilization caused by phenolic compounds extracted from supplementary seeds.

Table X. Effect of adding supplementary quantities of seeds on the content of catechins and procyanidins in Cabernet-Sauvignon wines made in different wineries

Winery	Seeds added[a]	(+)-catechin (mg/L)	(-)-epicatechin (mg/L)	Dimeric procyanidins (mg/L)
Novi Sad	0	81	42	20
	+ 100	147	104	75
	+ 200	241	165	149
Madrid	0	26	10	5
	+ 30	39	20	14
	+ 60	52	28	18

[a] % in relation to control

Table XI. Effect of adding supplementary quantities of seeds on the content of catechins, dimeric procyanidins and free anthocyanins in Tempranillo wines

Experiment	Catechins (mg/L)	Dimeric procyanidins (mg/L)	Free anthocyanins (mg/L)
0	6	19	207
+ 100	54	33	276
+ 200	97	50	207

SOURCE: Adapted from ref. 28

Most of wines made by the addition of supplementary quantities of seeds have been submitted to informal sensory evaluation by experts, prior to any stabilization or ageing process. Their opinion has been that the addition of a suplementary quantity of seeds which doubles the seeds naturally ocurring in grapes leads to wines with more pronounced variety characteristics and with more intense flavor and aroma than control wines. Of course, these wines contain a higher amount of catechins and procyanidins than control wines, and may be considered as more healthy than control wines.

Conclusions

The content of catechins and procyanidins in grapes is clearly affected by the four agroecological factors herein considered. Thus, depending on the cultivar, the year of production, the site of production and the degree of maturity, the amount of catechins and procyanidins in grapes may be quite different, and the levels of these molecules in wines made using the same technological practices, but different grapes, may be dramatically different.

The content of catechins and procyanidins in wines made with a shipment of grapes may be affected by several technological practices, like the length of maceration, the destemming of grapes clusters and the treatments with various fining agents. The addition of supplementary quantities of seeds during fermentation clearly modifies the levels of catechins and procyanidins in wines, and appears to be a promising technology to obtain red wines with better sensory characteristics and more healthy than some other made by a conventional technology.

Literature cited

(1) Flanzy, M.; Causeret, J. *C. R. Acad. Agric. Fr.* **1951**, *37*, 587-589.

(2) St. Leger, A.S.; Cochrane, A.L.; More, E. *Lancet* **1979**, *297*, 1017-1020.

(3) Renaud, S.; De Lorgeril, M. *Lancet* **1992**, *339*, 1523-1526.

(4) Artaud-Wild, S.M.; Connor, S.; Sexton, G.; Connor, W. *Circulation* **1993**, *88*, 2771-2779.

(5) Criqui, M.H.; Ringel, B.L. *Lancet* **1994**, *344*, 1719-1723.

(6) Singleton, V.L. In *Wine Analysis;* Linskens H.F.; Jackson J.F., Eds. Modern Methods of Plant Analysis, New Series, Volume 6; Springer-Verlag : Berlin, 1988, pp. 173-218.

(7) Masquelier, J. *Proc. Int. Symp. "L'Alimentation et la Consommation du Vin"*, Verona, Italy, 1982, pp. 147-155.

(8) Frankel, E.N.; Kanner, J.; German, J.B.; Parks, E.; Kinsella, J.E. *Lancet,* **1993**, *338*, 985-992.

(9) Whitehead, T.P; Robinson, D.; Allaway, S.; Syms, J.; Hale, A. *Clin. Chem.,* **1995**, *41*, 32-35.

(10) Demrow, H.S.; Slane, P.R.; Folts, J.D. *Circulation,* **1995**, *91*, 1182-1188.

(11) Uchida, S.; Edamatsu, R.; Hirazmatsu, M.; Mori, A.; Nonaka, G.; Nishioka, I.; Niwa, M.; Ozaki, M. *Med. Sci. Res.,* **1987**, *15*, 831-832.

(12) Moroney, M.A.; Alcaraz, M.J.; Forder, R.A.; Carey, F.; Hoult, J.R.S. *J. Pharm. Pharmacol.,* **1988**, *40*, 787-792.

(13) Griglewski, R.J.; Korbut, R.; Robak, J.; Swies, J. *Biochem. Pharmacol.,* **1987**, *36*, 317-322.

(14) Kimura, Y.; Okuda, H.; Arichi, S. *Biochim. Biophys. Acta,* **1985**, *834*, 275-278.

(15) Chung, M.I.; Teng, C.M.; Cheng, K.L.; Ko, F.N.; Lin, C.N. *Planta Med.,* **1992**, *58*, 294-296.

(16) Frankel, E.N.; Waterhouse, A.L.; Kinsella, J.E. *Lancet,* **1993**, *341*, 1103-1104.

(17) Siemann, E.H.; Creasy, L.L. *Am. J. Enol. Vitic,* **1992**, *43*, 49-52.

(18) Roggero, J.P.; Archier, P. *Sci. Aliment.,* **1994**, *14*, 99-107.

(19) Haslam, E.; Lilley, T.H. *Crit. Rev. Food Sci. Nutr.,* **1988**, *27*, 1-40.

(20) Somers, T.C.; Verette, E. In *Wine Analysis;* Linskens H.F.; Jackson J.F., Eds. Modern Methods of Plant Analysis, New Series, Volume 6; Springer-Verlag : Berlin, 1988, pp. 219-257.

(21) Hidalgo, L. *Tratado de Viticultura General;* Ediciones Mundi-Prensa: Madrid, 1993.
(22) Amerine, M.A.; Berg, H.W.; Kunkee, R.E.; Ough, C.S., Singleton, V.L.; Webb, A.D. *The Technology of Wine Making*; AVI Publishing Company, Inc.; Westport, CT, 1980.
(23) Kovac, V.; Bourzeix, M.; Heredia, N.; Ramos, T. *Rev. Franc. Oenol.*, **1990**, *125*, 7-14.
(24) Revilla, E.; Alonso, E.; Bourzeix, M.; Heredia, N. In *Flavors and Off-Flavors '89*, Charalambous G., Ed.; Elsevier Science Publishers: Amsterdam, 1990; pp. 53-60.
(25) Kovac, V.; Bourzeix, M.; Alonso E. *C. R. Acad. Agric. Fr.*, **1991**, *77*, 121-125.
(26) Kovac, V.; Bourzeix, M.; Heredia, N.; Alonso, E. *Jug. Vinogr. Vinarst.*, **1991**, *25*, 10-15.
(27) Kovac, V.; Alonso, E.; Bourzeix, M.; Revilla, E. *J. Agric. Food Chem.*, **1992**, *40*, 1953-1957.
(28) Kovac, V.; Alonso, E.; Revilla, E. *Am. J. Enol. Vitic.*, **1995**, *46*, 363-367.
(29) Revilla, E.; Escalona, J.M.; Alonso, E.; Kovac, V. In *Food Flavors: Generation, Analysis and Process Influence,* Charalambous G., Ed.; Elsevier Science Publishers: Amsterdam, 1995, pp. 1579-1596.
(30) Revilla, E.; Kovac, V.; Alonso E. In *Proc. 4th Int. Symp. "Innovations in Wine Technology"*, Sttutgart, 1995; pp. 132-141.
(31) Bourzeix, M.; Weyland, D.; Heredia, N. *Bull. OIV,* **1986**, *59*, 1171-1254.
(32) Revilla, E.; Bourzeix, M.; Alonso, E. *Chromatographia,* **1991**, *31*, 465-468.
(33) Singleton, V.L.; Esau, P. *Phenolic Substances in Grapes and Wines, and Their Significance;* Academic Press; New York, 1969.
(34) Ribéreau-Gayon, P. In *Anthocyanins as Food Colours,* Markakis P., Ed.; Academic Press: New York, 1982, pp. 209-224.
(35) Macheix, J.J.; Fleuriet, A.; Billot, J. *Fruit Phenolics;* CRC Press: Boca Raton, Fl., 1990.
(36) Cindric, P.; Jazic, L.J.; Ruzic, N. *Jug. Vinogr. Vinarst.*, **1983**, *17*, 55-67.
(37) Bourzeix, M. In *Polyphenolic Phenomena,* Scalbert A., Ed.; INRA Editions: Paris, 1993, pp. 187-197.
(38) Rapp, A.; Güntert, M.; Heinmann, W. *Z. Lebensm. Unter. Forsch.*, **1985**, *181*, 357-361.
(39) Czochanska, Z.; Foo, L.Y.; Porter, L.J. *Phytochemistry,* **1979**, *18*, 1818-1822.
(40) Romeyer, F.M.; Macheix, J.J.; Sapis, J.C. *Phytochemistry,* **1986**, *25*, 219-221.
(41) Kliewer, W.M. *Am. J. Enol. Vitic.*, **1972**, *23*, 71-77.
(42) Glories, Y. *Connaiss. Vigne Vin,* **1974**, *8*, 375-393.
(43) Kovac, V. *Bull. OIV,* **1979**, *52*, 560-572.
(44) Mennet, R.H., Nakayama, T.O.M. *Am. J. Enol. Vitic.*, **1969**, *20*, 169-175.
(45) Revilla, E.; Alonso, E. In *Food Flavors, Ingredients and Composition,* Charalambous G., Ed.; Elsevier Science Publishers: Amsterdam, 1993, pp. 455-468.

Chapter 8

The Structures of Tannins in Grapes and Wines and Their Interactions with Proteins

Véronique Cheynier, Corine Prieur, Sylvain Guyot[1], Jacques Rigaud, and Michel Moutounet

Institut Supérieur de la Vigne et du Vin, Institut National de la Recherche Agronomique, Unité de Recherche Polymères et Techniques Physico-Chimiques, 2 place Viala, 34060 Montpellier Cedex, France

> The structure of condensed tannins from grapes and wines was investigated by thiolysis followed by reversed-phase HPLC. Grape seed tannins consist of partly galloylated procyanidins whereas grape skins contain prodelphinidins in addition to procyanidins. Tannin average molecular weight is larger in skins than in seeds. Wine tannin composition depends on that of the grape from which the wine is made and on the wine-making conditions, which influence extraction of tannins from the solid parts of the cluster and their subsequent reactions. Tannin-like structures were also formed by enzymatic oxidation. Interactions of grape seed procyanidins with proteins increase with the degree of polymerization and number of galloyl substituents. The relative influence of each factor could not be determined as larger tannins were also more galloylated. Inhibitory effect of catechin dimers was tested on various polysaccharide hydrolases. Enzymatic inhibition by procyanidin B3 and by catechin dimers arising from oxidation were in the same range of magnitude but depended both on the enzymatic protein and on the tannin structure.

Grape and wine polyphenols show a great diversity of structures and properties. Among them, condensed tannins (i.e. proanthocyanidins) have attracted considerable interest because of their quantitative importance and major contribution to wine organoleptic properties (*1-5*), but also with respect to their high reactivity, in particular, as natural antioxidants (*5-7*). The term "tannins" refers to the ability of these molecules to complex with proteins, permitting their use in the production of leather from hide (*4*). It designates oligomeric derivatives of gallic and ellagic acid

[1]Current address: Station de Recherche Cidricole et de Biotransformation des Fruits, Légumes et Dérivés, Institut National de la Recherche Agronomique, BP 29, 35650 Le Rheu, France

© 1997 American Chemical Society

(hydrolysable tannins) and of flavanols (condensed tannins). Only members of the latter class occur in grapes but wine may also contain hydrolysable tannins extracted from oak cooperage in the course of barrel aging. Besides, transformation products of the original phenolic compounds may bind to proteins, and thus be regarded as tannins (4). The occurrence of specific tannins arising from oxidation (i.e. thearubigins and theaflavins) is well documented in black tea (8). As well, grape phenolics are known to proceed to polymeric pigments during wine making and aging (3,9,10). Although various products have been obtained in model solutions either by oxidation (11,12) or by tannin-anthocyanin complexation (13-15), the reactions actually taking place in wine as well as the structure and properties of the resulting products are unknown. The present paper summarizes our recent findings about the structure of tannins in grapes and wines and some results related to their interactions with proteins.

Structure of Proanthocyanidins (Condensed Tannins)

Proanthocyanidins are oligomers and polymers of flavan-3-ols. Several classes can be distinguished on the basis of the hydroxylation pattern of the constitutive units. Among them, prodelphinidins, consisting of (epi)gallocatechin units, and procyanidins, deriving from (epi)catechin, which are presented below, have been reported in grapes.

R = H : procyanidins
R = OH : prodelphinidins

Monomeric units may be linked by C4ÔC6 and/or C4ÔC8 bonds (B-type) or double linked, with an additional ether linkage (A-type). Besides, flavan-3-ol units may be encountered as 3-O-esters, in particular with gallic acid, or as glycosides (16). Finally, the degree of polymerization (DP) may vary greatly as proanthocyanidins have been described up to 20,000 in molecular weight (4).

The organoleptic properties and reactivity of tannins, including radical scavenging effects and protein-binding ability, largely depend on their structures. In particular, the number of active sites (phenolic and especially o-diphenolic groups) (17) increases with the degree of polymerization and with gallate esterification whereas their accessibility may be influenced by the position of C-C interflavanic linkages and that of the galloyl substituents. Therefore, determination of tannin structure and structure-activity relationships is a prerequisite to study their chemical properties and eventual health effect.

Methods to Determine Proanthocyanidin Structure

Formal identification of proanthocyanidins, including the determination of the C-C bond position, requires sophisticated NMR techniques as described by Ballas and Vercauteren (*18*). However, various acidolysis techniques give access to important structural information. In particular, a procedure based on partial thiolysis followed by reversed-phase HPLC analysis was developed to determine the nature and sequence of constitutive monomers of isolated oligomeric proanthocyanidins (*19*). It also enables formal identification of trimers and larger oligomers, provided that the linkage position in the released dimeric fragments can be unambiguously established. Application of the above mentioned identification methods is, however, restricted to pure compounds and thus implies tedious isolation procedures. In fact, purification of tannins becomes increasingly difficult as their molecular weight increases, owing to the larger number of possible isomers, smaller amounts of each individual compound, and poorer resolution of the chromatographic profiles. This is especially true in the case of grape products which contain a large diversity of tannin structures, based on several monomers, whereas some other plants synthesize essentially one series, *e.g.* (-)-epicatechin derivatives in the case of cacao (*20*).

Several methods have been developed to evaluate oligomeric and polymeric tannins. Some of them, including counter current chromatography (*21*), chromatography on Fractogel TSK HW-40 (*22,23*) or Sephadex LH20 (*24*) columns, normal phase TLC (*25*) or HPLC (*20,26*), aim to separate tannins on a molecular weight basis. Another group of methods, based on acid-catalyzed degradation in the presence of various nucleophilic agents, including toluene-α-thiol (*26-28*) and phloroglucinol (*29*), allow one to determine the monomeric composition and mean degree of polymerization of tannin extracts or fractions. The principle of these methods is as follows. Breakage of the interflavanic C-C bond under mild acidic conditions releases the terminal units as the corresponding flavanols and the upper and intermediate units as carbocations which react with nucleophiles to form stable adducts (*e.g.* benzylthioethers in the presence of toluene-α-thiol). The resulting solution can then be analyzed by HPLC (*19,30,31*) or NMR (*32*) and the mean DP calculated.

Grape and Wine Tannins

Characterization of Grape Tannins. About twenty dimeric and trimeric proanthocyanidins have been identified in grape seeds (*23*) and skins (*33*). Only B-type proanthocyanidins are present in grapes, with small amounts of dimers and trimers containing $4\bar{\text{O}}6$ linkages occuring along with the most common $4\bar{\text{O}}8$ linked oligomers. They usually consist of (+)-catechin, (-)-epicatechin and (-)-epicatechin-3-O-gallate units, although a catechin-3-O-gallate derivative has also been reported in non-*vinifera* varieties (*34*).

The major oligomeric procyanidins have been quantified individually in various grape extracts by reversed-phase HPLC (*34-37*). However, concentration of oligomers in plant tissues is usually relatively low compared to that of larger molecular weight tannins (*38*).

Chromatography on a Fractogel column was carried out on various grape skin and seed extracts in order to separate flavanol monomers, dimeric procyanidins and larger molecular weight tannins (DP>2). Seed extracts were fractionated as described by Ricardo da Silva *et al.* (*23*) and skin extracts also, following an adaptation of this procedure developed for wine tannins (*26*). Monomers and dimers were assayed by reversed-phase HPLC analysis of the first two fractions. The polymeric fractions were submitted to complete thiolysis (*26,28*) and the amounts of tannins were calculated by summing the concentrations of monomer units (and of the corresponding benzylthioethers) thus released. Polymeric tannins were much more abundant than monomers and dimers both in seeds and in skins. An example of distribution among these three groups is presented in Table 1.

Table 1 : Amounts of flavanol monomers, procyanidin dimers and larger molecular weight tannins (DP >2) in *Vitis vinifera* (var. Cabernet franc)

	skins	seeds
monomers	13.8	188
dimers	7.2	66
polymers (DP>2)	312	3600

expressed in mg catechin equivalent per kg berries

Reversed-phase HPLC analysis of the fragments released by thiolysis of the polymeric fractions (DP>2) showed that grape seed tannins consist of partly galloylated procyanidins whereas grape skins also contain prodelphinidins, detected as the (-)-epigallocatechin benzylthioether derivative arising from upper and intermediate units. Grape seeds contained larger amounts of tannins and larger proportions of galloylated units than grape skins but the average molecular weight was higher in skins than in seeds for all studied varieties. Monomeric composition of seed and skin tannins determined for two *Vitis vinifera* varieties is presented in Figure 1.

Wine Tannin Composition. Wine tannin composition depends on the grape from which the wine is made but also, as tannins are mostly confined to the solid parts of the cluster (*36*), on the wine-making conditions influencing extraction of tannins from pomace. Moreover, once extracted, tannins undergo various types of reactions, themselves depending on the presence of other wine components as well as on the storage conditions.

Red wine samples (*Vitis vinifera*, var. Carignane) were taken after 0, 3, 9, and 20 days of fermentation and submitted to chromatography on Fractogel as described by Prieur (*26*). Thiolysis of the tannin fractions (DP>2) thus obtained, Figure 2, showed that prodelphinidins were extracted faster than procyanidins whereas diffusion of galloylated procyanidins was slower. This may indicate that tannins diffuse more easily from skins than from seeds. But it may also be due to differences in water solubility, with lower polarity compounds such as gallates being gradually extracted as the ethanol level increases throughout fermentation. Larger molecular weight tannins also diffused later than smaller oligomers, presumably owing to their poorer solubility. Note that, in the case of grape seed tannins, the proportion of galloylated units was shown to increase with the degree of polymerisation (*28*).

Analysis of the wines after four months showed that losses of all proanthocyanidins, Figure 3, but especially of prodelphinidins and to a lesser extent of galloylated compounds, Figure 2, had occurred. This probably reflects the higher reactivity of trihydroxylated molecules. In particular, procyanidin gallates were shown to complex more easily with proteins (*5,39*) and, when oxidized, to proceed to condensation products faster (*5*) than the corresponding non-galloylated molecules. The average degree of polymerisation also decreased from 13.5 to 9 during this period, meaning that larger molecular weight tannins were more easily degraded. This can be partly due to their hydrolysis to smaller molecules in the acidic wine environment (*3*). Besides, losses of larger molecular weight tannins may result from insolubilisation, in particular following complexation with proteins. However, the amount of total phenols in the polymeric fraction increased within the first months of wine aging, Figure 3, suggesting that tannins had been partly converted to other phenolic polymers rather than precipitated out. Formation of anthocyanin-tannin complexes (*9,10,13-15*) may be responsible for part of these changes, as polymeric red pigments also accumulated. In fact, half of the anthocyanins originally present in red wine were shown to be converted to polymeric pigments within the first year of ageing (*9*). Oxidative coupling is another possible mechanism since catechin dimers generated by enzymatic oxidation were resistant to thiolysis (*12,40*).

In any case, all derivatives formed from grape phenolics in the course of processing may participate in wine organoleptic properties and eventual health effects. In particular, both genuine tannins (*i.e.* proanthocyanidins) and related tannin-like structures (*e.g.* oxidation products, tannin-anthocyanin complexes) should be involved in interactions with proteins, which are responsible for astringency, haze formation, and perhaps, antibiotic or antiviral properties.

Interactions with Proteins

Studies of protein-tannin interactions were performed using two different approaches. In the first series of studies, the extent of interaction was estimated by assaying tannins remaining in solution after removal of the insoluble protein-tannin complexes (*5,26,41*). In the second one, various catechin dimers were tested with regards to their inhibitory effects on enzymes degrading polysaccharides.

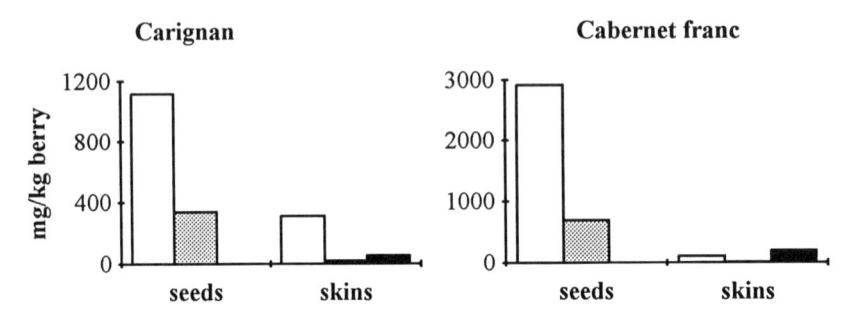

Figure 1. Composition of polymeric tannins (degree of polymerisation>2) in the seeds and skins of two *Vitis vinifera* varieties as determined by thiolysis (□ : procyanidins, ▨ : galloylated procyanidins, ■: prodelphinidins)

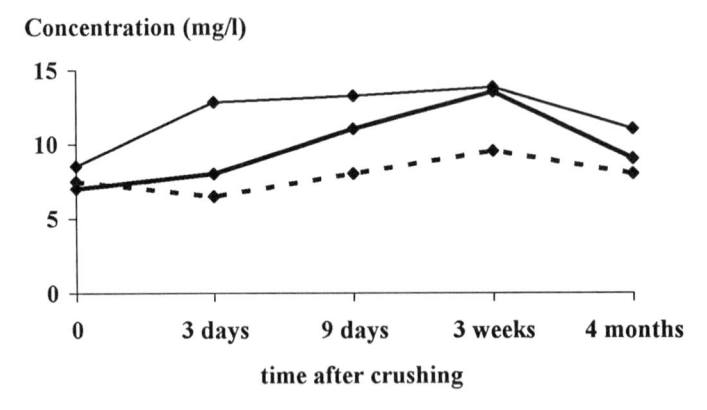

Figure 2. Changes of tannin composition (degree of polymerisation >2) during vinification of Carignane grapes as determined by thiolysis (——— : prodelphinidins (%); - - - - : galloylated units (%); ——— : mean degree of polymerisation).

Interactions of Procyanidin Oligomers with Proteins. The influence of procyanidin structure on their interactions with various proteins, including classical enology fining agents, a grape arabinogalactan protein (*42*) and poly(L-prolines) was investigated in wine-like model solutions (*5,41*). Among the proteins tested, poly(L-prolines) showed the highest affinity for all procyanidins, as expected from other works which clearly established the role of proline in the mechanism of tannin bonding to proteins (*43-45*). The affinity of procyanidins towards polyprolines, casein and gelatins appeared essentially determined by the number of o-dihydroxyphenyl groups, increasing primarily with the number of galloyl substituents and also with the degree of polymerisation. The influence of the interflavanic linkage position was also important, as larger losses of oligomers containing a C4-C6 bond were measured (*41*). This presumably indicates that the shape and flexibility of these molecules allowed easier access of the proteins to the o-dihydroxyphenyl reactive sites. Complexation with grape arabinogalactan-protein increased as a function of procyanidin molecular weight, suggesting that the carbohydrate moiety contributed substantially to the interaction (*46*), as shown earlier in the case of salivary glycoproteins (*47*). When applied to a red wine (*Vitis vinifera*, Mourvèdre variety), the protein fining treatments did not modify the levels of catechin, epicatechin and procyanidin oligomers, although absorbances at 280, 420, 520 and 620 nm were lower in all treated wines (*41*). Thus, it seems that the lower molecular weight flavanols were protected by other wine components, presumably polymeric tannins and/or tannin-derived molecules.

Interactions of Grape Seed Procyanidin Fractions with PVP. A crude grape seed tannin extract (40 mg/l in synthetic wine) was treated with increasing amounts of polyvinylpyrrolidone (PVP), a polymer interacting strongly with tannins in the same way as proteins, owing to the proline-like structure of its vinylpyrrolidone constitutive units (*48*). Normal-phase HPLC analysis (*28*) of the supernatants obtained after centrifugation showed that, with the lower PVP concentrations, the proportion of tannins insolubilised increased with the molecular weight, Figure 4. At 40 mg/l PVP, most oligomers and polymers (DP >3) were precipitated out whereas dimers and trimers remained totally soluble. Thiolysis of the supernatants showed that the average degree of polymerisation decreased as the amount of PVP was increased from 0 to 98 mg/l. This confirms that larger molecular weight tannins interact more readily with proteins, thus protecting oligomers. The proportion of galloylated units in the soluble tannins also decreased with increasing amounts of PVP, meaning that galloylated procyanidins were selectively precipitated. However, in the grape seed extract tested, larger molecular weight tannins were also more galloylated (*28*) so that the respective influence of DP and galloylation cannot be distinguished.

Enzymatic Inhibition Studies. In the second series of experiments, the inhibitory effects of (+)-catechin and of several catechin dimers on polysaccharide hydrolases were compared. The dimers studied included procyanidin B3 (catechin-(4α$\tilde{O}$8)-catechin) and dimeric oxidation products, showing biphenyl or ether interflavanic

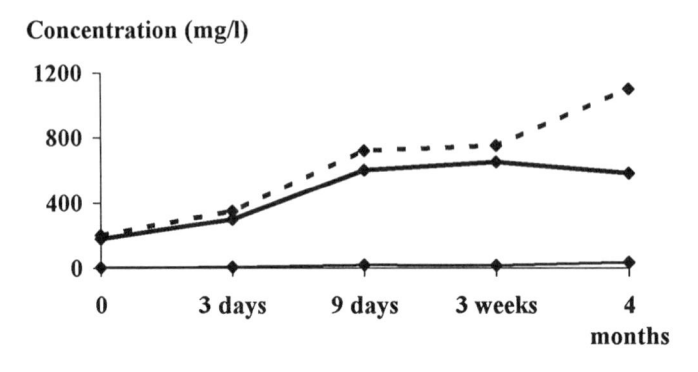

Figure 3. Changes of phenolic polymers during vinification of carignane grapes (- - - - : total phenols in the polymeric fraction estimated from 280 nm absorbance in eq. catechin) ; ——— : polymeric pigments estimated from 520 nm absorbance (in eq. malvidin-3-glucoside) ; ——— : total proanthocyanidins determined by thiolysis (in eq. catechin).

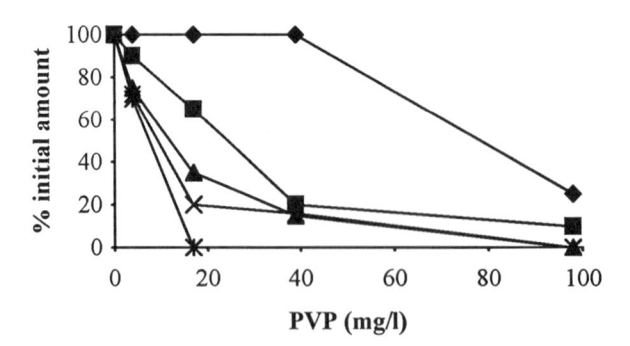

Figure 4. HPLC analysis of procyanidins remaining in solution following addition of PVP to a grape seed tannin extract. ◆ : dimers and trimers (mean degree of polymerisation = 2.3); ■, ▲, × : oligomers (mean degree of polymerisation = 3.6, 5.4 and 7.8, respectively); ✶ : polymers (mean degree of polymerisation = 15).

linkages, identified by Guyot (12). Colorless and yellow solutions containing mostly catechin dimers, obtained by enzymatic oxidation of catechin respectively at pH 3 and pH 6 (12,40) were also tested. Among the four enzymes studied, *Aspergillus niger* endo-polygalacturonase and almond (*Amygdalae dulces*) β-glucosidase were significantly inhibited by tannins.

β-glucosidase activity was assayed by measuring the glucose released from *p*-nitrophenyl-β-D-glucose using high performance ionic chromatography (49). Inhibition of *A. dulces* β-glucosidase by catechin oxidation products was non-competitive, as shown earlier for other tanning substances (17,50). A Ki of 2.6 mM (in catechin equivalent) was calculated for the mixture of colorless products obtained by enzymatic oxidation of catechin at pH 3.

Endopolygalacturonase activity was measured by viscosimetry using orange polygalacturonic acid (Sigma) as the substrate. All catechin dimers tested (at 0.5 g/l each) exhibited similar inhibitory effects, Figure 5. Preincubation of the enzyme with the inhibitor significantly enhanced the inhibitory effect, as would be expected from the kinetics of tanning reactions (44). Comparison of individual colorless dimers showed no obvious structure-activity relationship, and in particular no marked role of *o*-dihydroxyphenyl moieties. In fact, one of the C-O linked dimers was a more powerfull inhibitor than both C-C linked dimers, although it had only one *o*-diphenolic group, whereas the other one was less inhibitory. However, the solution containing yellow oxidation products was more active than the colorless solution obtained by oxidation at pH 3 (respectively 93% and 65% inhibition at 0.5g/l).

Catechin itself was inhibitory at 3g/l but this effect disappeared after purification by liquid chromatography on Fractogel, although the original commercial sample was chromatographically pure. As well, the solution containing colorless catechin dimers was more inhibitory than its main components, meaning that most of its activity was actually due to minor compounds. This points out that contaminants in trace amounts can exert powerfull effects which may be wrongly attributed to the major product tested.

The other two enzymes studied, namely β-mannanase and β-galactosidase from *Aspergillus niger*, were totally unaffected at the concentrations used (up to 3 g/l). The various results obtained strongly suggest that inhibition is related to protein-tannin interactions and depends both on the protein and on the tannin structure.

Conclusions

The data presented point out the complexity of wine tannin composition and the difficulties likely to be encountered when studying the structures and properties of wine phenolics.

Grape tannins consist essentially of proanthocyanidins, which are partly galloylated procyanidins in seeds, procyanidins and prodelphinidins in skins. Wine tannin composition is influenced by the fermentation conditions (e.g. skin contact duration, temperature) as rather polar tannins from skins (prodelphinidins) are more

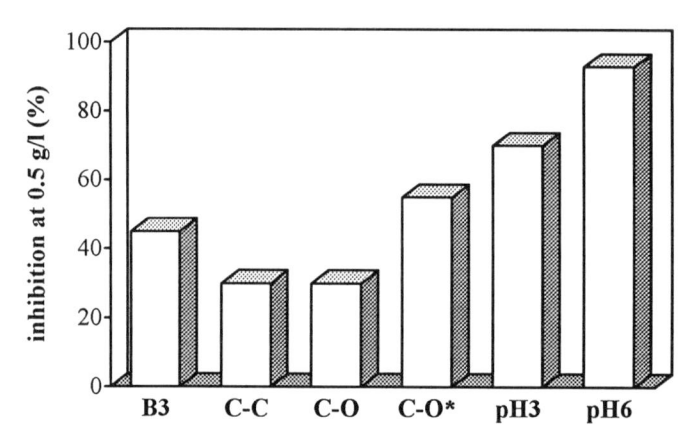

Figure 5. endopolygacturonase inhibition by catechin dimers. B3 : procyanidin B3; C-C : catechin dimer formed by enzymatic oxidation with a biphenyl linkage; C-O and C-O* : catechin dimers arising from enzymatic oxidation, showing ether linkages; pH3, pH6 : mixtures of catechin oxidation products obtained at pH 3 and pH 6, respectively.

readily extracted than less polar –and presumably also less accessible– seed components (galloylated procyanidins). In addition to grape proanthocyanidins, wine tannins include non-proanthocyanidin tannin-like structures, formed in increasing amounts as the wine ages. Trihydroxylated compounds (i.e. prodelphinidins and gallates) and larger molecular weight tannins, which are also more galloylated, seem to proceed to such derivatives faster than oligomeric procyanidins.

Larger molecular weight tannins were also selectively precipitated by protein fining agents. In fact, tannin-protein interactions increase both with the degree of polymerisation and with galloylation but also depend on the protein structure as only some of the enzymes tested were inhibited by tannins. Structural isomers of procyanidin dimers arising from catechin oxidation showed tanning effects similar to that of procyanidin B3 whereas yellow oxidation products were more active. Enzymatic inhibition studies will be continued using a larger number of isolated tannins, including in particular the yellow oxidation products. Better knowledge of the enzyme structure is also needed to interpret inhibition data in terms of structure-activity relationships. Finally, the structure of tannin-like compounds in wine will be investigated further and their properties compared to that of genuine grape proanthocyanidins.

Literature Cited

1. Singleton, V.L.; Noble, A.C. In *Phenolic Sulfur and Nitrogen Compounds in Food Flavors;* Charalambous, G.; Katz, I., Eds.; *A.C.S. Symp. Series,* **1976**, *26*, 47-70.
2. Lea, A.G.H.; Bridle, P.; Timberlake, C.F.; Singleton, V.L. *Am. J. Enol. Vitic.* **1979**, *30*, 289-300.
3. Haslam, E. *Phytochemistry* **1980**, *19*, 2577-2582.
4. Haslam, E.; Lilley, T.H. *Crit. Rev. Food Sci. Nutr.* **1988**, *27*, 1-40.
5. Cheynier, V.; Rigaud, J.; Ricardo da Silva, J.M. In *Plant Polyphenols.* Hemingway, R.W.; Laks, P.E., Eds.; Plenum Press, New York, 1992; 281-294.
6. Uchida, S.; Edamatsu, R.; Hiramatsu, M.; Mori, A.; Nonaka, G.I.; Nishioka, I.; Niwa, M.; Ozaki, M. *Med. Sci. Res.* **1987**, *15*, 831-832.
7. Okuda, O.; Yoshida, T.; Hatano, T. In *Phenolic Compounds in Food and their Effects on Health;* Ho, C.H.; Lee C.Y.; Huang, M.T., Eds.; *ACS Symp. Series* **1992**, *507*, 87-97.
8. Roberts, E.A.H. *J. Sci. Food Agric.* **1958**, *9*, 212-216.
9. Somers, T.C. *Phytochemistry* **1971**, *10*, 2175-2186.
10. Ribéreau-Gayon, P. in *Anthocyanins as Food Colors;* Markakis, P., Ed. Academic Press, New York, 1982; 209-244.
11. Cheynier,V.; Fulcrand, H.; Guyot, S.; Oszmianski, J.; Moutounet, M. in *Enzymatic Browning and its Prevention;* Lee C.Y.; Whitaker, J.R., Eds.; *ACS Symp. Series* **1995**, *600*, 130-143.
12. Guyot, S.; Vercauteren, J.; Cheynier, V. *Phytochemistry* **1996** *42*, 1279-1288.

13. Jurd, L. *Am. J. Enol. Vitic.* **1969**, *20*, 191-195.
14. Timberlake, C. F.; Bridle, P. *Am. J. Enol. Vitic.* **1976**, *27*, 97-105.
15. Liao, H.; Cai, Y.; Haslam, E. *J. Sci. Food Agric.* **1992**, *59*, 299-305.
16. Porter, L.J. In *The Flavonoids. Advances in Research since 1980* Harborne, J.B., Ed.; Chapman and Hall, London, 1988, 21-62.
17. Haslam, E. *Biochem. J.* **1974**, *139*, 285-288.
18. Balas, L.; Vercauteren, J. *Magn. Res. Chem.* **1994**, *32*, 386-393.
19. Rigaud, J.; Perez-Ilzarbe, J.; Ricardo da Silva, J.M.; Cheynier, V. *J. Chromatogr.* **1991**, *540*, 401-405.
20. Rigaud, J.; Escribano-Bailon, M.T.; Prieur, C.; Souquet, J.M.; Cheynier, V. *J. Chromatogr.* **1993**, *654*, 255-260.
21. Putman, L.J.; Butler, L.G. *J. Chromatogr.* **1985**, *318*, 85-93.
22. Derdelinckx, G.; Jerumanis, J. *J. Chromatogr.* **1984**, *285*, 231-244.
23. Ricardo da Silva J.; Rigaud, J.; Cheynier, V.; Cheminat, A.; Moutounet, M. *Phytochemistry,* **1991**, *30*, 1259-1264.
24. Lea, A.G.H.; Timberlake, C.F. *J. Sci. Food Agric.* **1974**, *25*, 1537-1545.
25. Lea, A.G.H. *J. Sci. Food Agric.* **1978**, *29*, 471-477.
26. Prieur, C. Dissertation Université de Montpellier II, 1994.
27. Thompson, J.; Tanner, D.; Haslam, E.; Tanner, R.J.N. *J. Chem. Soc. Perkin Trans I*, **1972**, 1387.
28. Prieur, C.; Rigaud, J.; Cheynier, V.; Moutounet, M. *Phytochemistry* **1994**, *36*, 781-784.
29. Foo, L.Y.; Porter, L.J. *J. Chem Soc. perkin Trans I 1978,* 1186-?.
30. Shen, Z.; Haslam, E.; Falsham, C.P.; Begley, M.J. *Phytochemistry* **1986**, *25*, 2629-2635.
31. Koupai-Abyazani M.R.; McCallum, J.; Bohm, N.A. *J. Chromatogr.* **1992**, *594*, 117-123.
32. Cai, Y.; Evans, F.J.; Roberts, M.F.; Phillipson, J.D.; Zenk, M.H.; Glebas, Y.Y. *Phytochemistry* **1991**, *30*, 2033-2040.
33. Escribano-Bailon, M.T.; Guerra, M.T.; Rivas Gonzalo, J.C.; Santos Buelga, C. *Polyphenols 94*; Ed. INRA, Paris, 1995, 225-226.
34. Lee, C.Y.; Jaworski, A.W. *Am. J. Enol. Vitic.* **1990**, *41*, 87-89.
35. Czochanska Z.; Foo, L.Y.; Porter, L. *Phytochemistry* **1979**, *18*, 1819-1822.
36. Bourzeix, M.; Weyland, D.; Heredia, N. *Bull. OIV* **1986**, *59*, 1171-1254.
37. Ricardo da Silva, J.M.; Rosec, J.P.; Bourzeix, M.; Heredia, N. *J. Sci. Food Agric.* **1990**, *53*, 85-92.
38. Czochanska Z.; Foo, L.Y.; Newman, R.H. Porter, L. *J. Chem. Soc. Perkin Trans I* **1980**, 2278-2286.
39. Okuda, T.; Mori, K.; Hatano, T. *Chem. Pharm. Bull.* **1985**, *33*, 1424-1433.
40. Guyot, S.; Cheynier, V.; Souquet, J.M.; Moutounet, M. *J. Agric. Food Chem.* **1995**, *43*, 2458-2462.
41. Saulnier, L.; Brillouet, J.M. *Carbohydr. Res.* **1989**, *188*, 137-144.
42. Ricardo da Silva, J.M.; Cheynier, V.; Souquet, J.M.; Moutounet, M.; Cabanis, J.C.; Bourzeix, M.; *J. Sci. Food Agric.* **1991**, *57*, 111-125.

43. McManus, J.P.; Davis, K.G.; Beart, J.E.; Gaffney, S.H; Lilley, T.H.; Haslam, E. *J. Chem. Soc. Perkin Trans 2*, **1985**, 1429-1438.
44. Hagerman, A.E.; Butler, L.G. *J. Biol. Chem.* **1981**, *256*, 4494-4497.
45. Murray, N.J.; Williamson, M.P.; Lilley, T.H.; Haslam, E. *Eur. J. Biochem.* **1994**, *219*, 923-935.
46. Ya, C.; Gaffney, S.H.; Lilley, T.H.; Haslam, E. In *Chemistry and Significance of Condensed Tannins*. Hemingway, R.W.; Karchezy, J.J., Eds.; Plenum Press, New York, 1989; 307-322.
47. Asquith,T.N.; Uhlig, J.; Mehansho, H.; Putman, L.; Carlson, D.M.; Butler, L. *J. Agric. Food Chem. 1987,35*, 331-334.
48. Loomis, W.D.; Battaile, J. *Phytochemistry* **1966**, *5*, 423-438.
49. Guyot, S.; Pellerin, P.; Brillouet, J.M.; Cheynier, V. *Biosci. Biotechnol. Biochem.* **1996**, 60, 1131-1135.
50. Dick, A.J.; Williams, R.; Bearne, S.L.; Lidster, P.D. *J. Agric. Food Chem.* **1985**, *33*, 798-800.

Chapter 9

Enantiomeric Analysis of Linalool for the Study of the Muscat Wine Flavorings Composition

Fernando Tateo, E. Desimoni, and M. Bononi

Dipartimento di Fisiologia delle Piante Coltivate e Chimica Agraria, Sezione di Chimica Analitica Agroalimentare ed Ambientale, Facoltà di Agraria, Università degli Studi di Milano, Via Celoria 2, 20133 Milano, Italy

Enantiomer separation is fundamental in the field of flavours analysis and also in the analytical control of wines because it gives access to biogenetic information concerning some flavouring compounds and very often, as a consequence, the corresponding matrix: it makes possible to determine the enantiomeric excess (ee) and to identify possible adulterations.

In the "muscat wine flavourings", not necessary those produced for the flavouring of wines, but also those designed for the flavouring of sauces, seasonings and other semi-finished products, one of the most useful, and therefore quantitatively preponderant, components for flavouring impact, is linalool. Generally, this compound is not employed as such in formulation: for that purpose, essential oils and herbs extracts containing an amount of it sufficient to the aim, are preferably used.

The study on natural enantiomeric distribution of linalool has been carried out by several authors on different matrices (essential oils, vegetable extracts, etc.) (1-10).

Enantiomers distribution has turned out to be widely differentiated in examined diverse natural sources, but distinctive for each of them, with "ee" values referable to a predominance of R (-) form for some of them, and of S (+) form for the other ones.

On the contrary, neither data concerning enantiomeric distribution of linalool in "muscat wine" are to be found in bibliography, nor information about the composition of the

© 1997 American Chemical Society

"muscat wine flavourings" present on the market, designed to enhance low-quality wines, proves to be published somewhere.

In this paper two "muscat wine flavourings", which can be considered as classical reference flavourings, present on the international market and conventionally named "E" and "F", which many others, come onto the same market, draw their inspiration from, have been examined through chiral analysis by HRGC serial coupling between non-chiral Easy Wax column and chiral Beta-Dex column. In a parallel way, the enantiomeric distribution of linalool in two essential oils, Coriander oil and Salvia sclarea essential oil, which in most cases represent the fundamental raw material for the formulation of the "muscat wine flavourings", has been examined.

The aim of this work is to evaluate if, from HRGC analysis carried out by serial coupling, as from "ee" values of the "muscat wine flavourings", it is possible to obtain any information about the use of the above-mentioned essential oils, known as fundamental raw materials for the formulation of the flavourings themselves.

As for the quantitative resolution of linalool enantiomers within the adopted analytical conditions, it has been deemed useful to apply techniques of peak-shape analysis, which have turned out to be particularly helpful in case of unsufficient resolution of enantiomeric peaks.

Peak-shape analysis of overlapping peaks is a slowly growing field in chromatography (see reference 11 and 12 for recent literature information) even if, in principle, it represents a good alternative to more complex experimental separation, from both the points of view of speed and economy. The simplest data analysis systems should allow:

    1) chromatogram display and expansion

    2) baseline removal

    3) addition and subtraction of peaks

    4) integration and area measurement

    5) chromatographic synthesis

Each of the above points can be implemented by different approaches but all can profit of previous experience in the field of data analysis. X-ray photoelectron spectroscopy (XPS), in particular, is a technique in which peak-shape analysis of overlapping peaks is routinely perfomed (see for example reference 13). As far as we know, even if XP spectra analysis must necessarily take into account specific aspects of the photoelectron emission from a solid surface, many of the practical solutions developed for XPS data system (13-16) can be fruitfully exploited in chromatographic peak analysis.

Some points on which attention was focused in the course of preliminary tests (17) performed to evaluate the main problems involved in the resolution of overlapping chromatographic peaks due to linalool enantiomers, are discussed in this paper.

EXPERIMENTAL

Samples

The "muscat wine flavourings" E and F correspond to products present on the international market of flavourings.

The muscat wine analysed by SPME (solid phase micro extraction) is absolutely a genuine "moscato reale", wine-made and transformed in Puglia (Cantele srl - Lecce).

GC/MS analysis

HRGC - analysis has been carried out within the following operating conditions:

Column: SPB-5 (30 m x 0,32 mm, 0,25 μm film)
Column temp.: isot.80°C x 10 min, incr. 1°C/min to 120°C,
isot.120°C x 10 min, incr. 3°C/min to 260°C

HRGC - chiral analysis has been carried out within the following operating conditions:

Serial Columns:

1) Deactivated column (1 m x 0,32 mm i.d.)

2) Easy Wax (25 m x 0,25 mm i.d., 0,25 μm film)

3) Beta-Dex 120 (30 m x 0,25 mm i.d., 0,25 μm film)

Column temp.: 60°C x 10 min, incr. 1.5 °C/min to 120°C, 120°C x 5 min, incr. 3°C/min to 240°C

The SPME has been carried out using a 100 μm polydimethylsiloxane fiber (Supelco).

Peak shape analysis

Data analysis concerning linalool was carried out by temporarily adapting the routines at a homebuilt data station for X-ray photoelectron spectroscopy data (14-16). The goodness of fit was evaluated using the χ^2 test specified in reference (13).

RESULTS AND DISCUSSION

HRGC - Chiral Analysis

The comparison between the GC chromatogram concerning Salvia sclarea oil and the GC chromatogram referring to one of the two "muscat wine flavourings" which have been discussed in the introduction: (E), allows to point out interesting composition affinities in particular, a quantitative predominance of linalool and linalil acetate, a significant presence of α-terpineol and geranyl acetate, a presence of other minor components (for instance, neryl acetate and β-caryofillene).
The comparison is shown in Figure 1.
Chiral analysis performed on E flavouring, as shown by the comparison of the chromatograms in Figure 2, points out, as far as linalool is concerned, a quantitative predominance of S (+) enantiomer, and therefore a enantiomeric distribution substantially

different from that concerning linalool derived from Salvia sclarea essential oil, in which, on the contrary, R (-) is quantitatively preponderant.

The columns serial coupling system described in the experimental section, among other things, allows to compare, as shown in Figure 3, the enantiomeric distribution of some terpenes (α-pinene, limonene), and, moreover, to emphasize the presence of camphor as a component much better represented in the "muscat wine flavouring E", than in Salvia sclarea oil.

Verified that Coriander oil presents a enantiomeric distribution characterized by "ee" S(+)=54,8 , once "ee" value in Salvia sclarea oil has been calculated, it is possible to calculate the percentage of linalool derived from the two oils in a muscat wine flavouring like "E".

It is plain that the predominant sources of linalool are basically the above-mentioned essential oils. The presence of camphor, among other things, confirms the presence of Coriander oil.

For the calculation of the enantiomeric ratio of linalool in Salvia sclarea oil, deduced from peak in Figure 2, see the section "Peak Shape Analysis".

Table 1 contains some data about "ee" values concerning linalool derived from different mixtures of the two mentioned oils. As to linalool in the "muscat wine flavouring E", with the same criteria adopted in "Peak Shape Analysis" , the enantiomeric ratio has been calculated as equivalent to

$$R(-) = 45,9 \qquad S(+) = 54,1 \qquad "ee" = S (+) \; 8,2$$

From the comparison of the data contained in Table 1, it follows that the percentage of linalool derived from Coriander oil is about 33-35% against 65-67% of linalool derived from Salvia sclarea oil.

On the contrary, the analysis of "muscat wine flavouring F" (Figure 4), shows an enantiomeric distribution of linalool of the kind of Coriander oils, with a predominance of S(+) form, according to a "ee" value which is fairly near to that concerning this oil, as

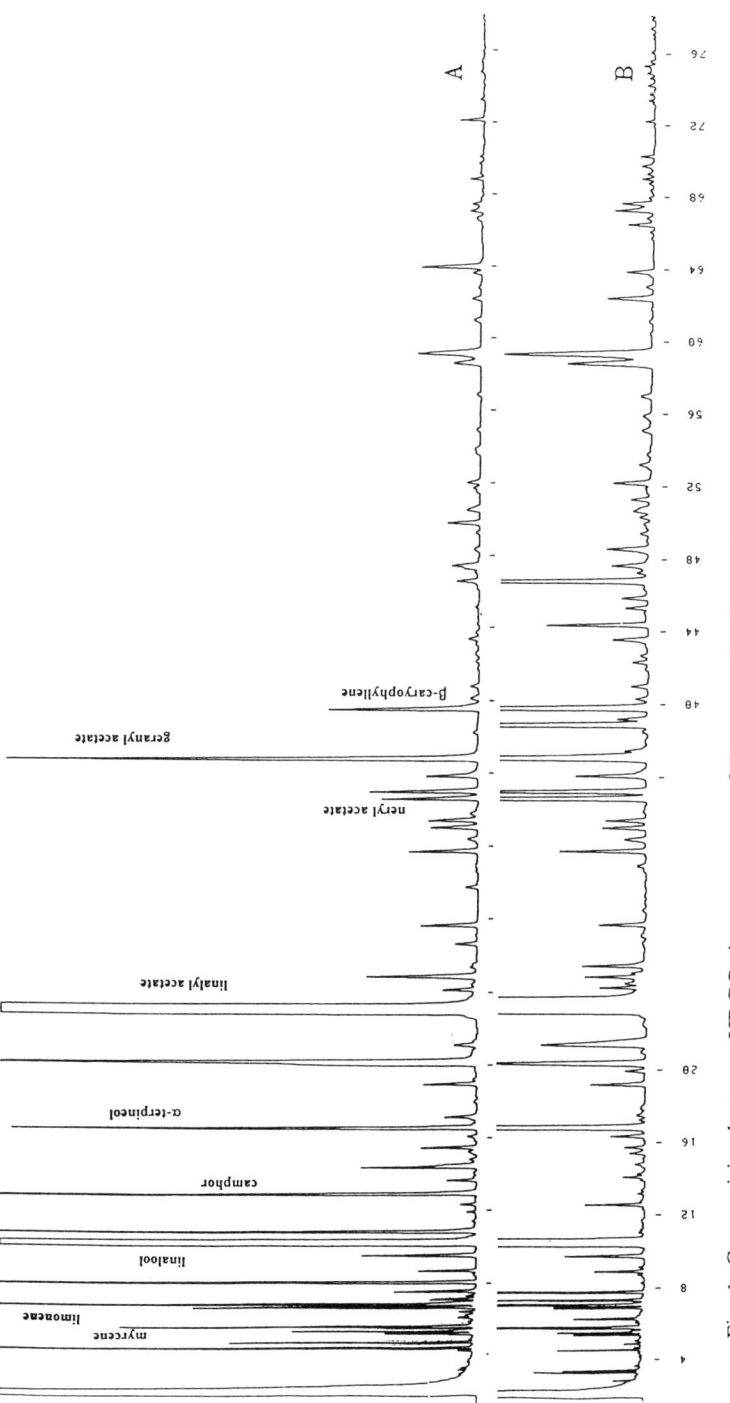

Fig. 1. Comparision between HRGC chromatograms of "muscat wine flavouring E" (A) and *Salvia sclarea* essential oil (B).

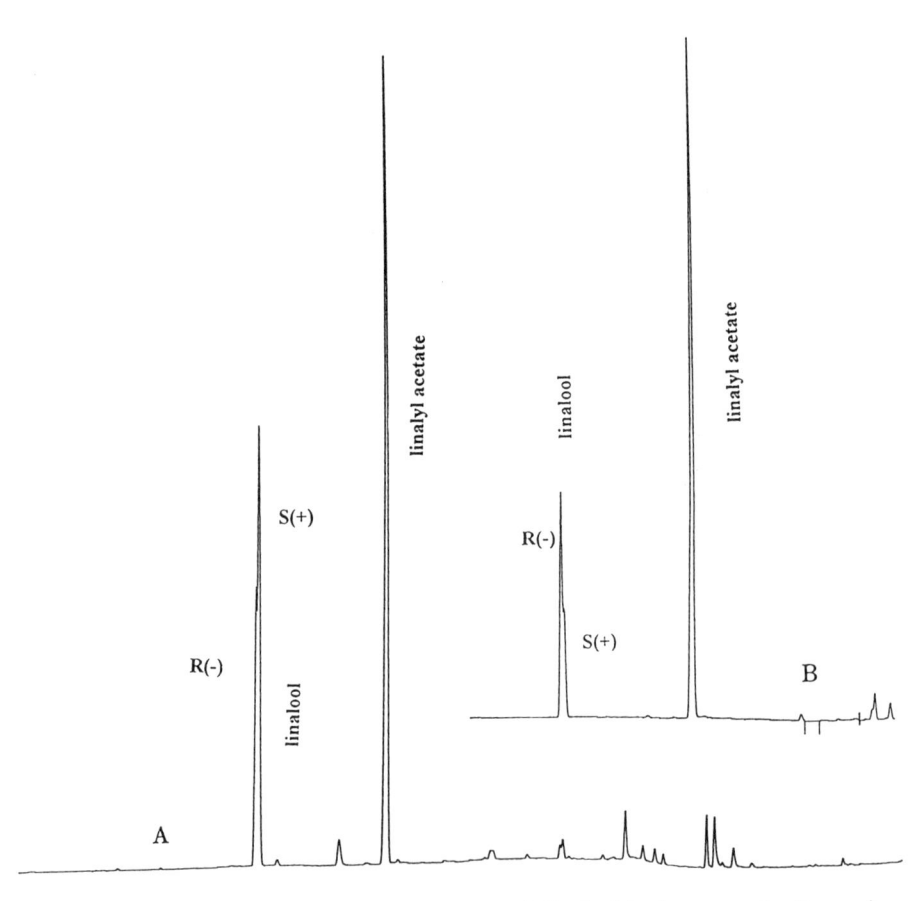

Fig. 2. Comparison of enantiomeric distribution of linalool in "muscat wine flavouring E" (A) and in *Salvia sclarea* essential oil (B).

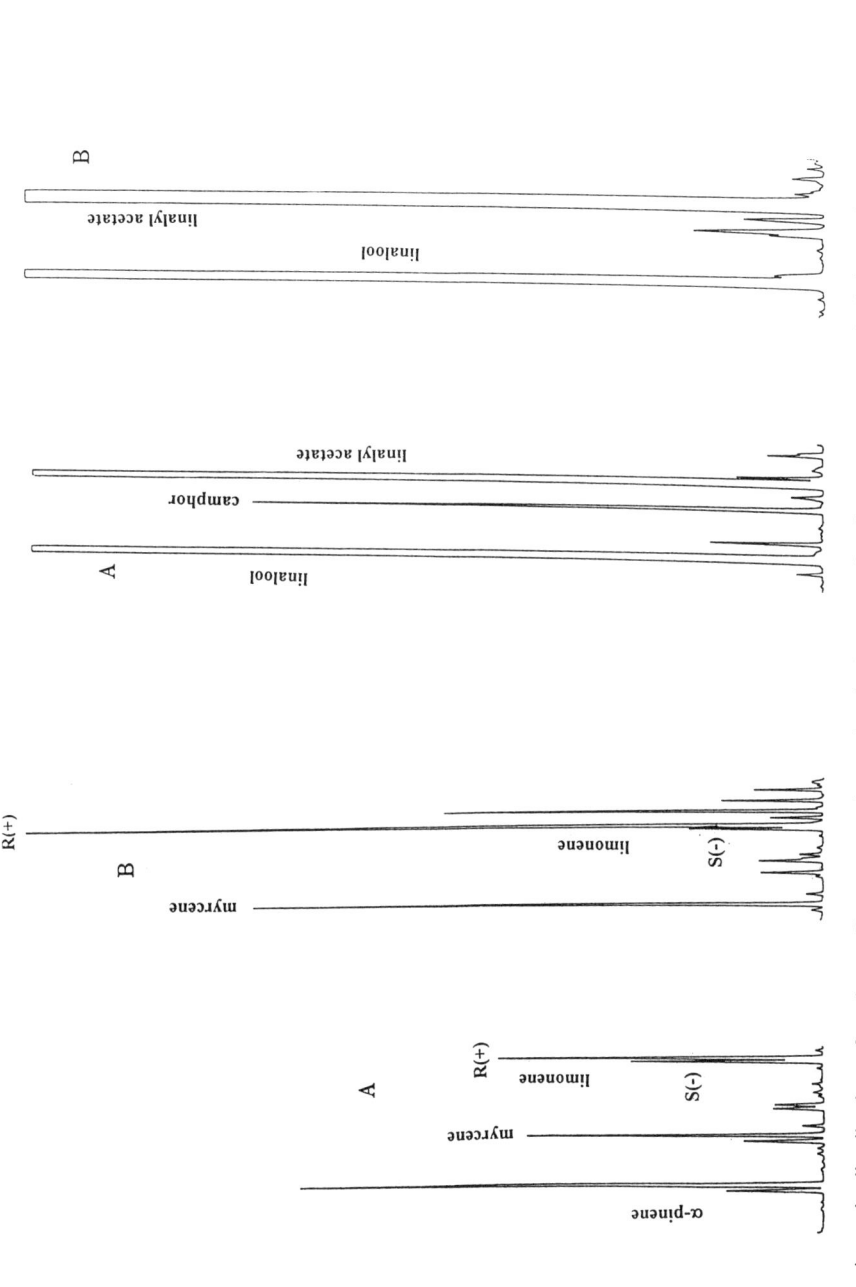

Fig. 3. Enantiomeric distribution of α-pinene, limonene and camphor in "muscat wine flavour E" (A) and in *Salvia sclarea* essential oil (B).

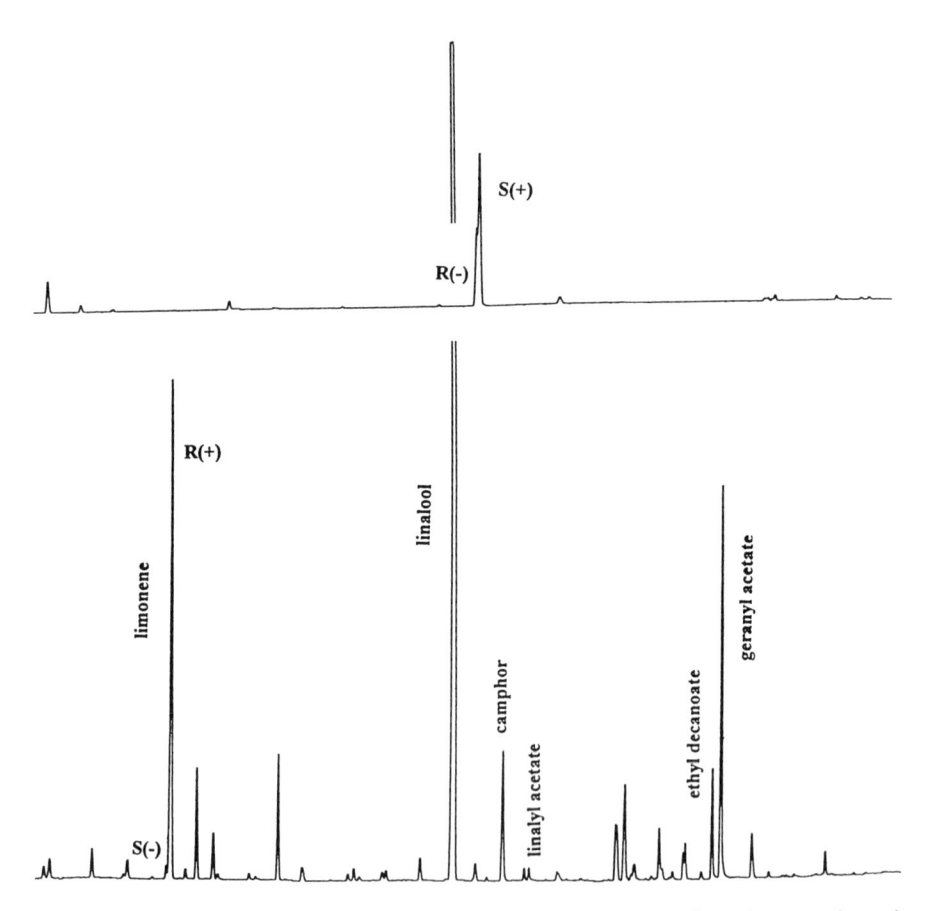

Fig. 4. Chiral Analysis of "muscat wine flavouring F", showing the enantiomeric distribution of linalool.

reported in Table 1. In such a flavouring, neither an appreciable amount of Salvia sclarea oil, nor other high sources of linalool besides Coriander oil, have turned out to be employed.

Table 1. To see these "ee" values correspond different "C/S" ratios between percentages of linalool derived from Coriander oils and percentages of linalool derived from Salvia sclarea. The excess of S (+) is evident from percentages over 23% of linalool derived from Coriander oils.

	R(-)	S(+)	"ee"
CORIANDER OIL (C)	22,6	77,4	S(+) 54,8
SALVIA sclarea (S)	58,1	41,9	R(-) 16,2
C 23 / S 77	49,8	50,2	S(+) 0,4
C 50 / S 50	40,3	59,7	S(+) 19,4
C 70 / S 30	33,2	66,8	S(+) 33,6
C 90 / S 10	26,1	73,9	S(+) 47,8

Another aim of this work is to verify if and to what extent an analysis carried out by SPME can be useful for the analytical control of the muscat wine flavourings and, therefore, for a judgement of genuinity about the wine itself.

Figure 5 shows a comparison between two chromatograms concerning to SPME extracts: one referring to a white wine first deflavoured and then flavoured with "muscat wine flavouring "E", the other concerning a genuine "moscato reale". It follows that:

- the absorption turns out to be selective; within the adopted conditions linalil acetate turns out to be extracted to a greater extent that linalool;

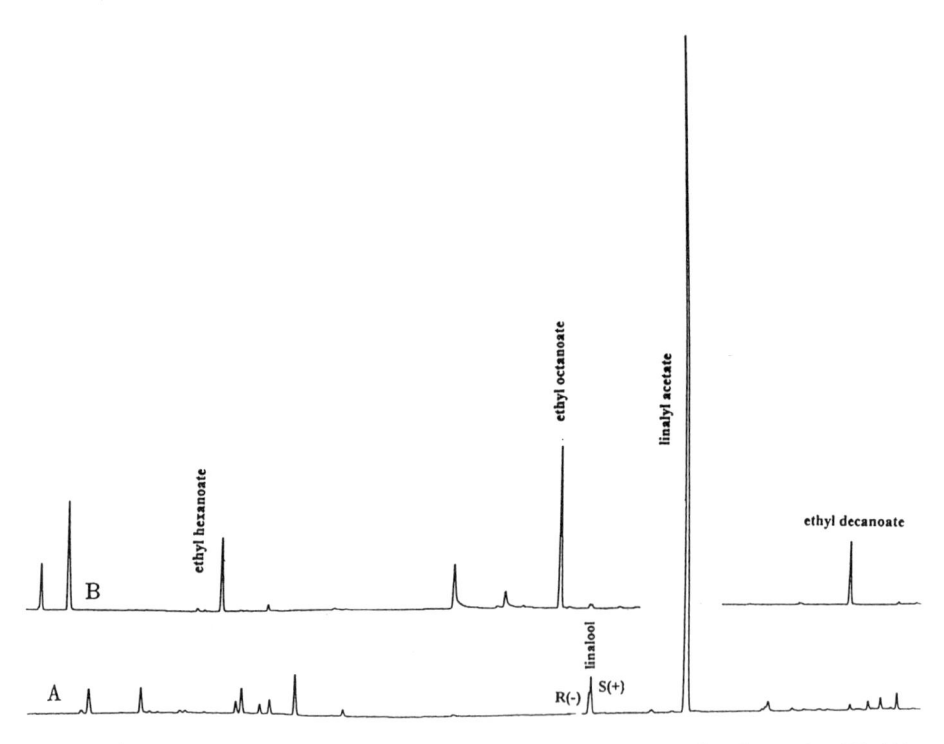

Fig. 5. Comparison between SPME extracts refering to "muscat wine flavouring E" (A) and to "moscato reale" (B).

- the enantiomeric ratio of linalool turns out to be still calculable, but to an extent which depends on the quantity;
- the "moscato reale" does not happen to contain linalil acetate in any appreciable amount;
- the "moscato reale" happens to contain linalool, but the enantiomeric distribution does not seen to be similar to that of the flavourings "E" and "F".

Peak shape analysis

A first problem in chromatographic peak analysis is the choice of the *right* peak-shape. Non-Gaussian peak-shapes can be obtained (12) in chromatographic systems with non-linear isotherms or slow retention kinetics or can result from deliberate attempts to overload the column, while asymmetrical peak-shapes can be observed when using too high sample sizes or because of distortions produced by the elution of the initially symmetrical peak. In our opinion, until specific investigations will make available a generally applicable model, a peak-shape must stem from an optimal compromise between flexibility and ease of use. This means that a peak-shape must be defined by a sufficient number of parameters to allow for eventual asymmetries and for an easy calculation of peak-width and area. A possible choice is the Gaussian-Lorentzian sum (GLS) function

$$y = H \, (GLR \cdot e^{-4Q\ln 2} + (1 - GLR)/(1-4Q))$$

in which H is the peak height, GLR the Gaussian-Lorentzian mixing ratio (GLR=1 means a pure Gaussian, while GLR=0 means a pure Lorentzian), $Q = [(x-T_r)/FWHM]^2$, $(x-T_r)$ is the distance from the peak maximum, T_r is the retention time, and FWHM the full width at half maximum. According to previous results (14) the GLS function offers the following advantages:

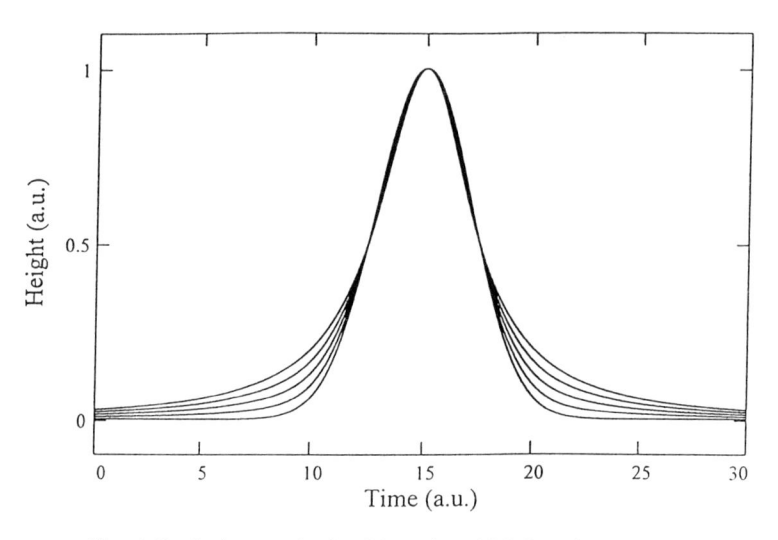

Fig. 6. Peak-shapes obtained by using GLS functions having different GLR values at constant FWHM.

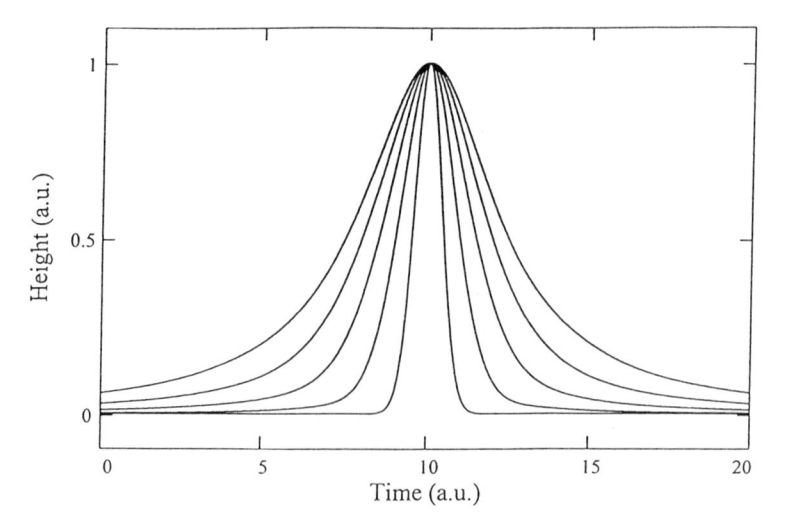

Fig. 7. Peak-shapes obtained by using GLS functions having different FWHM and GLR values.

i) symmetrical peaks require the definition of only four parameters (T_r; H; FWHM; GLR);

ii) asymmetrical peaks can be obtained by using different half widths at half maximum and Gaussian-Lorentzian mixing ratios on the left and right wing of the GLS function. This can be done by using six parameters (T_r; H; left-HWHM, right-HWHM, left-GLR, right-GLR) i.e. by using left-HWHM and left-GLR when (x-T_r) is negative and right-HWHM and right-GLR when (x-T_r) is positive; in this way peak is made from two half-peaks and FWHM = left-HWHM + right-HWHM;

iii) the peak asymmetry factor (AF) can be easily obtained from the same input parameters (AF = right-HWHM/ left-HWHM).

iv) the GLS function parameters of a given peak can be easily read by inspection of the experimental chromatograms while for example when using the Gaussian-Lorentzian product function, the FWHM has to be calculated by using iterative methods; see reference 13.

Some examples of GLS functions obtained by changing GLR at constant FWHM are reported in Figure 6. Other examples of GLS functions obtained by changing GLR and FWHM are reported in Figure 7. Any combination of left and right half-peaks is possible (14-16).

A second major point is the baseline subtraction, which should be performed in such a way not to modify peak and areas. A versatile software should allow the subtraction of linear, s-shapes or curved baselines (polynomial, exponential, gaussian or lorentzian tails, etc): a synthetic example is shown in Figure 8, where two partially resolved peaks are overlapped to a polynomial baseline (b=a + bx + cx^2, etc). This Figure shows that peak area measurements can be heavily affected by the use of improper baseline functions: a linear baseline between points A and B (used for both peaks) or between points A and C (for peak 1) and points C and B (for peak 2) significantly underestimate both peak areas.

A third point is the availability of an efficient test to evaluate the goodness of fit, essential to minimize the difference between synthetic (baseline plus peaks) and experimental chromatogram through subsequent iterations. This is particularly crucial in iterative routines (see below). A well-known but simple criterion is the chi-square, (χ^2), statistical test (13, 15, 16), which allows to estimate the confidence interval of the fit on properly considering the degrees of freedom in the fitting procedure (16). The χ^2 is easily obtained by the equation

$$\chi^2 = \Sigma[F(i, p_1,...,p_n) - Y_{exp}(i)]^2/Y_{exp}(i)$$

that is by evaluating the sum of the squared differences between the fitting function F (i, $p_1,..., p_n$), which is function of the single channel, i, and of the fitting function parameters ($p_1,..., p_n$), and the experimental data, $Y_{exp}(i)$, each squared difference being weighted by $Y_{exp}(i)^{-1}$. The lower the χ^2, the better the fit.

Additional help in finding out systematic errors in peak-fitting can be obtained (15) by evaluating the surface difference percentage [100 x (fitted area - experimental area)/experimental area] and by plotting the residuals [F(i, $p_1,..., p_n$) - $Y_{exp}(i)$] below the peak-fit: systematic errors are easily noticed by non-random fluctuations of the residuals. Figure 9 B shows the two peaks assigned to linalool enantiomers after the subtraction of the linear baseline (in this case a linear baseline was selected because the background was clearly constant: see Figure 2 B). The figure shows the best fit of the real chromatogram. As it can be seen, the S (+) enantiomer was fitted by a practically symmetrical line shapes while, in order to minimise the χ^2 value, an asymmetrical line shape was necessary for the R(-) enantiometer peak.

The "ee" value estimated in this case was R(-) 16,2.

This preliminary experiment on peak shape analysis has been made by interactive routines. A much useful and time-saving approach should use iterative analysis, which only can lead to automation and minimize personal bias of the operator. Iterations are driven by parameters selected for the goodness of the fit. A comparison of some algorithms used in chromatography is reported in reference 11 but many different approaches are detailed in specialised reviews (see for example reference 18). However,

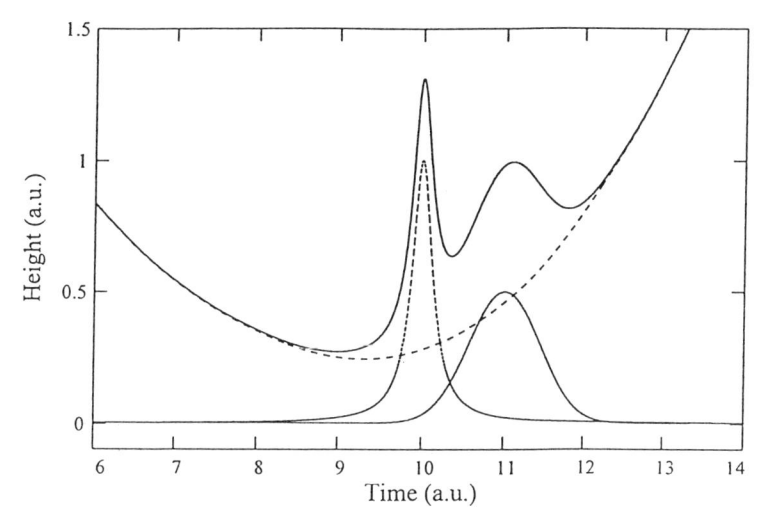

Fig. 8. The overlapping of two partially resolved peaks on a polynomial baseline (dashed curve) and erroneous linear baseline.

as shown in a recent paper (16) dealing with a non-linear least squares refinement method for XPS data analysis, the recovery of the effective peak-shapes in the presence, for example, of Poisson-distributed noise can be very difficult. This aspect of the problem will be fronted as soon as a reliable interactive software will be developed in our laboratory but, according to our experience in spectroscopy data systems, satisfactory results can be more easily obtained by using iterative routines to refine curve syntheses obtained by interactive analysis. This approach can be sometime slower that fully automatic, iterative one, but can help in rejecting *non-physical* solutions by exploiting the *chemical sense* in driving mathematical operations. Work is in progress in this direction.

Conclusion

Once more this work has allowed to emphasise the usefulness of carrying out the determination of some molecules by chiral analysis. In this case the enantiomeric distribution of linalool has been examined in order to get information about the nature of the most common essential oils for the production of the "muscat wine flavourings". Besides, the present research has pointed out the opportunity of critical evaluations about the results reached by SPME analysis. Moreover, the possibility and the opportunity of adopting a method of "peak shape analysis" for the evaluation of "ee" values for enantiomers, even in case of strong overlapping, have been proved.

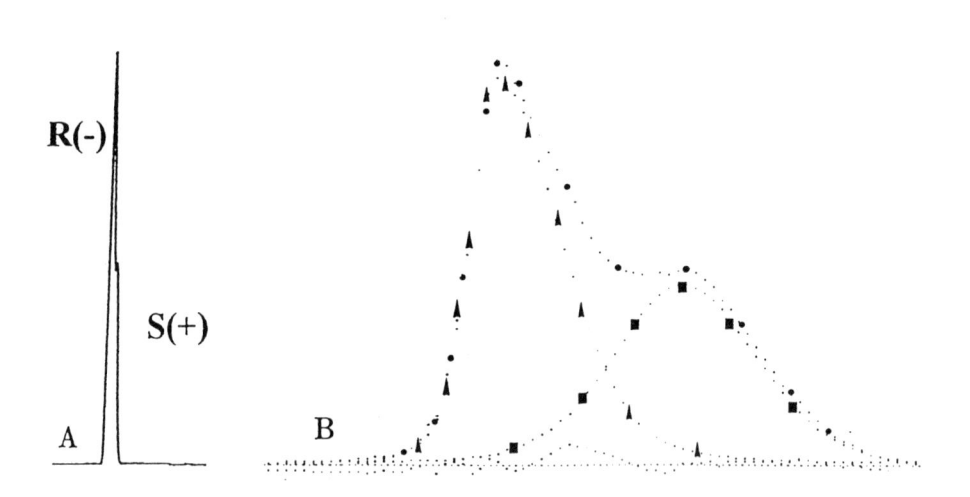

Fig. 9. Comparison of experimental (A) and digitized (B) peaks of linalool in Salvia sclarea essential oil.
(•): digital peaks after linear baseline subtraction;
(▲ and ■): synthesized peaks.
Peak parameters are:

Peak R(-)		Peak S(+)
38,075	P' (s)	38.2
3550	H (q.u.)*	1650
0,0527	r-HWHM (s)	0,0589
0,8	r-GLR	0,85
0,0176	l-HWHM (s)	0,0530
0,6	l-GLR	0,7
0,0703	FWHM (s)	0,119
289.22	Area (s.q.u.)	208.99

q.u.* arbitrary units.

Acknowledgments

We wish to thank Paula Constantino Chagas Lessa (UNICAMP-Brasil) for the collaboration.

References

1. P. Kreis and A. Mosandl, *Flavour Frag. J.*, **8**, 161 (1993).
2. U. Hener, R. Braunsdorf, P. Kreis, A. Dietrich, B. Maas, E. Euler, B. Schlag and A. Mosandl, *Chem. Mikrobiol. Technol. Lebensm.*, **14**, 129 (1992).
3. A. Mosandl, U. Hener, H.-G. Schmarr and M. Rautenschlein, *HRC*, **13**, 528 (1990).
4. A. Monsandl, U. Hagenauer-Hener, U. Hener, D. Lehman, P. Kreis and H.-G. Schmarr, *Flavour Science and Technology*, 6th Weurman Symp., p.21 (1990).
5. G. Dugo, A. Verzera, A. Trozzi, A. Cotroneo, L. Mondello and K. Bartle, Poster presented at the 15th International Symposium on Capillary Chromatography, Riva del Garda (Italy), 24-27 May (1993).
6. V. Schurig, M. Jung, D. Schmalzing, M. Schleimer, J. Duvekot, J. C: Buyten, J. A. Peene, and P. Mussche, *HRC*, **13**, 470 (1990).
7. V. Schubert and A. Mosandl, *Phytochem. Anal.*, **2**, 171 (1991).
8. Y. Ueyama, S. Hashimoto, H. Nii and K. J. Furukawa, *Ess. Oil Res.*, **4**, 15 (1992).
9. A. Controneo, I. S. d'Alcontres and A. Trozzi, *Flav. Frag. J.*, **7**, 49 (1992)
10. K. Bauer, D. Garbe, H. Surburg, *Common Fragrance and Flavor Materials*, VCH Verlagsgesellschaft: Weinheim (1990).
11. E. Reh, Trends *Anal. Chem.*, **14**, 1 (1995).
12. E.V. Dose, G. Guiochon, *Anal. Chem.*, **62**, 174 (1990).
13. P.M.A. Sherwood in *Practical Surface Analysis*, D. Briggs and M.P. Seach Editors, 2nd edition Appendix III, p 555. (1990).

14. E. Desimoni, G.I. Casella, T.R.I. Cataldi and C. Malitesta, *J. Electron Spectrosc. Relat. Phenon.*, **49**, 247 (1989).
15. E. Desimoni, U. Biader Ceipidor, *J. Electron Spectrosc. Relat. Phenon.*, **56**, 221(1991).
16. U. Biader Ceipidor, T.R.I. Cataldi, E. Desimoni and A.M. Salvi, *J. Chemometrics*, **8**, 221 (1994).
17. F. Tateo, E. Desimoni and M. Bononi, Paper presented at the 210th ACS National Meeting Chicago (IL), 20-24 August 1995.
18. P Gans, *Data Fitting in Chemical Sciences*, J. Wiley & Sons, Chichester (1992).

Chapter 10

Monitoring Authenticity and Regional Origin of Wines by Natural Stable Isotope Ratios Analysis

Giuseppe Versini, A. Monetti, and F. Reniero[1]

Centro Sperimentale, Istituto Agrario di San Michele all'Adige, 38010 San Michele all'Adige, Italy

The effectiveness of stable isotopes ratios of hydrogen (D/H, for the methyl (D/H$_I$) and the methylene (D/H$_{II}$) sites of ethanol), carbon ($^{13}C/^{12}C$ of ethanol) and oxygen ($^{18}O/^{16}O$ of water) to detect adulterations like chaptalization or watering and to assess the geographical origin of wines is affected by the natural variability of these parameters. Their usefulness in wine origin identification improves when they are used jointly. The factors which determine their effectiveness in the Italian conditions are being studied. D/H$_I$ and $^{18}O/^{16}O$ ratios depend on latitude but, in the meantime, $^{18}O/^{16}O$ is noticeably modified by the meteorological course during grape ripening. $^{13}C/^{12}C$ and D/H$_{II}$ show interesting patterns over regions which modify their relationship with latitude. On a single variable basis, the most powerful ratios to discriminate between regions are D/H$_I$ and $^{18}O/^{16}O$. Quadratic discriminant analysis improves the possibility of origin identification and, at the same time, is useful to limit adulterations.

Research of the last three decades on stable isotope ratios of some of the elements involved in organic biosynthetic pathways and particularly represented in plant photosynthesis main products and in vegetal water like D/H, $^{13}C/^{12}C$ and $^{18}O/^{16}O$ has made really appliable the possibility of detecting adulterations in fruit juices and derivates (1-12). These adulterations are mainly watering and illegal addition of exogenous sugars from other C$_3$ and C$_4$ plants. Most of this work has been performed through isotope ratio mass spectrometry (IRMS) and, at the same time, the possibility of using these results for geographical origin characterization was guessed (8,12,14,15).

More recently, the attention focused on grape products, especially wines, through an important application of nuclear magnetic resonance investigation of site-specific natural isotope fractionation (SNIF ^{2}H-NMR) of the deuterium in the methyl and methylene sites of ethanol. The method, developed by Martin et al. (10,16), has been

[2]Current address: EC Joint Research Centre, TP 540, 21020 Ispra, VA, Italy

recognized in 1987 by the Office International de la Vigne et du Vin (O.I.V.) (*17*) and in 1990 by the European Community (EC) (*18*) as the official method for ascertaining the chaptalization of the musts (i.e. the increase of the natural potential alcoholic proof through the addition of foreign sugar) with beet sugar or to confirm the addition of C_4 plant sugars (e.g. corn or cane). The latter is also detectable by ^{13}C-IRMS on the whole ethanol molecule (*19,20*). In the EC, foreign sugar addition to the musts (*21-22*) is generally not allowed in those countries which have a favourable climate like Italy, Spain, Portugal and Greece and only limited additions of grape must concentrate or of a very pure grape sugar solution - concentrated rectified must - are allowed. The chaptalization is restrictedly allowed in other countries where the climate is less favourable like France, Germany, Belgium, Luxembourg and the United Kingdom. In both the situations, the aim is to control production and quality of grape and wine through different economic policies.

In the SNIF ^2H-NMR method, the ratio of D/H at the isotopomer CH_2D-CH_2-OH (D/H$_I$) of ethanol gives the most useful information about the botanic source of sugar while the variation at the other isotopomer CH_3-CHD-OH (D/H$_{II}$) is more influenced by the deuterium content of the fermentation medium (*16*). The watering of the medium, often combined with the addition of sugar, can be detected by NMR analysis of the deuterium content of water, D/H$_w$. The natural variability of D/H in both positions and that of their ratio R=2(D/H$_{II}$)/(D/H$_I$) can be derived from reference data banks. The Italian one has gathered about 500 samples per annum since 1987 and these data have been validated from 1991 onwards by a specific EC committee (*23*). In the Italian wines, D/H$_I$ and D/H$_{II}$ range between 98 and 107 ppm and from about 124 to 137 ppm (*24*) respectively. Their standard deviations per region are between less than 0.5 and 1.9 ppm for D/H$_I$ and from less than 1 up to 4 ppm for D/H$_{II}$, similar to those observed in some French areas (*25*). The mean D/H$_I$ value of beet alcohols is about 92 ppm while that of C_4 plants is about 110 ppm (*18*). Limited frauds with sugar solutions from a single type or from mixtures of different plants can be easily detected if the corresponding non-adulterated samples are available for comparison (*26*). The assessment of the chaptalization becomes more difficult without them and when the changes of the isotopic parameters remain within the range of natural variability of the reference frame such as the data bank values for a certain growing area. In this case, the EC method suggests to control the $^{13}C/^{12}C$ ratio (δ‰) of ethanol which could be modified through addition of C_4 plant sugar mixed up with beet sugar to mime the natural D/H values. On the other hand, differently from what happens for the D/H$_I$ values of ethanol, beet represents no exception among the C_3 plants for the $\delta^{13}C$. In this respect, the natural variability of $\delta^{13}C$ level in ethanol - as for wine, see (*27*), whose values are strongly correlated with the $\delta^{13}C$ content of the starting sugar - was deeply investigated (e.g. see the final report of EC-supported project AIR3-ST92-005). To overcome the difficulties of detecting sophisticated adulterations, further researches have been addressed to find out inter and intramolecular isotopic correlations which can involve the isotopic elements usually investigated (*28*). In orange juices, but also in grape products (*29*), a linear correlation between the $\delta^{13}C$ content of certain organic acids and sugar has been established. In the grape products without acids like the concentrated rectified musts, the $\delta^{13}C$ content of the sugar is correlated to that of glucose of the heterosides (*27*).

The $^{18}O/^{16}O$ ratio of water has been already proposed to detect the watering of unfermented or fermented not rediluted juices (*8,30*). Its variability in grape products was studied and the importance of some climatic factors which, differently from D/H and $^{13}C/^{12}C$ ratios in sugar and ethanol (*25,31-33*), can determine its variation during grape ripening was highlighted. Long term data banks of the $^{18}O/^{16}O$ (δ‰) content in wine water have been set up and investigated.

All the above isotopes are influenced by latitude or by certain general climatic peculiarities of the growing areas (8,14,25,34) so it was obvious to extend the analyses from adulteration detection to geographical origin control of grape derivates, both with univariate and multivariate approaches (14,24,25,34-36). The stable isotope ratio of an inorganic element determined by the soil characteristics, $^{87}Sr/^{86}Sr$, was also used to support the wine origin control (37).

With respect to the natural variability which exists in the Italian context, in this paper the practical problems of both adulterations and geographical origin control are being studied through the analysis of samples of the last three vintages available from our data bank.

Experimental Section

1496 samples of wines and their distillates were provided by the peripheral offices of the Control Service against Adulterations in Foods of the Italian Ministry of Agriculture to set up the national data bank. The samples refer to every region for the vintages 1992-1994 and were collected at technological ripeness and then crushed, fermented and distilled in standard conditions at about 93° proof (18,38).

Chemical Analysis. The site-specific quantitative analysis of deuterium in ethanol was carried out with an AMX 400 Bruker NMR instrument, in accordance with the EC method (18) and with a line broadening of 0.5 Hz as previously detailed (24); the results were expressed as ppm. $δ^{13}C$ of ethanol and $δ^{18}O$ of wine water were measured with a SIRA II VG mass spectrometer according to the Italian official method (39) and literature references (1,40) respectevely; the results were expressed as ‰ scale against international standards PDB for carbon and V-SMOW for oxygen isotopes.

Statistical Analysis. Statistical analyses were performed with SAS 6.06 (41) on a computer DEC VAX 4000-610 AXP with o.s. VMS 1.5. Univariate analysis of variance (ANOVA) with subsequently multiple comparisons (Tukey test) have been used to investigate the regional pattern and the interannual variability of the four isotopic parameters. This univariate approach was introductory, in order to understand the behaviour of the variables. Once statistically significant differences were found, a quadratic discriminant analysis (QDA, 42) was performed to verify the possibility of regional characterization. This technique has been chosen considering that the normal-based quadratic rule relative to the linear improves as the covariance matrices become more disparate and the separation between the groups become smaller (43).

Adulterations and natural variability of D/H_I, D/H_{II}, $δ^{13}C$ and $δ^{18}O$ content in wines: the case of Italian products

Vinegrowing in Italy is a continuum so the evaluation of the isotopic ratios according to a segmentation into geopolitical regions or areas could oversimplify reality. Among all the possible splits (e.g. the 20 political regions or the Northern, Central and Southern areas or those provided by EC regulations (23) like the so-called CIb in the North, CIIIb in the South and CII), in this work the subdivision into 20 regions (Figure 1) has been adopted because authenticity declarations usually refer to areas within regions.

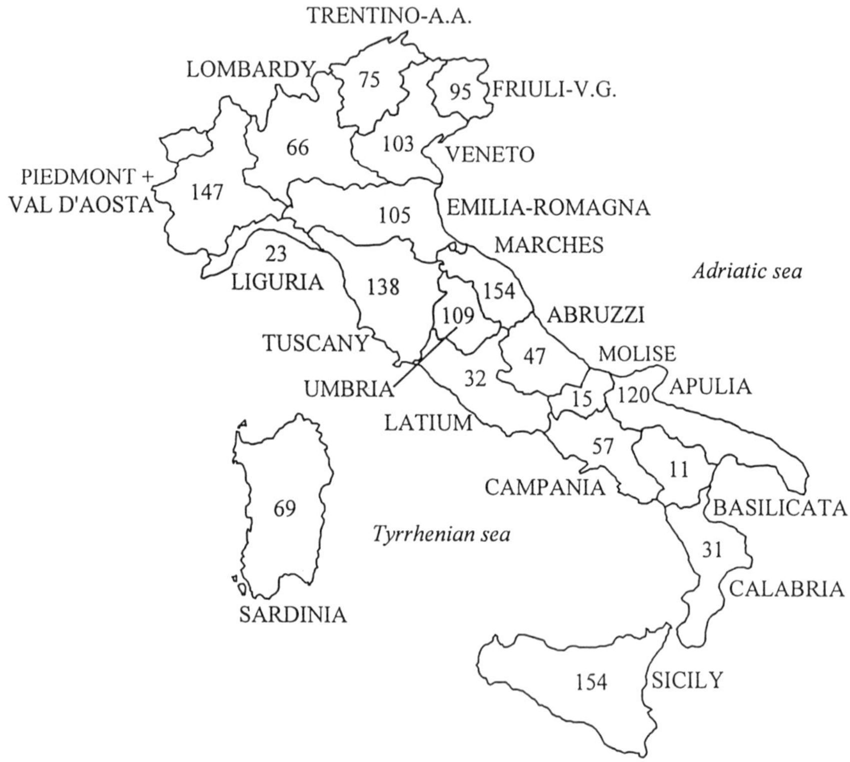

Figure 1. Samples by Italian Regions for the Period 1992-1994.

Examining the frequency distribution of the isotopic ratios both at the national and at the regional level, a normal-shaped distribution for the D/H$_I$ and D/H$_{II}$ values was confirmed (25,34) as well as for $^{13}C/^{12}C$. $^{18}O/^{16}O$ was different because, also in regions with many samples, its distribution had a more irregular behaviour. The $^{13}C/^{12}C$ values of ethanol show a rather high variability ranging from about −23 ‰ in the South up to −28.5 ‰ in the North; this corresponds (27) to a level in sugar from about −21.5 up to −27 ‰. At the same time, standard deviations per region range between 0.6 and 1.4 ‰. If we consider a mean value of about −11.5±1.5 ‰ for C$_4$ plant alcohol (44), the possible chaptalization with this sugar could be used to adjust the corresponding D/H$_I$ value that has to be evaluated in relation with the variability of a peculiar area. This worsen with a mixture containing C$_3$ sugar (e.g. with beet sugar where the δ^{13}C average is about −27±2 ‰ (44) for relevant alcohol). The $^{18}O/^{16}O$ parameter has a wide range also, approximately from −3 ‰ in the North up to 9 ‰ in the South, with standard deviations similar to those of D/H$_I$ with the exception of the Northern regions where they are greater. In the meantime, recalling that the $^{18}O/^{16}O$ into Italian tap water ranges from −10 ‰ in the North up to −6 ‰ in the South (35), watering limits can be computed.

Correlation between Isotopic Ratios and Latitude. The seasonal differences among regions (Table I) often are statistically significant but not powerful. The multiple comparisons test applied to each variable for the period 1992-1994 (Table II: regions joined by the same segment are not significantly different) allows us to confirm some previous results (24,36). D/H$_I$ and $^{18}O/^{16}O$ show the highest discriminating power because, in spite of the North-South gradient, the regional overlapping is less emphasized than for the other parameters. The lowest mean values are in alpine, inland and at higher latitude regions. The correlation of D/H$_I$ with latitude (Figure 2) is approximately linear every year while for δ^{18}O this correlation is not so. In Figure 3 it is possible to see that δ^{18}O in the Southern regions, which are between 36° and 41° North latitude, have a similar mean level. The other two variables, D/H$_{II}$ and $^{13}C/^{12}C$, generate more overlapped subgroups including a larger number of regions and in their North-South gradient there are several exceptions.

Figure 4 shows the relationship between the regional mean values of D/H$_I$ and δ^{18}O and it is also possible to appreciate the ordination along latitude. On the other hand, D/H$_I$ with δ^{13}C (Figure 5) show a poor correlation due to many exceptions: Calabria is different from Sicily, Apulia and Basilicata which are all Southern neighbouring regions with almost the same D/H$_I$ mean values but with differences of about 2 ‰ in their δ^{13}C; Abruzzi, located in Central Italy, shows the same δ^{13}C differences from some of its neighbouring regions like Umbria, Marches and Tuscany. D/H$_{II}$ with δ^{18}O (Figure 6) again have a complex pattern where some Adriatic regions like Apulia, Molise and Abruzzi have D/H$_{II}$ mean values lower than others at the same latitude as well as Trentino-Alto Adige with Piedmont.

Once a precise geographical origin is declared, a multivariate statistical analysis of the isotopic ratios allows to evaluate product genuineness regarding sugar addition and/or watering, even though with some limitations. For instance, the difference among the D/H$_I$, D/H$_{II}$ and δ^{13}C levels within regions next to each other such as the ones in North-Eastern Italy (Trentino-Alto Adige, Veneto and Friuli-Venezia Giulia), which does not allow a good discrimination among them on the basis of the wine data bank, is effective for other grape products like the marc distillates ("grappa") (45). Probably, in this case, the production process levels the variability by mixing lots of raw materials so the average values are close to those of the data bank but the standard deviations per

Regional Values and Variability of the Isotope Ratios by Vintage

Table I. Means (first row) and Standard Deviations (second row) of Hydrogen Isotopes Ratios

	D/H I (ppm)			D/H II (ppm)		
Regions	1992	1993	1994	1992	1993	1994
Abruzzo	101.37	102.35	102.93	126.54	130.09	131.13
	0.86	1.28	0.96	2.23	1.56	1.77
Apulia	103.89	103.91	103.47	130.35	131.24	131.13
	1.27	1.20	1.03	3.48	2.43	2.56
Basilicata	104.86	104.83	103.92	133.40	134.08	132.59
	1.76	0.54	0.42	1.73	0.05	1.31
Calabria	104.04	104.03	103.22	134.26	133.85	133.98
	0.91	0.66	1.00	2.73	2.45	1.00
Campania	103.04	103.18	102.40	132.93	135.71	130.99
	1.00	1.25	0.78	1.22	1.46	2.53
Emilia-Romagna	100.39	101.00	101.18	129.67	132.17	130.21
	1.13	0.79	1.11	2.15	1.49	2.09
Friuli-V.G.	101.37	102.12	101.74	128.57	132.88	132.12
	1.04	1.86	1.21	2.10	1.89	1.52
Latium	102.75	103.24	103.09	132.99	133.77	133.08
	1.15	1.64	1.34	1.94	1.97	2.03
Liguria	102.26	102.20	101.01	132.08	132.19	130.95
	0.70	0.72	0.86	3.48	1.43	0.94
Lombardy	99.96	100.31	100.19	131.55	131.74	129.96
	1.02	0.84	0.89	1.79	2.10	1.27
Marches	102.04	102.40	101.52	129.60	133.60	131.29
	1.34	1.04	0.99	2.08	1.94	1.55
Molise	102.61	103.32	102.69	127.77	130.02	131.96
	0.34	0.87	1.05	1.04	3.23	1.47
Piedmont	99.92	100.09	99.96	128.88	130.07	130.07
	1.23	1.31	1.11	2.61	1.31	2.09
Sardinia	103.00	102.79	103.27	131.28	132.14	132.59
	1.4	1.35	1.15	1.36	2.53	2.41
Sicily	104.50	104.67	104.21	132.85	133.97	133.68
	1.39	1.55	1.49	2.77	2.15	2.64
Trentino-A.A.	99.43	100.08	100.88	126.28	128.24	128.96
	0.93	1.05	0.65	1.54	1.60	1.69
Tuscany	101.71	101.63	101.74	131.94	131.80	131.88
	1.49	1.23	1.42	2.01	2.33	1.97
Umbria	101.31	101.85	101.78	133.15	103.93	133.90
	1.29	1.48	1.23	1.87	1.47	2.32
Veneto	101.14	101.67	101.81	128.93	132.61	131.27
	1.31	1.20	1.23	2.57	2.13	2.60

Table I (cont.). Means (first row) and Standard Deviations (second row) of Carbon and Oxygen Isotopes Ratios

Regions	δ 13C (‰) 1992	1993	1994	δ 18O (‰) 1992	1993	1994
Abruzzo	-24.97	-24.04	-24.93	3.41	5.16	5.14
	0.96	0.81	0.86	1.32	0.85	1.66
Apulia	-24.64	-24.98	-24.87	6.46	7.05	6.75
	0.87	0.78	1.00	1.78	1.28	1.05
Basilicata	-25.09	-25.61	-25.39	n.a.*	3.88	5.43
	1.28	0.48	1.21	n.a.*	0.88	1.87
Calabria	-25.43	-26.45	-26.61	5.22	7.06	6.67
	0.67	0.58	0.99	1.04	0.71	0.95
Campania	-25.92	-26.05	-26.37	2.41	4.40	3.34
	1.12	1.04	1.13	1.07	0.88	1.48
Emilia-Romagna	-26.55	-26.73	-26.89	1.11	3.31	1.72
	0.87	0.58	0.67	2.21	1.21	1.50
Friuli-V.G.	-25.55	-25.39	-25.81	2.64	2.07	1.43
	0.60	0.87	0.99	2.05	1.55	1.03
Latium	-25.44	-25.20	-25.77	5.33	5.05	4.80
	0.64	0.79	0.84	1.13	1.17	1.01
Liguria	-26.80	-26.07	-26.04	3.02	3.07	2.02
	1.03	0.81	0.95	1.76	1.09	0.79
Lombardy	-26.69	-26.66	-26.50	1.25	1.69	1.12
	0.65	0.98	1.42	3.01	1.52	1.90
Marches	-25.86	-25.87	-26.42	1.38	3.90	2.61
	1.10	1.02	1.01	0.97	0.91	1.34
Molise	-25.20	-24.90	-26.12	4.02	5.66	5.30
	1.06	1.17	0.41	1.04	1.31	1.15
Piedmont	-26.31	-26.90	-26.52	-0.54	0.82	0.72
	1.07	0.90	1.05	2.81	1.51	1.42
Sardinia	-24.87	-25.63	-25.51	5.13	6.30	6.34
	1.07	0.77	1.09	1.6	1.29	1.71
Sicily	-25.07	-24.76	-25.32	6.12	7.07	7.54
	0.83	0.90	0.79	0.95	1.34	1.55
Trentino-A.A.	-26.97	-27.34	-26.96	-0.50	0.83	0.52
	0.94	0.78	0.80	2.87	2.05	1.16
Tuscany	-26.14	-26.05	-25.91	3.84	4.07	4.15
	1.23	1.19	1.15	1.63	1.34	1.01
Umbria	-26.25	-26.30	-26.79	3.53	4.15	3.65
	0.91	0.89	0.89	1.93	1.12	1.36
Veneto	-25.81	-25.68	-26.06	1.76	2.53	1.00
	0.95	0.92	1.08	2.32	1.89	1.14

*n.a.: not available

Multiple Comparisons among Geographical Regions

Table II. Tukey Test for the Regional Means (regions joined by the same segment are not significantly different; α=5%)

(D/H) I	(D/H) II
Sicily	Calabria
Calabria	Umbria
Apulia	Sicily
Basilicata	Latium
Latium	Campania
Sardinia	Tuscany
Molise	Basilicata
Campania	Sardinia
Abruzzi	Liguria
Marches	Friuli-V.G.
Liguria	Veneto
Friuli-V.G.	Lombardy
Tuscany	Marches
Umbria	Apulia
Veneto	Emilia-R.
Emilia-R.	Molise
Trentino-A.A.	Piedmont
Lombardy	Abruzzi
Piedmont	Trentino-A.A.

$\delta 13C$	$\delta 18O$
Abruzzi	Sicily
Apulia	Apulia
Basilicata	Calabria
Sicily	Sardinia
Sardinia	Latium
Molise	Molise
Latium	Basilicata
Friuli-V.G.	Abruzzi
Veneto	Tuscany
Tuscany	Umbria
Campania	Campania
Marches	Liguria
Calabria	Marches
Liguria	Emilia-R.
Umbria	Friuli-V.G.
Lombardy	Veneto
Piedmont	Lombardy
Emilia-R.	Piedmont
Trentino-A.A.	Trentino-A.A.

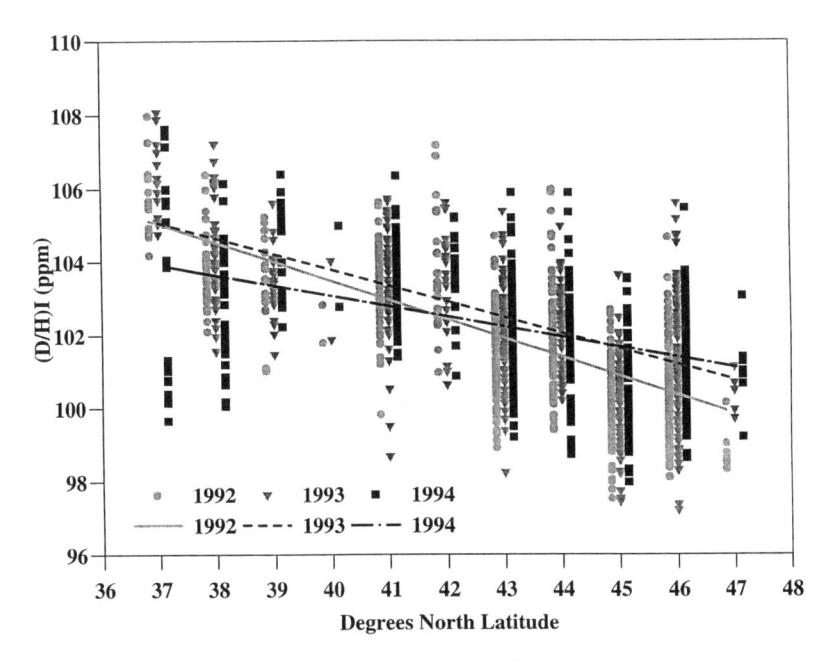

Figure 2. Correlation between D/H$_I$ and Latitude.

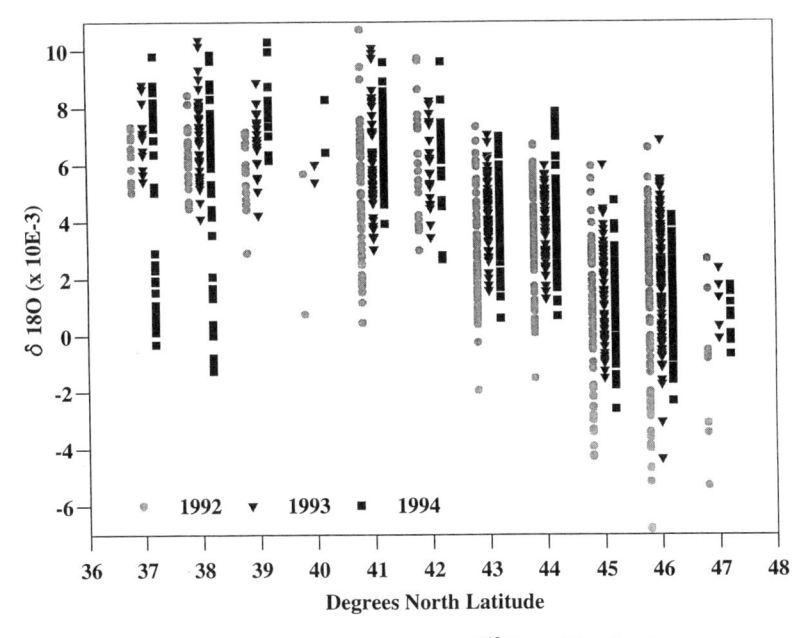

Figure 3. Correlation between $\delta^{18}O$ and Latitude.

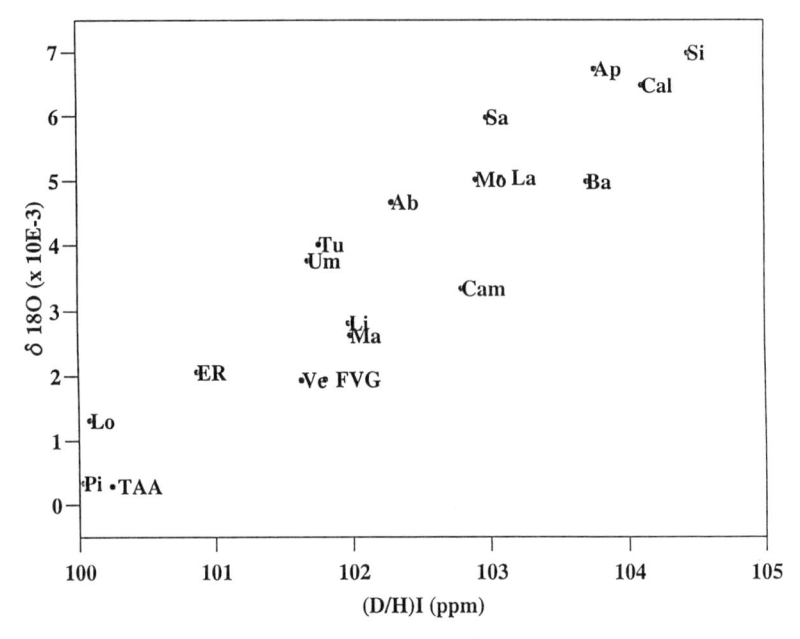

Figure 4. Correlation between D/H$_I$ and δ^{18}OMean Values for the Italian Regions (for abbreviations see Table III).

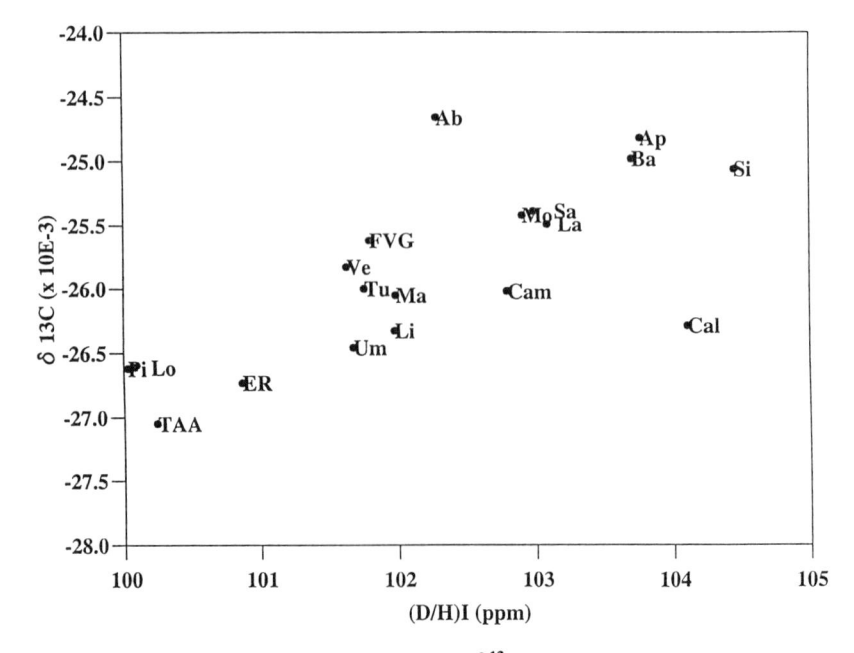

Figure 5. Correlation between D/H$_I$ and δ^{13}C Mean Values for the Italian Regions (for abbreviations see Table III).

region are smaller and make possible the characterization. Being the distillation techniques overall similar, a possible distillation effect on this discrimination (46) can be ruled out.

$\delta^{18}O$ **and Wheather.** A peculiar source of variation for $\delta^{18}O$ is rainfall during grape ripening. The consequences are probably stronger than those observed by Dunbar (32), who supposed a consequent dilution effect on the fruit. This phenomenon is more evident in the Northern part of Italy, where it often rains at the beginning of autumn: variations of even 3-4 ‰ were observed in a few days' time (Figure 7 shows the case of Piedmont in 1992 and 1993). Furthermore, following the evolution of D/H, $\delta^{13}C$ and $\delta^{18}O$ contents in grape picked in two wineyards of Trentino during the rainy 1992 vintage (47), we observed only the expected limited reduction of the sugar level but no variations for D/H and $\delta^{13}C$ values, as well as for magnesium and sodium contents (unpublished data). This fact excludes that $\delta^{18}O$ variation simply depends on a dilution effect in the berry juice and it would instead suggest the presence of intensive and rapid exchanges of water between berries and environment. Such observations support previous results by Förstel (15) who noticed that it is not the variety but the harvesting time that implies a different $\delta^{18}O$ content in musts. The same author widely discussed about the connections between the isotopic situation of berries, other vegetative parts of the plant and the soils at different depths, as well as the air humidity (14). What here reported could be explained considering that an isotopic layering of the soil according to the evaporation is present and can be noticebly modified by heavy rains as deep as where the layer of the preferential water adsorption by the vine roots takes place. It is also interesting to notice in Figures 6 and 7 that, for a rain of similar intensity in both vintages, a different mean decrease of $\delta^{18}O$ is observable. Finally, a further source of variation that is worth considering is vine irrigation (48).

Considering all the aspects above outlined, the interpretation of $\delta^{18}O$ (35) to discover a potential watering of wine requires carefulness, possibly taking into consideration the usual grape harvesting time for that variety in that region and the rainfall situation.

Identification of the wine geographical origin by means of multi-isotopic analysis

The information provided by the different isotopes is often complementary so, to verify the geographical origin of the Italian wines, the analysis has been multivariate. A previous study carried out by applying linear discriminant analysis (LDA) to the deuterium variables only was poor of effectiveness because only few regions, the farthest, do not overlap.

Introducing also the $\delta^{13}C$ and $\delta^{18}O$ variables in the analysis of the 1992 vintage data (36), it was possible to improve considerably the geographical identification with an apparent error rate of misclassification of about 25%. In that case, and in the present work too, to reflect the continuum which exists between vine growing areas, a sample attribution is considered correct if it is assigned to its known region or to a region which adjoin the true one. For the data here considered, with a LDA the apparent error rate was about 50%; in this case, the previously missing data of Lombardy were also considered. To improve identifiability, a quadratic discriminant analysis was used. The apparent error rates for every vintage are presented in Table III where it is possible to see that about 75% of the samples were correctly assigned. On the whole, most of the regions are better recognized with some exceptions like Liguria, Veneto and Friuli among the Northern

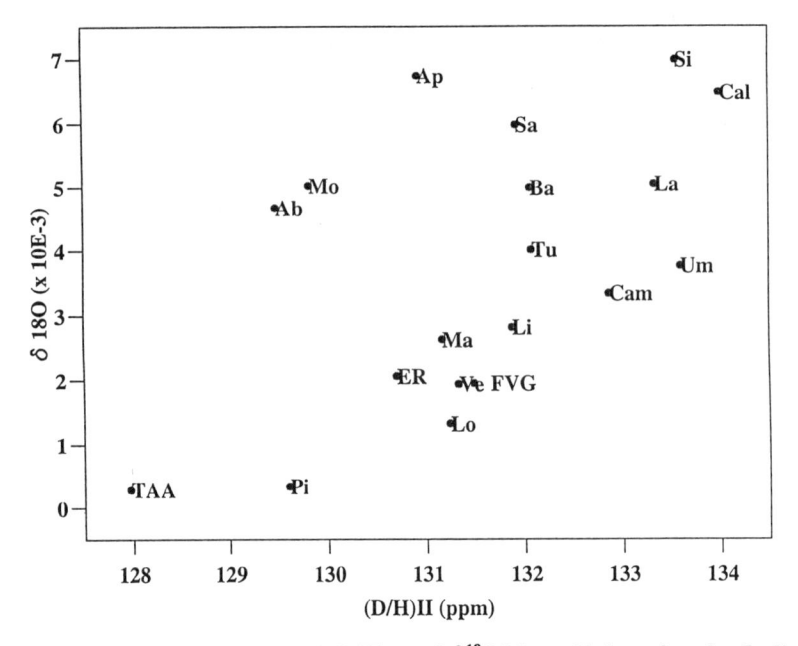

Figure 6. Relationship between D/H_{II} and $\delta^{18}O$ Mean Values for the Italian Regions (for abbreviations see Table III).

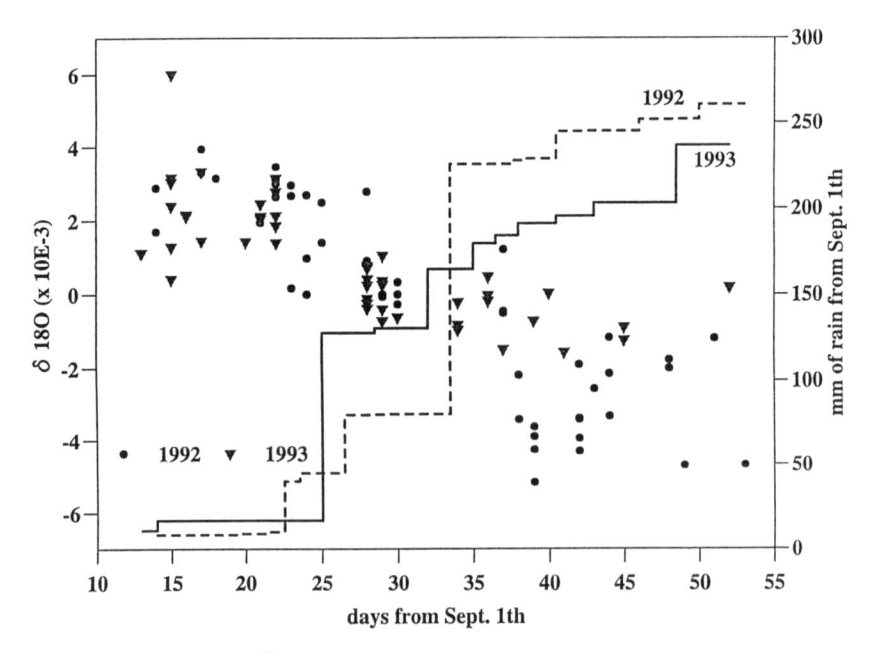

Figure 7. Decrease of $\delta^{18}O$ Content in Grape Berries after Rainfall in Piedmont in Vintages 1992 and 1993.

Table III. Re-classification of the Samples in 1992 Vintage

Identifiability of the Geographical Origin through Quadratic Discriminant Analysis

From Region	Ab	Cal	Cam	ER	FVG	La	Li	Lo	Ma	Mo	Pi	Ap	Sa	Si	TAA	Tu	Um	Ve
Abruzzo	8	0	0	0	2	0	0	0	0	0	1	1	0	0	0	0	0	1
Calabria	0	6	0	0	0	0	0	0	0	0	0	0	0	0	0	1	0	0
Campania	0	0	13	0	0	0	0	0	3	0	0	0	0	0	0	1	1	0
Emilia-Romagna	0	0	0	12	1	0	0	0	0	0	0	0	2	0	3	0	2	0
Friuli-V.G.	2	0	0	0	7	0	0	0	3	0	1	0	0	0	3	4	1	0
Latium	0	1	0	0	0	5	0	0	0	0	0	0	0	1	0	0	0	0
Liguria	0	0	0	0	0	0	7	0	0	0	0	2	0	0	0	0	2	0
Lombardy	0	0	0	1	0	0	0	26	0	0	0	1	0	0	0	6	5	0
Marches	0	0	1	0	0	0	0	1	44	0	2	0	0	0	2	0	0	1
Molise	0	0	0	0	0	0	0	0	0	5	0	0	0	0	0	0	0	0
Piedmont	0	0	0	0	1	0	0	0	2	0	37	0	0	0	3	3	0	1
Apulia	1	0	0	0	2	1	0	0	1	0	0	35	2	0	0	3	0	0
Sardinia	0	0	0	0	1	0	0	1	1	0	0	2	12	0	0	2	1	0
Sicily	0	0	0	0	0	2	0	0	0	1	0	0	0	35	0	3	0	0
Trentino-A.A.	0	0	0	0	0	0	0	0	2	0	2	0	0	0	19	0	0	0
Tuscany	0	0	1	0	2	0	0	4	0	1	0	3	3	2	1	36	0	1
Umbria	0	0	2	0	0	0	0	3	0	0	0	0	0	2	0	0	29	0
Veneto	2	0	1	0	0	0	0	0	5	0	3	1	0	0	0	2	2	9

continued on next page

Table III (cont.). Re-classification of the Samples in 1993 Vintage

From Region	Ab	Cal	Cam	ER	FVG	La	Li	Lo	Ma	Mo	Pi	Ap	Sa	Si	TAA	Tu	Um	Ve
Abruzzo	15	0	0	0	0	0	0	0	0	0	0	0	1	0	0	0	0	0
Calabria	0	11	0	0	0	0	0	0	0	0	0	0	0	0	0	0	0	0
Campania	0	0	11	0	1	0	0	0	1	0	0	0	0	2	0	0	1	0
Emilia-Romagna	0	0	0	18	0	0	0	0	0	0	1	0	0	0	0	0	1	0
Friuli-V.G.	0	0	0	2	25	1	1	0	2	0	0	0	0	0	0	1	1	0
Latium	0	0	0	0	0	7	0	0	0	0	0	1	0	2	0	0	0	1
Liguria	0	0	0	1	0	0	2	0	4	0	0	0	0	0	0	0	0	1
Lombardy	0	0	0	0	0	0	0	14	0	0	0	0	0	1	0	0	1	0
Marches	0	0	1	0	0	0	0	0	46	0	0	0	0	0	0	0	0	3
Molise	0	0	0	0	0	0	0	0	0	6	0	0	0	0	0	0	0	0
Piedmont	0	0	0	0	0	0	0	0	1	0	45	0	0	3	0	0	0	2
Apulia	1	0	0	0	0	1	0	0	0	0	0	30	4	0	0	1	0	0
Sardinia	0	0	0	1	0	0	0	0	0	0	0	6	11	2	0	1	0	0
Sicily	0	0	1	0	0	2	0	0	1	0	0	0	0	46	0	0	3	0
Trentino-A.A.	0	0	0	0	0	0	0	0	0	0	8	0	0	0	10	0	0	0
Tuscany	0	0	0	0	0	0	0	1	0	0	0	0	0	2	0	20	0	4
Umbria	0	0	5	3	0	0	1	0	0	0	1	0	0	0	0	0	20	3
Veneto	0	0	1	0	0	2	1	0	13	0	5	1	0	1	0	1	0	25

Table III (cont.). Re-classification of the Samples in 1994 Vintage

From Region	Ab	Cal	Cam	ER	FVG	La	Li	Lo	Ma	Mo	Pi	Ap	Sa	Si	TAA	Tu	Um	Ve
Abruzzo	5	0	0	0	1	0	0	0	0	0	0	5	0	1	0	5	1	0
Calabria	0	13	0	0	0	0	0	0	0	0	0	0	0	0	0	0	0	0
Campania	0	0	6	1	4	0	0	0	3	0	0	0	0	0	1	4	4	0
Emilia-Romagna	0	0	0	18	1	0	0	0	0	0	0	0	0	0	1	0	0	0
Friuli-V.G.	0	0	0	0	27	0	0	1	3	0	4	0	0	0	1	2	0	0
Latium	0	0	0	0	0	9	0	0	0	0	0	1	0	1	0	0	0	0
Liguria	0	0	0	0	2	0	2	0	0	0	0	0	0	0	1	0	0	0
Lombardy	0	0	0	0	2	0	0	8	1	0	0	0	0	0	0	2	0	1
Marches	0	0	1	0	7	0	0	0	38	0	3	0	0	0	2	0	0	0
Molise	0	0	0	0	0	0	0	0	0	4	0	0	0	0	0	0	0	0
Piedmont	0	0	0	0	7	0	0	0	5	0	29	0	0	0	6	0	1	0
Apulia	0	0	0	0	0	0	0	0	0	0	0	35	0	0	0	4	0	0
Sardinia	0	0	0	1	0	0	0	0	1	0	0	7	13	0	0	3	3	0
Sicily	0	0	0	0	1	0	0	0	0	0	0	0	0	53	0	3	3	0
Trentino-A.A.	0	0	0	1	1	0	0	0	1	0	4	0	0	0	27	0	0	0
Tuscany	1	0	3	0	0	0	0	0	0	0	1	2	1	1	0	48	0	0
Umbria	0	0	2	0	3	0	0	0	0	0	0	2	1	1	1	0	30	0
Veneto	0	0	1	0	0	0	0	0	4	0	3	0	0	0	0	0	1	19

regions, Latium, Umbria and Abruzzi among the Central ones and Campania and Sardinia among the Southern ones. This fact could be partially justified by the limited number of samples from Liguria and Latium but in most cases it probably depends on close climatic similarities among even non-bordering politically defined regions. In particular, we emphasize that the wines of the southern CIIIb regions (Apulia, Sardinia, Calabria and Sicily) are quite all validated in the same area.

Conclusion

The results derived from the Italian wine pluriannual and multi-isotopic data bank show an almost stabilized situation that allows us to have a complete idea about the interregional variability of the isotopic ratios here considered. Especially for D/H_I and $^{18}O/^{16}O$, latitude is the most important factor which determines the isotopic variability while for D/H_{II} and $^{13}C/^{12}C$ there are some interesting peculiarities in their distribution along the peninsula. The discriminant contribution of each isotope to the geographical origin is also stressed. The odd sensitivity of $\delta^{18}O$ to rainfall intensity as the main climatic factor during vintage is also discussed and emphasized to judge the potential watering of wines.

The reduction of the uncertainty through a quadratic discriminant analysis with the four isotopes, expressed by the apparent error rate of the reclassification of about 25%, offers a real possibility of limiting adulterations like wine chaptalization and/or watering. Clearly, this is possible when the geographical origin is officially declared or ascertained.

These results are even more important considering the vine growing continuum of Italy, which differs from other European countries.

Aknowledgements

The research was developed in collaboration with the Control Service against Adulterations in Food of the Italian Ministry of Agriculture.
Technical support of M. Simoni and L. Ziller is thankfully recognized.

Literature Cited

1. Epstein, S.; Mayeda, T. *Geochim. Cosmochim. Acta* **1953**, *4*, 213-224.
2. Bender, M.M. *Phytochemistry* **1971**, *10*, 1239-1244.
3. Smith, B.N.; Epstein, S. *Plant Physiol.* **1971**, *47*, 380-384.
4. Smith, B.N. *Naturwissenschaften* **1975**, *62*, 390-391.
5. Bricout, J. *J. Ass. Anal. Chem.* **1973**, *56*, 739-742.
6. Schmid, E.R.; Fogy, I.; Schwarz, P. *Z. Lebensm. Unters.-Forsch.* **1978**, *166*, 89-92.
7. Rauschenbach, P.; Simon, H.; Stichler, W.; Moser, H. *Z. Naturforsch.* **1979**, *34c*, 1-4.
8. Bricout, J. In *Stable isotopes*; Schmidt, H.-L.; Förstel, H., Keinzinger, K. Eds.; Elsevier, Amsterdam, 1982, pp. 483-493.
9. Dunbar, J. In *Stable isotopes*; Schmidt, H.-L.; Förstel, H., Keinzinger, K. Eds.; Elsevier, Amsterdam, 1982, pp. 495-501.
10. Martin, G.J.; Martin, M.L.; Mabon, F. *Anal. Chem.* **1982**, *54*, 2380-2382;
11. Dunbar, J.; Schmidt, H.-L.; Woller, R. *Vitis* **1983**, *22*, 375-386.

12. Förstel, H.; Hützen, H. *Weinwirtschaft-Technik* **1984**, *120/3*, 71-76.
13. Rossmann, A.; Schmidt, H.-L. *Z. Lebensm. Unters.-Forsch.* **1989**, *188*, 434-438.
14. Förstel, H. *Naturwissenschaften* **1985**, *72*, 449-455.
15. Förstel, H. *Weinwirtschaft-Technik* **1986**, *122/5*, 202-208.
16. Martin, G.J.; Zhang, B.L.; Naulet, N.; Martin, M.L. *J. Am. Chem. Soc.* **1986**, *108*, 5116-5122.
17. Martin, G.J.; Brun, S. *Bull. OIV* **1987**, *671-672*, 131-145.
18. EC Regulation n° 2676/90, *Official Jurnal of the European Communities* **1990**, *L 272*, 64-73.
19. Bricout, J.; Fontes, J.C.; Merlivat, L. *Ind. Alim. Agric.* **1975**, *92*, 375-378.
20. Bricout, J.; Koziet, J. In *D.G.R.S.T. Compte-rendu de fin de contrat N° 75-70-370*, **1979**.
21. EC Regulation n°822/87, modified on the 19 June 1989 (2043-2048/89), *Official Journal of the European Communities* **1987**, *L 84*, 1-68 and **1989**, *L 202*, 1-40.
22. EC Regulation n°1594/70, *Official Journal of the European Communities* **1970**, *L 173*, 23-26.
23. EC Regulation n°2348/91, *Official Journal of the European Communities* **1991**, *L 214*, 39-43.
24. Monetti, A.; Reniero, F.; Versini, G. *Z. Lebensm. Unters.-Forsch.* **1994**, *199*, 311-316.
25. Martin, G.J.; Guillou, C.; Martin, M.L.; Cabanis, M.-T.; Tep, Y.; Aerny, J. *J. Agric. Food Chem.* **1988**, *36*, 316-322.
26. Martin, G.J.; Guillou, C.; Naulet, N.; Brun, S.; Tep, Y.; Cabanis, J.-C.; Cabanis, M.T.; Sudraud, P. *Sci. Aliments* **1986**, *6*, 385-405.
27. Versini, G. In *Proceed. 10th Intern. Oenol. Symposium*; Lemperle, E., Ed.; Intern. Assoc. Winery Technol. Management; Breisach, 1992, pp. 440-450.
28. Schmidt, H.-L.; Butzenlechner, M.; Rossmann, A.; Schwarz, S.; Kexel, H.; Kempe, K. *Z. Lebensm. Unter.-Forsch.* **1993**, *196*, 105-110.
29. Schmidt, H.-L.; Rossmann, A.; Gensler, M. In *Progress in the authenticity-assurance for fruit juices*; Funk, P.M.; Rieth, W. Eds.; Schutzgemeinschaft der Fruchtsaft-Industrie, Zornheim, 1994, pp. 203-217.
30. Bricout, J.; Fontes, J.C.; Merlivat, L. *Conn. Vigne Vin* **1974**, *2*, 161-170.
31. Martin, G.J.; Martin, M.L. In *Modern methods of plant analysis. Wine analysis*; Linskens, H.F.; Jackson, J.F. Eds.; Springer Verlag, Berlin, 1988, pp. 258-275.
32. Dunbar, J. *Z. Lebensm. Unters.-Forsch.* **1982**, *175*, 253-257.
33. Di Marco, G.; Grego, S.; Tricoli, D.; Turi, B. *Physiol. Plant.* **1977**, *41*, 139-141.
34. Reniero, F.; Monetti, A.; Scienza, A.; Simoni, M. *Bull. CIDEAO* **1991**, *11*, 49-54.
35. Holbach, H.; Förstel, H.; Otteneder, H.; Hützen, H. *Z. Lebensm. Unters.-Forsch.* **1994**, *198*, 223-22.
36. Monetti, A.; Versini, G.; Reniero, F. In *Food flavors: generation, analysis and process influence*; Charalambous, C. Ed.; Elsevier Science, Amsterdam, 1995, pp. 1723-1730.
37. Horn, P.; Schaaf, P.; Holbach, B.; Hölzl, S.; Eschnauer, H. *Z. Lebensm. Unters.-Forsch.* **1993**, *196*, 407-409.
38. EC Regulation n°2347/91, *Official Journal of the European Communities* **1991**, *L 214*, 32-38.
39. *Gazzetta Ufficiale della Repubblica Italiana*, Serie generale n°95, 24 Aprile 1993, Decreto del 16 febbraio 1993, pp. 18-19.

40. Office International de la Vigne et du Vin, FV N°919, 1955/220792.
41. SAS Institute Inc. *SAS/STAT User's Guide, Version 6*; SAS Institute Inc., Cary, NC, 1989.
42. Krzanowsky, W.J. *Principles of multivariate analysis*; Clarendon Press, Oxford, 1988.
43. Mc Lachlan, G.J. *Discriminant analysis and statistical pattern recognition*; Wiley, New York, 1992.
44. Martin, G.J. *Revue Franç. Oenol.* **1988**, *114*, 23-60.
45. Reniero, F.; Versini, G.; Simoni, M.; Ziller L. *Riv. Sc. Alim.* (in press).
46. Martin, G.J. *Economia Trentina* **1994**, *43, Suppl. 2*, 94-105.
47. Reniero, F.; Versini, G.; Simoni, M.; Ziller, L. In *Atti Convegno CBA: Metodologie analitiche innovative in enologia*; Intern. Serv. Meeting, Ischia, 1994, pp. 85-86.
48. Tardaguila, J. Ph.D. Thesis, University of Padua, Italy, 1995.

HEALTH BENEFITS

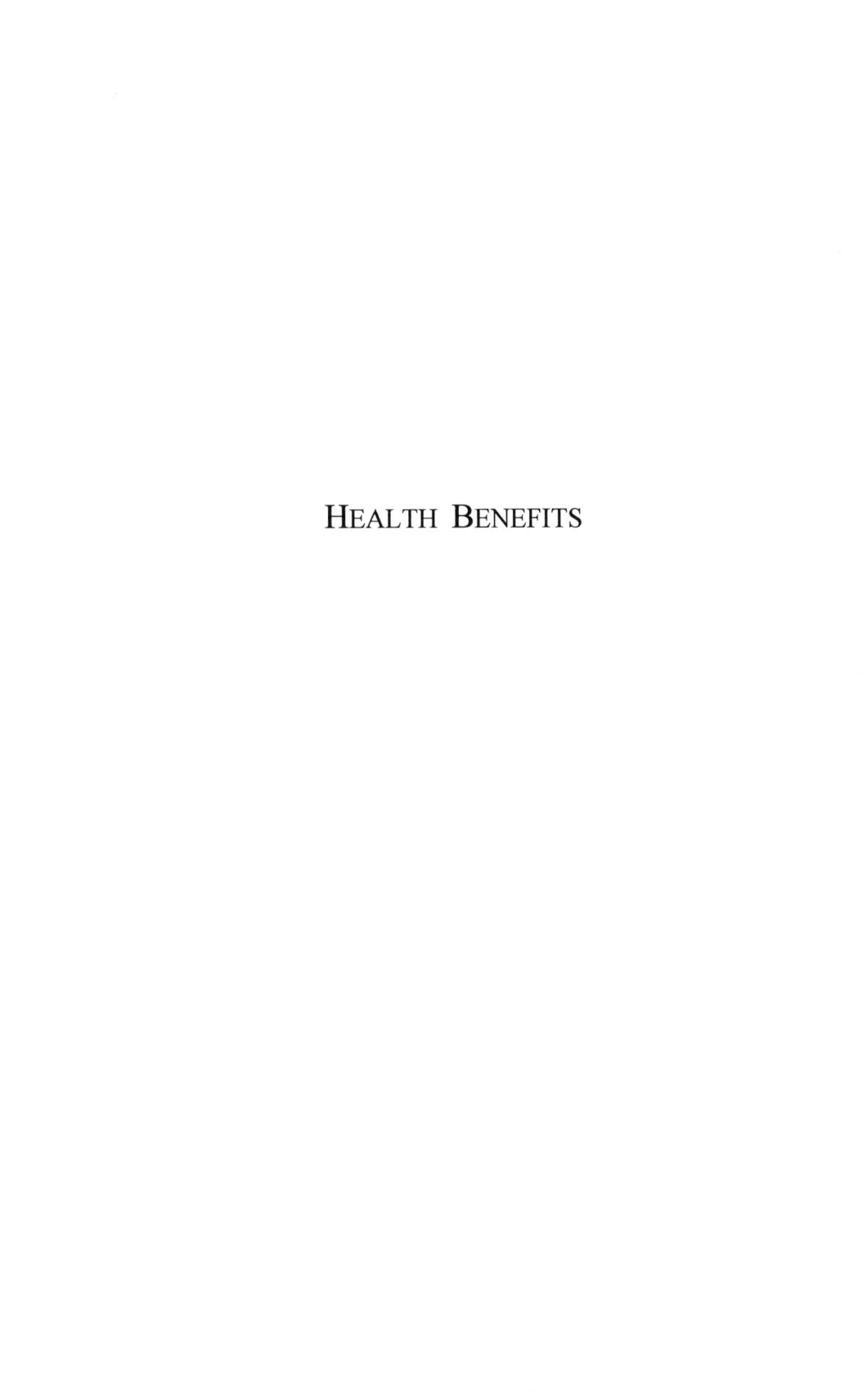

Chapter 11

The Epidemiology of Alcohol and Cardiovascular Diseases

Arthur L. Klatsky

Kaiser Permanente Medical Center, 280 West MacArthur Boulevard, Oakland, CA 94611

Disparities in the relations of alcohol consumption to various cardiovascular (CV) conditions have become evident. Heavier drinking is related to higher prevalence of cardiomyopathy, hypertension (HTN), hemorrhagic stroke, and cardiac dysthythmias. Lighter drinking is related to lower prevalence of coronary artery disase (CAD), occlusive stroke, and sudden cardiac death. The composite of these relations in several population studies of overall CV mortality is a U-shaped curve (lighter drinkers at lower risk than abstainers or heavier drinkers), although several other studies show all drinkers, lighter and heavier, at lower CV mortality risk than abstainers. Increased non-cardiovascular mortality among heavier drinkers is found in all studies, with a J-curve for the total alcohol-mortality relation.

Alcoholic Cardiomyopathy (ACM)

The concept of an independent direct cardiotoxic effect of alcohol has become accepted. The circumstantial evidence is substantial, but the absence of specific markers continues to impede epidemiologic study. Alcohol-associated CM cannot be distinguished clinically or pathologically from dilated CM of unknown cause(s). Historical episodes suggest synergistic myocardial toxicity of alcohol with arsenic and cobalt; other cofactors in alcoholic heart disease remain speculative. A role for thiamine deficiency in low .output chronic heart

© 1997 American Chemical Society

failure has never been established, although an interaction with alcohol cardiotoxicity might exist in malnourished persons.

The most convincing circumstantial evidence for ACM is the extensive data, in animals and humans, of nonspecific cardiac abnormalities related to alcohol. These include structural abnormalities in autopsy and biopsy studies and demonstration of acute and chronic functional and metabolic derangements by several techniques. Two recent reports deserve special mention: (1) A possible nonoxidative metabolic pathway for alcohol has been reported by Lapasota and Lange (1) in the heart, muscle, pancreas, and brain, related to fatty acid metabolism. Accumulation of fatty acid ethyl esters was shown to be related to blood alcohol levels and to mitochondrial metabolism. (2) A report by Urbano-Marquez et al. (2) showed a clear relation in alcoholics of lifetime alcohol consumption to structural and functional myocardial and skeletal muscle abnormalities. The amounts of alcohol were large -- the equivalent of 120 grams alcohol/day for 20 years.

As of 1995, a large proportion (~50%) of all cases of CM are considered to be of unknown cause. The proportion of CM attributed to alcohol varies markedly in reports, probably due mostly to differences in the alcohol habits of the populations under study. Thus, recent reports include alcohol-attributable proportions ranging from 3.4% at Johns Hopkins Hospital (3) to 41.9% at the Philadelphia VA Hospital (4).

The lack of specific markers for ACM necessitates exclusion of other CV conditions for diagnosis. However, the probability of synergistic damage includes cardiotoxicity additive to other myocardial damage. For this reason, persons with heart muscle impairment or major arrhythmias should be especially strongly advised to limit alcohol intake to < 3 drinks/day.

Hypertension (HTN)

An association between heavier alcohol consumption and HTN

Figure 1.
Age-adjusted mean systolic and diastolic blood pressure according to reported alcohol consumption by race and sex.

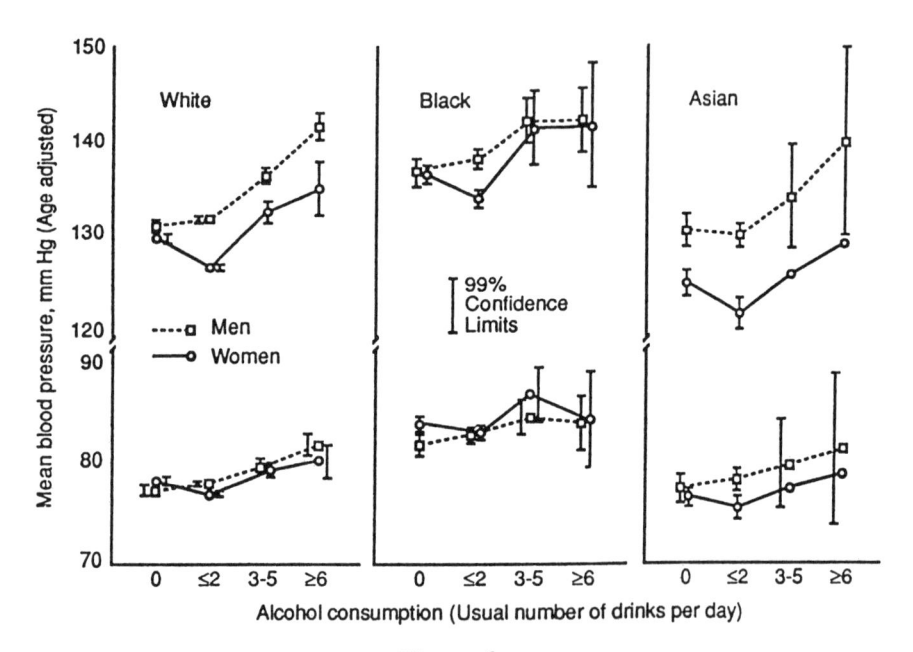

Reprinted with permission from The New England Journal of Medicine; 296: 1194-1200; Copyright 1977 Massachusetts Medical Society.

reported by Lian in French servicemen in 1915 was largely ignored for the next 60 years. Since the mid-1970s, largely because of epidemiologic studies in developed countries, alcohol ingestion has joined other correlates of hypertension, such as obesity and salt intake, as a major focus in research about possible HTN risk factors. An alcohol-HTN link has been shown in almost all of >50 cross-sectional and 10 prospective population studies in ambulatory persons in a number of countries (5,6). Studies differ about whether the alcohol-HTN link is linear or nonlinear (i.e., is a consumption threshold present) in men; in women the relation is J-shaped or present only at higher alcohol intake. Studies of hospitalized alcoholics or problem drinkers have been conflicting with respect to HTN. It is possible that chronic alcohol-related conditions such as malnutrition, cirrhosis, and cardiomyopathy modulate HTN in these persons.

Two Kaiser Permanente studies are among the largest of the cross-sectional population surveys. The first (Figure 1) showed a J-curve in women and a threshold relation in men, with higher blood pressures at 3+ drinks per day in both sexes. The findings were independent of age, sex, and race and, by direct cross-classification, of smoking, coffee intake, reported past heavy drinking, education, adiposity and habitual salt use. HTN ($\geq$160/95 mm Hg) prevalence was doubled in white men and women reporting 6+ drinks per day. The second Kaiser Permanente study showed similar findings in an analysis adjusted simultaneously for age, adiposity, smoking, coffee, tea, and seven blood tests (Figure 2). Exdrinkers did not have higher blood pressure than lifelong abstainers. Study of drinking variability and intake in the week before examination suggested rapid regression of alcohol-associated HTN with abstinence.

Several intervention studies suggest a short-term pressor effect of 3-8 alcoholic drinks per day, with short-term drops in blood pressure upon abstention or marked reduction in alcohol intake. No elevations of blood pressure due to withdrawal have been seen in these studies. A few studies present data showing independence

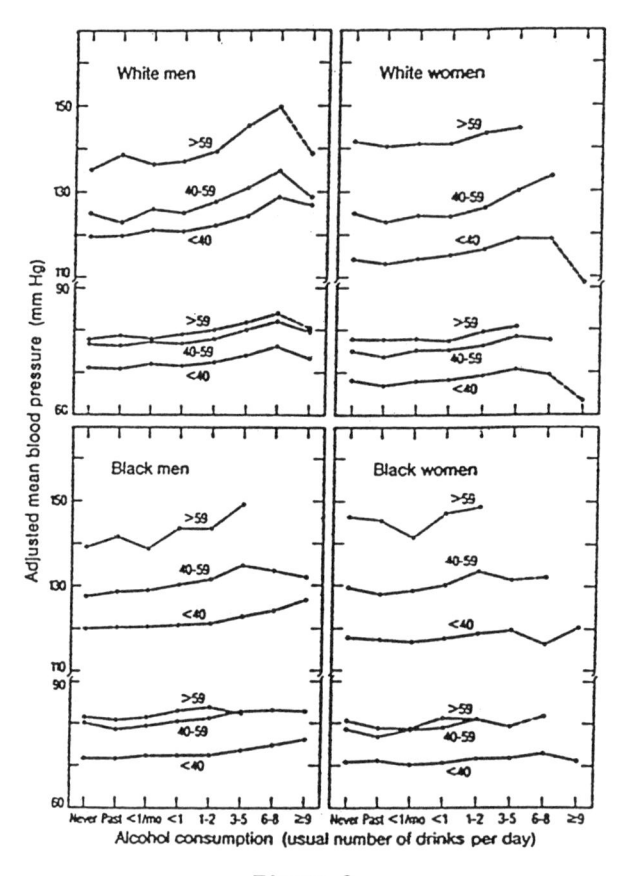

136   WINE: NUTRITIONAL AND THERAPEUTIC BENEFITS

Figure 2.
Adjusted mean systolic and diastolic blood pressures (mm Hg) according to alcohol consumption by three age groups (top left, white men; lower left, black men; top right, white women; lower right, black women). Dashed lines and open circles indicate 10< n <25. Data omitted from figure for categories with n<11 (white women age 40 to 59 years, nine or more drinks/day and age >59 years, six to eight and nine or more drinks/day; black men age >59 years, six to eight and nine or more drinks/day; black women age 40 to 59 years, nine or more drinks/day and age >59 years, three to five, six to eight, and nine or more drinks/day).

Reproduced with permission from Circulation; 73: 628-636; Copyright 1986 American Heart Association.

of the alcohol-blood pressure association from intake of salt, physical activity, and psychosocial stress. Even without confirmation in long-term trials, the intervention studies support a causal hypothesis between alcohol intake and HTN. Estimates of possible population attributable risk range from 5% to 30%. Even if only 5% of HTN is attributable to alcohol, this may be the commonest cause of reversible HTN in developed societies.

The reported acute effects of alcohol on blood pressure in human and animal studies are inconsistent and may not be directly relevant to the epidemiologic relation in humans. There is no known animal model for chronic studies. There is no proof of a sustained effect in humans via the renin-angiotensin mechanism, cortisol, catecholamines, increased cardiac output, a "hypermetabolic state," central nervous system actions, or autonomic nervous system effects. A recently reported experiment (7) in normal humans used intraneural microelectrodes to demonstrate increased sympathetic activation in response to i.v. alcohol with a delayed (2nd hour) blood pressure rise. Inhibition by dexamethasone suggested a central mechanism via corticotropin-releasing hormone. There is some current interest on a possible direct effect upon peripheral vascular tone via a calcium transport mechanism. Explanations for the alcohol-HTN association remain speculative; this fact is the major deficiency in the case for causality. Studies of HTN sequellae (coronary disease, stroke, congestive heart failure, renal insufficiency, etc.) are greatly complicated by the independent relations of alcohol use to several common hypertension sequellae.

It is likely that the alcohol-HTN is causal. Reduction of intake in some heavier drinkers is probably therapeutic, and avoidance of heavier drinking will probably prove to have an important role in primary prevention of HTN (8).

Coronary Artery Disease (CAD)

Data showing that major CAD events are more likely to develop in abstainers than in alcohol drinkers include

Figure 3.
Relative Risk of Coronary Artery Disease Hospitalization* According to Alcohol Use and Other Traits

Trait	RR†	95% CI	p Value
Drinking category			
Nondrinkers			
Abstainer (reference)	1.00	—	—
Exdrinker	0.99	(0.72, 1.36)	0.93
Drinkers			
<1/month	0.93	(0.74, 1.18)	0.57
<1/day, >1/month	0.65	(0.51, 0.82)	<0.001
1–2/day	0.55	(0.42, 0.72)	<0.0001
3–5/day	0.54	(0.38, 0.76)	<0.001
6–8/day	0.52	(0.26, 1.05)	0.07
≥9/day	0.47	(0.15, 1.49)	0.20
Age (per 10 years)	2.14	(2.02, 2.27)	<0.001
Race (black vs white)	1.02	(0.85, 1.22)	0.84
Sex (male vs female)	2.90	(2.46, 3.40)	<0.001
Cigarettes (per 10/day)	1.28	(1.19, 1.37)	<0.001
Coffee (cups/day)	1.08	(1.01, 1.15)	0.03
College degree (yes vs no)	0.86	(0.72, 1.03)	0.10

* First for any CAD diagnosis (n = 756).
† Computed from coefficients estimated by Cox proportional hazards model.
CAD = coronary artery disease; CI = confidence interval; RR = relative risk.

Figure 4.
Relative Risk of Any Coronary Artery Disease Hospitalization According to Alcohol Use Among Persons Free of Clinical Coronary Artery Disease or Recent Major Illness*

Drinking Category	RR†	95% CI	p Value
Nondrinkers			
Abstainer (reference)	1.00	—	—
Exdrinker	0.94	(0.58, 1.55)	0.82
Drinkers			
<1/month	0.88	(0.62, 1.25)	0.48
<1/day, >1/month	0.61	(0.43, 0.87)	<0.01
1–2/day	0.48	(0.33, 0.70)	<0.001
3–5/day	0.50	(0.30, 0.83)	<0.01
6–8/day	0.66	(0.23, 1.84)	0.42
≥9/day	0.51	(0.07, 3.74)	0.51

* n = 336 cases.
† Computed from coefficients estimated by Cox proportional hazards model.
CAD = coronary artery disease; CI = confidence interval; RR = relative risk.

Reprinted with permission from reference 12.
Copyright 1986 by Excerpta Medica Inc.

international comparisons, time-trend analyses, case-control studies, and longitudinal studies (9,10). Most studies of CAD hospitalizations show heavier drinkers at similar or lower risk of CAD hospitalization than lighter drinkers (i.e., no U-shaped curve). Several population studies using CAD mortality as an endpoint also show a progressive inverse relation to amount of alcohol consumption, but others show a U-shaped curve. Those studies which separate lifelong abstainers from past drinkers suggest that both subsets of nondrinkers are at higher risk of CAD than drinkers, but some would still dispute this. Many population studies were not able to distinguish these subsets of nondrinkers. Where available, data about choice of type of alcoholic beverage suggest that beverage choice is a minor factor in CAD risk. Studies of sudden cardiac death, due mostly to CAD, also show an inverse relation to alcohol use.

There are plausible mechanisms by which alcohol drinking might protect against CAD (9,10). These include a favorable effect upon HDL cholesterol concentration, a similar favorable effect upon apolipoproteins, and an antithrombotic action. Controversy about protection persists, however, on the grounds that correlates of abstinence and lighter drinking could explain the higher risk of abstainers. For example, a much publicized hypothesis advanced by Shaper et al.(11) suggested that movement of persons at high CAD risk into the abstainer referent group could explain the U-shaped curve in their work and that of other investigators.

Our most recent study of alcohol habits in relation to CAD hospitalizations (12) showed that exdrinkers and infrequent (<1/month) drinkers were at risk similar to that of lifelong abstainers. A lower CAD risk was present among all other drinkers with no U-shaped curve, independent of a number of potential confounders (Figure 3). These relations were independent of baseline CAD risk (Figure 4) and beverage choice. The data suggested a protective effect of alcohol against risk of hospitalization for CAD.

In a prospective mortality study of total CV

Figure 5.

Relative risk of death* from various cardiovascular conditions and cirrhosis according to alcohol use.

	RR for each drinking category vs. lifelong abstainers					
Condition (n deaths)	Exdrinkers	<1/mo	<1/day,>1/mo	1-2/day	3-5/day	6+/day
All CAD (600)	1.0	0.9	0.8	0.7‡	0.6§	0.8
AMI (284)	1.0	0.7	0.8	0.6§	0.5§	0.6
Other CAD (316)	0.9	1.0	0.7	0.8	0.7	1.0
Cerebrovascular (138)	1.0	0.8	0.8	0.8	0.7	1.4
Hemorrhagic (41)	1.4	1.5	1.6	1.8	1.3	4.7
Occlusive (34)	0.9	0.5	0.5	0.3	0.4	--‖
Nonspecific (63)	1.1	0.7	0.9	1.0	1.0	1.2
Hypertension (64)	2.8	2.4	1.9	1.3	2.2	2.1
Cardiomyopathy (24)	3.4	8.5‡	4.0	5.6	2.4	8.0
Syndromes (82)¶	0.6	0.6	0.5	0.4‡	0.6	1.0
Arterial (41)**	--‖	1.1	1.6	0.4	1.7	--‖
Cirrhosis (42)	10.8§	1.4	1.0	4.3	8.1‡	22.0††

*Computed from coefficients estimated by Cox proportional hazards models controlled for age, sex, race, smoking, body mass index, marital status, education. †p<0.05; ‡p<0.01; ††p<0.001.
‖ Unable to calculate RR due to insufficient number of cases.
¶ Includes symptomatic heart disease (n=32), other disorders of heart rhythm (n=22), and ill-defined heart disease (n=28).
** Includes arteriosclerosis (n=15), aneurysms (n=23), peripheral vascular disease (n=2), and arterial embolism and thrombosis (n=1).

AMI = acute myocardial infarction; CAD = coronary artery disease; mo = month; RR = relative risk

Reprinted with permission from reference 13.
Copyright 1990 by Excerpta Medica Inc.

mortality (*13*), exdrinkers had higher age-adjusted CAD and overall CV mortality risk than lifelong abstainers, but the difference disappeared when adjusted for other traits. Among drinkers, there were U-shaped mortality curves relating amounts of alcohol and both CV and CAD, with a nadir at 1-2 and 3-5 drinks/day. Subsets free of baseline risk had similar alcohol-CAD and alcohol-CV mortality curves. The study demonstrated the expected disparities between alcohol and various CV conditions (Figure 5). A number of features of the analysis argued against a spurious inverse alcohol-CAD relation, including: 1) independence from baseline lifetime CAD risk, 2) absence of higher CAD risk among persons reducing alcohol intake for medical reasons, 3) evidence that the higher unadjusted CAD risk of exdrinkers is due to confounding, 4) absence of a relation among exdrinkers of CAD risk to maximal past intake, 5) absence of a relation of infrequent (<1/month) drinking to CAD risk, and 6) similar reduction of CAD risk among drinkers of wine, liquor, and beer.

Another large recent prospective study among women free of baseline CAD (*14*) showed a progressive inverse relation of alcohol use to major CAD events, independent of prior reduction in alcohol intake and of nutrient intake (the latter was analyzed in detail). The relative risk of CAD events in women reporting daily alcohol intake of 25+ grams/day was 0.4, similar to the findings for women in the Kaiser Permanente study. Another prospective study in women showed similar findings (*15*), and demonstrated that net beneficial effects of moderate alcohol use in women was limited by adverse effects to persons clearly at above-average CAD risk (i.e., those above 50 years of age). Increased susceptibility of women (vs. men) to alcohol effects could include greater reduction of CAD risk.

Two large prospective studies in men confirm the lower CAD risk of drinkers, independent of confounders or baseline disease (*16,17*). The American Cancer Society Study (*16*) was a 12 year prospective mortality study of 276,802 white men; there was a U curve for CAD mortality, with a RR of 0.8 (vs. abstainers) at 1-2 drinks/day. The

Health Professional Followup Study of 51,529 men (17) was well controlled for dietary habits; newly diagnosed CAD was inversely related to increasing alcohol intake. A study in both sexes, the Auckland Heart Study (18), was designed to study the hypothesis that persons at high CAD risk are likely to become nondrinkers; the analysis showed that moderate drinkers had lower CAD risk than both lifelong abstainers and exdrinkers, thus supporting the hypothesis that alcohol protects against CAD.

Reduced risk of CAD is present at various ages, although the impact upon total mortality is clearest in older age brackets and the adverse effects of alcohol are greater among younger persons (19). Among persons > 60 years of age, overt or latent CAD may play a role in risk of death from causes other than CAD (19).

The hypothesis that the apparent protective effect of alcohol against CAD is mediated by higher HDL cholesterol levels in drinkers has been examined quantitatively in three separate studies (20-22). All three analyses yielded similar findings suggesting that higher HDL levels in drinkers mediated about half of the lower CAD risk. One of these studies (22) suggests that both HDL2 and HDL3 are involved. HDL3 may be more strongly related to lighter alcohol intake, but is probably related as strongly as HDL2 to lower CAD risk. There are no similar data about protective mechanisms other than the HDL link, but some data support several possible antithrombotic mechanisms (9,10,22). Thus, multiple mechanisms may play a role.

International comparison studies (23-25) suggest that wine confers more protection against CAD than beer or liquor. The "French paradox" concept has arisen from these data; it refers to the fact that France tends to be an outlier on graphs of mean dietary fat intake vs. CAD mortality, unless adjusted for wine alcohol intake (26). Reports of nonalcohol antioxidant phenolic compounds (27-29) or antithrombotic substances (30-33) in wine, especially red wine, have appeared. Inhibition of oxidative modification of low-density-lipoprotein cholesterol is probably anti-atherogenic, although prospective clinical trials of anti-oxidant supplements are not yet conclusive (34). Thus, antioxidant substances in wine are an attractive hypothetical explanation for CAD protection. However, the prospective population studies provide no consensus that wine has additional benefits, and various studies show benefit for wine, beer, liquor, or all three major beverage types (9,10). In Kaiser Permanente studies, all three major beverage types show evidence of protection against CAD (12,13); wine drinkers fare best with respect to CAD mortality, but drinkers of red and non-red wine fare equally well (35). Since the beverage differed in user traits, with wine drinkers having the most favorable CAD risk profile (36), a noncausal explanation was favored for the lower CAD risk of wine drinkers. Drinking pattern differences among the beverage types are another hypothetical factor. The wine/liquor/beer issue is unresolved at this time, but it seems likely that ethyl alcohol is the major factor with respect to lower CAD risk.

It remains theoretically possible that lifelong abstainers could differ from drinkers in psychological traits, dietary habits, physical exercise habits, or some other way which could be related to CAD risk, but there is no good evidence for such a trait. The various studies indicate that such a correlate would need to be present in persons of both sexes, various countries, and multiple racial groups. A causal, protective effect of alcohol is a simpler and more plausible explanation (9,10,37,38).

Cerebrovascular Disease

Several reports suggest that alcohol use, especially heavier drinking, is associated with higher risk of stroke. Some studies examined only drinking sprees; some others did not differentiate between hemorrhagic and occlusive strokes. Several studies have suggested that alcohol was related only to hemorrhagic stroke. The Nurse's Health Study (14) showed drinkers to be at higher risk of subarachnoid hemorrhage, but lower risk of occlusive stroke.

A Kaiser Permanente study looked at the relations between reported alcohol use and the incidence of

Figure 6.

Relative Risk of Cerebrovascular Disease Hospitalization According to Alcohol Use and Other Characteristics

Characteristic	Hemorrhagic stroke (n=69) RR	95% CI	Occlusive stroke (n=292) RR	95% CI
Alcohol use,				
Abstainers	1.00	—	1.00	—
Former drinkers	0.78	0.21–2.93	0.97	0.58–1.61
<1/day	0.85	0.41–1.77	0.63*	0.45–0.88
1–2/day	0.75	0.30–1.87	0.54*	0.36–0.82
≥3/day	1.38	0.53–3.59	0.44*	0.25–0.76
Age (per 10 years)	1.68*	1.37–2.06	2.38*	2.12–2.68
Sex (female vs. male)	0.83	0.49–1.38	0.57*	0.45–0.74
Race (black vs. white)	2.35*	1.39–4.00	1.01	0.75–1.35
Coffee (≥4 cups/day)	0.89	0.71–1.12	0.90	0.80–1.01
Smoking (≥1 pack/day vs. never)	1.85	0.82–4.14	3.13*	2.04–4.78
Quetelet index (per 0.1 unit)	0.97	0.93–1.01	0.99	0.97–1.01
Systolic blood pressure (per 10 mm Hg)	1.21*	1.07–1.37*	1.17*	1.10–1.24
Baseline disease (yes vs. no)	1.21	0.74–1.98	1.76*	1.40–2.22

RR, relative risk computed from coefficients estimated by Cox proportional hazards model; CI, confidence interval.
*Significantly different ($p<0.05$) from 1.0.

Reproduced with permission from reference 39.
Copyright 1989 American Heart Association.

Figure 7.

Relative Risk of Supraventricular Arrhythmia in Persons with High Versus Low Daily Alcohol Intake

Rhythm	Persons with SVA 6+ (n=1,322) %	No.	<1 (n=2,644) %	No.	Relative Risk for 6+ vs <1	p Value
Atrial fibrillation	1.1	15	0.5	13	2.3	0.02
Atrial flutter	0.6	8	0.2	6	3.0	0.05
SVT	0.4	5	0.1	2	5.0	0.03
Premature atrial beats	3.3	43	1.3	32	3.0	<0.01
Fibrillation, flutter or SVT	1.6	21	0.7	19	2.3	<0.01

* Relative risks and p values estimated using McNemar's method for matched pairs.
SVA = supraventricular arrhythmia; SVT = supraventricular tachycardia; <1 = <1 drink per day; 6+ = >6 drinks per day.

Reprinted with permission from reference 41.
Copyright 1988 by Excerpta Medica Inc.

hospitalization for several types of cerebrovascular disease (39). Daily consumption of 3 or more drinks, but not lighter drinking, was related to higher hospitalization rates for hemorrhagic cerebrovascular disease, especially intracerebral hemorrhage. Higher blood pressure appeared to be a partial mediator of this relation. Alcohol use was associated with lower hospitalization rates for occlusive cerebrovascular disease; an inverse relation was present in both sexes, whites and blacks, and for extracranial and intracerebral occlusive lesions (Figure 6). Our data suggest that heavier drinking increases the risk of hemorrhagic cerebrovascular events, but that alcohol use may lessen the risk of occlusive lesions.

At this time there is no consensus about the relations of alcohol drinking to the various types of cerebrovascular disease and agreement only that more study of this important are is needed (40).

Cardiac Dysrhythmias

Increased ventricular ectopic activity has been documented after ingestion of substantial amounts of alcohol, although epidemiologic studies have not shown a higher risk of sudden death in drinkers. Various atrial dysrhythmias have been reported to be associated with spree drinking. A Kaiser Permanente study (41) compared atrial dysrhythmias in 1,322 persons reporting 6+ drinks per day to dysrhythmias in 2,644 light drinkers. The relative risk in the heavier drinkers was at least doubled for atrial fibrillation, atrial flutter, supraventricular tachycardia, and atrial premature complexes (Figure 7).

Conclusion

This brief survey documents the evidence for disparity in the relations of alcohol and CV disorders. Published reviews are available (42,43). Figure 8 summarizes the relations in tabular form. The figure also emphasizes the

Figure 8.

THE RELATIONS OF ALCOHOL DRINKING TO VARIOUS CV CONDITIONS

	amount of alcohol	
condition	small	large
cardiomyopathy	none	? toxic in susceptibles
beri-beri	none	? none (thiamine deficiency)
(arsenic) cobalt beer disease	none	? synergistic toxicity
hypertension	? 0,↓,↑	↑ in susceptibles
coronary artery disease	↓	? ↓
dysrhythmia	?	↑ in susceptibles
hemorrhagic stroke	? 0	↑
occlusive stroke	↓	? ↓

disparity between the relations of lighter drinking, with overall favorable relations and heavier drinking, with overall unfavorable relations.

Literature cited.

1. Lapasota, E.A.; Lange, L.G. *Science* 1986, *231*, pp.497-9.
2. Urbano-Marquez, A,; Estrich, R.; Navarro-Lopez, F.; Grau, J.M.; Mont, L.; Rubin, E. *N Engl J Med* 1989, *320*, pp.409-15.
3. Kasper, E.K.; Willem, W.R.P.; Hutchins, G.M.; Deckers, J.W.; Hare, J.M.; Baughman, K.L. *J Am Coll Cardiol* 1994, *23*, pp.586-90.
4. Wang, R.Y.; Alterman, A.I.; Searles, J.S.; McLellan, T. *Arch Int Med* 1990, *150*, pp.1079-87.
5. Klatsky, A.L. In *Hypertension Primer;* Izzo, J.L.; Black, H.L. Eds. American Heart Association: Dallas, TX, 1993; pp.164-76
6. Klatsky AL. In *Hypertension: Pathophysiology, Diagnosis and Management;* Laragh, J.H.; Brenner, B.M. Eds. Raven Press: New York, NY, 1995, 2nd ed., pp.2649-2667.
7. Randin, D.; Vollenweider, P.; Tappy, L.; Jequier, E.; Nicod, P.; Scherrer, U. *N Engl J Med* 1995, *332*, pp. 1733-1737.
8. Joint National Committee on Detection, Evaluation, and Treatment of High Blood Pressure (JNC-V). *Arch Int Med* 1993, *153*, pp. 158-83.
9. Klatsky, A.L. *Alcohol Clin Exp Res* 1994, *18*, pp.88-96.
10. Renaud, S.; Criqui, M.H.; Farchi, G.; Veenstra, J.; In *Health Issues Related to Alcohol Consumption;* Verschuren, P.M. Ed. ILSI Press, Washington, DC, 1993, pp. 81-124.
11. Shaper, A.G.; Wannamethee, G.; Walker, M. *Lancet* 1988*(2)*, pp. 1267-73.
12. Klatsky, A.L,; Armstrong, M.A.; Friedman GD. *Am J Cardiol* 1986, 58, pp.710-14.
13. Klatsky, A.L.; Armstrong, M.A.; Friedman, G.D. *Am J Cardiol.* 1990, *66*, pp.1237-42.
14. Stampfer, M.J.; Colditz, G.A.; Willett, W.C.; Speizer, F.E.; Hennekens, C.H. *N Engl J Med* 1988, *319*, pp.267-73.
15. Fuchs, C.S.; Stampfer, M.J.; Colditz, G.A.; et al. *N Engl J Med* 1995, *332*, pp.1245-50.

16. Boffetta, P.; Garfinkle, A. *Epidemiology* 1990, *1*, pp. 342-48.
17. Rimm, E.B.; Giovannucci, E.L.; Willett, W,C.; et al. *Lancet* 1991, *388*, pp.464-68.
18. Jackson, R,; Scragg, R,; Beaglehole, R. *Br Med J* 1991, *303*, pp.211-16.
19. Klatsky, A.L.; Armstrong, M.A.; Friedman, G.D. *Ann Intern Med* 1992, *117*, pp. 646-54.
20. Criqui, M.H.; Cowan, L.D.; Tyroler, H.A.; Gangdiwala, S.;, Heiss, G.; Wallace, R.B.; Cohn, R. *Am J Epidemiol* 1987, *126*, pp. 629-37.
21. Suh, I.; Shaten, J.; Cutler, J.A.; Kuller, K.H. *Ann Intern Med* 1992, *116*, pp 881-7.
22. Gaziano, J.M.; Buring, J.E.; Breslow, J.L.; et al. *N Engl J Med* 1993, *329*, pp. 1829-34.
23. St. Leger, A.S.; Cochrane, A.L. Moore, F. *Lancet* 1979 *(1)*, pp. 1017-20.
24. Renaud, S.; de Lorgeril, M. *Lancet* 1992, *339*, pp. 1523-26.
25. Criqui, M.H.; Ringel, B.L. *Lancet* 1994, 344, pp. 1719-23
26. Renaud, S.; de Lorgeril, M. *Lancet* 1992, *339*, pp. 1523-26
27. Siemann, E.H.; Creasy, L.L. *Am J Enol Viticulture* 1992, *43*, pp. 1-4.
28. Frankel, E.N.; Kanner, J.; German, J.B.; Parks, E.; Kinsella, J.E. *Lancet* 1993, *342*, pp. 454-57.
29. Maxwell, S.; Cruickshank, A.; Thorpe, G. *Lancet* 1994, *344*, pp. 193-4.
30. Fitzpatrick, D.F.; Hirschfield, D.L.; Coffey, R.G. *Am J Physiol* 1993, 265, H774-78.
31. Kluft, C.; Veenstra, J.; Schaafsma, G.; Pikaar, N.A. *Fibrinolysis* 1990, 4 *(suppl 2)*, pp.69-70.
32. Demrow, H.S.; Slane, P,R.; Folts, J.D. *Circulation* 1995, *91*, pp. 1182-8.
33. Seigneur, M.; Bonnet, J.; Dorian, B.; et al. *J Appl Cardiol* 1990, 5, pp. 215-22.
34. Hoffman, R.M.; Garewal, H.S. *Arch Int Med* 1995, *155*, pp. 241-6.
35. Klatsky, A.L.; Armstrong, M.A. *Am J Cardiol* 1993, 71, pp. 467-9.
36. Klatsky, A.L.; Armstrong, M.A.; Kipp, H. *Br J Addict* 1990, 85, pp. 1279-89.
37. Marmot, M.; Brunner, E. *Br Med J* 1991, *303*, pp. 365-8.

38. Friedman, G.D.; Klatsky, A.L. N Engl J Med 1993, *329*, pp. 1882-3.
39. Klatsky, A.L.; Armstrong, M.A.; Friedman, G.D. Stroke 1989, *20*, pp.741-6.
40. Van Gign J, Stampfer MJ, Wolfe C, Algra A. In *Health Issues Related to Alcohol Consumption*. Verschuren, P.M. Ed. ILSI Press, Washington, D.C., 1993, pp. 43-80.
41. Cohen, E.J.; Klatsky, A.L.; Armstrong, M.A. Am J Cardiol 1988, *62*, pp. 971-3.
42. Davidson, D.M. West J Med 1989, *151*, pp. 430-9.
43. Klatsky, A.L. Scientific American Sci and Med 1995, *2*, pp. 28-37.

Chapter 12

Wine Antioxidants and Their Impact on Antioxidant Activity In Vivo

Simon R. J. Maxwell

Division of Clinical Pharmacology, Clinical Sciences Building, Leicester Royal Infirmary, Leicester LE2 7LX, United Kingdom

There has been considerable interest in the role of dietary antioxidants such as flavonoids in retarding the development of cardiovascular disease in human populations. Red wine is a rich source of flavonoid antioxidants. These compounds have been demonstrated to have potent antioxidant properties *in vitro* but their role as antioxidants *in vivo* remains to be proven. We have recently developed an enhanced chemiluminescent assay for antioxidant activity in biological fluids. This chapter describes the use of this technique to examine changes in serum antioxidant activity following the ingestion of red wine by healthy human volunteers.

Cardiovascular disease, principally coronary artery disease and stroke, is the major cause of premature death and disability in the developed world. Atherosclerosis in the large arteries supplying blood to the heart or brain is the major pathology underlying most serious cardiovascular events. Atherosclerosis refers to the progressive deposition of cholesterol in the vessel wall which in turn leads to blockage of the vessel, restriction of blood flow to the tissues downstream (ischaemia) and eventually death of those tissues (infarction). In many cases the final event that precipitates blockage is the formation of a blood clot (thrombosis) in the diseased vessel. After cell death has occurred regeneration of cells is impossible and there is irreversible damage to the function of the heart or brain. A reduction in such cardiovascular events will be necessary to produce any significant improvement in life-expectancy in the developed world.

The last thirty years have seen an enormous increase in our understanding of the development of atherosclerosis. Four major risk factors - hypercholesterolaemia, hypertension, smoking and diabetes - have been identified. Since smoking, the major lifestyle risk factor, is now declining increasing interest is being focused on other aspects of lifestyle such as nutrition and exercise that might influence the rate of

© 1997 American Chemical Society

development of vascular disease. Wine is a popular beverage in the Western world. This article will briefly review some of the evidence to suggest that wine flavonoids might have an influence on the development of atherosclerotic vascular disease by acting as antioxidants. In particular, it will examine whether their potent antioxidant effects in vitro may be manifest in vivo and whether wine can be considered as an important source of dietary antioxidants in human nutrition.

Oxidative Stress and Atherosclerosis

Oxidative stresses are ubiquitous throughout the body and arise primarily from oxidants produced endogenously (e.g. by mitochondrial electron transport or phagocytic cells) or exogenously by environmental pollution including cigarette smoke or the products of ionising radiation (1). The four electron reduction of molecular oxygen by mitochondria is essential to life in all aerobic organisms. Unfortunately, the process is not completely efficient allowing leakage of the superoxide radical ($O_2^{\bullet -}$) which is a precursor for the formation of more potent oxidants such as the peroxide ion (O_2^{2-}) and the hydroxyl radical (OH•). The latter can initiate the peroxidation of lipids and so disrupt biological membranes and render lipoproteins more atherogenic (2). These processes are accelerated in the presence of free transition metal ions such as Fe^{2+}.

This sequence of events is of particular relevance to development of atherosclerosis (Figure 1). A characteristic feature of atherosclerosis is the presence of lipid-laden macrophages within the intima of arteries. Macrophages in culture are unable to accumulate significant amounts of *native* low-density lipoprotein (LDL) because of the low number and affinity of LDL receptors on these cells and their down regulation by accumulated intracellular cholesterol (3). In contrast, the uptake of *oxidized* LDL is rapid and not subject to down-regulation. Oxidized LDL is also chemotactic for macrophages (4) and cytotoxic to the vascular endothelium (5). Although oxidative mechanisms are clearly not the only pathophysiological events relevant to atherogenesis (6) it is clear that oxidation of lipoproteins represents a significant biological threat and should ideally be prevented.

A number of natural antioxidant mechanisms exist to protect against the everpresent threat of oxidation of LDL. These include proteins such as transferrin, caeruloplasmin and albumin that limit the availability of metal ions. Another very important protective influence is the presence of scavenging antioxidant molecules that are readily sacrificed (oxidized) in preference to more important targets such as LDL. Most of the important sacrificial antioxidants are derived from the diet and include vitamins such as ascorbate (vitamin C) and alpha-tocopherol (vitamin E) and polyphenolic flavonoids derived from sources such as wine, tea and vegetables. The potent antioxidant properties of dietary flavonoids have stimulated interest in whether flavonoid-rich diets might offer any protection against diseases such as atherosclerosis and cancer where oxidation is thought to play an important role. Preliminary evidence from epidemiological studies suggests that high dietary antioxidant intake may indeed be protective against the development of vascular disease (7-9).

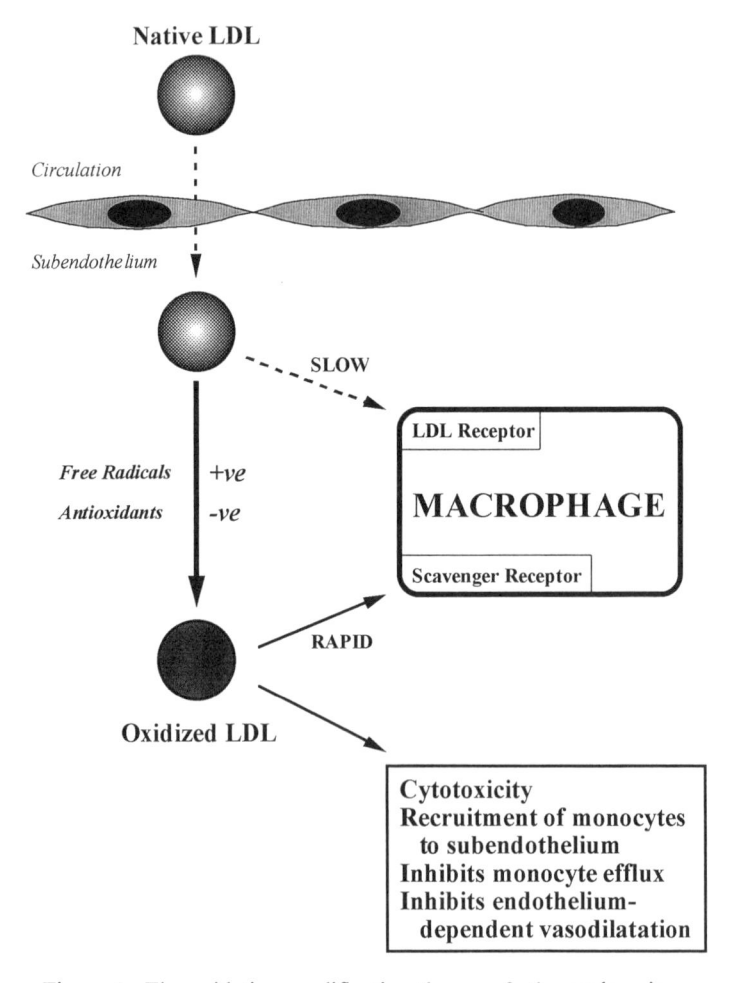

Figure 1. The oxidative-modification theory of atherosclerosis.

Do flavonoids Protect Against Heart Disease?

Although most of these studies have concentrated on the better known antioxidants such as vitamin C and vitamin E more recent epidemiological studies have focused on the role of flavonoids. The Zutphen Elderly Study (*10*) assessed the flavonoid intake of 805 men aged 65-84 years in 1985 and followed them up for 5 years. Flavonoid intake analysed in tertiles was significantly inversely associated with death from coronary heart disease (p=0.015) and showed a trend towards an inverse association with myocardial infarction (p=0.08). The relative risk of coronary heart disease in the highest versus the lowest tertile of flavonoid intake was 0.42 (95% CI 0.20-0.88). This relationship persisted after controlling for all other relevant coronary risk factors. Hertog et al (*11*) also retrospectively reviewed the flavonoid intake of 16 cohorts originally entered into the Seven Countries Study in 1960 calculated from the original dietary questionnaire. Over 25 years of follow-up the flavonoid intake was significantly inversely associated with coronary heart disease mortality and explained 25% of its variance. The only stronger predictor of coronary mortality was saturated fat intake.

Knekt et al (*12*) studied 5133 Finnish men and women aged 30-69 years recruited between 1967 and 1972. The flavonoid intake was calculated from the reported dietary recall of subjects for the year prior to entry into the study and then related to coronary and total mortality over the subsequent 26 years. For women there was a significant inverse gradient of risk for coronary and total mortality with flavonoid intake. The relative risk between the highest and lowest quarters of intake after adjusting for other coronary risk factors was 0.69 (95% CI 0.53-0.90) for total mortality and 0.54 (95% CI 0.33-0.87) for coronary mortality. For men the corresponding values were 0.76 (95% CI 0.63-0.93) and 0.78 (95% CI 0.56-1.08). It was suggested that since the intake of vitamin C in the Finnish diet was low dietary flavonoids may offer an alternative source of antioxidants.

Red Wine Protects against Heart Disease : the French Paradox

Flavonoids are derived from many sources in the human diet including fruit, vegetables, red wine and tea. Red wine is a particularly rich source of flavonoids. Previous calculations have suggested that the addition of two glasses of red wine to the Western diet will increase its flavonoid content by 40% (*13*). Studying the potential impact of red wine flavonoids on coronary heart disease is complicated by the presence of other wine constituents such as alcohol and sugars. Alcohol in particular may have a significant protective effect against vascular disease in its own right (*14-18*). These effects can probably be attributed to the potential for alcohol to increase protective HDL cholesterol levels and decrease platelet aggregation.

However, there have been many claims that there may be benefits associated with the flavonoid content of red wine over and above the effect of alcohol. One of the earliest experiments to suggest this examined the effect of feeding rabbits a high cholesterol diet for three months while also administering alcohol, beer, white wine, red wine or water. These beverages reduced the atherosclerotic lesions over the subsequent 3 months to 75%, 83%, 67% and 40% respectively of those found in the water drinking controls (*19*).

The epidemiological evidence for a specific protective effect of flavonoid-rich alcoholic beverages is rather more confused (20). In most countries intakes of saturated fat are directly associated with mortality from coronary heart disease. However, some countries appear to defy this general association. The most notable exception is France where high fat intakes, serum cholesterol and smoking remain associated with a low incedence of coronary heart disease (18). This circumstance has come to be known as the 'French Paradox' and has stimulated interest in local lifestyle factors that may protect the French against heart disease. A likely candidate was the preference of the French for regular consumption of red wine which offers not only the benefits of moderate alcohol consumption but also the potential benefits of a high flavonoid intake. Indeed, it has been reported that wine consumption in several countries shows a remarkable inverse correlation to local rates of coronary heart disease mortality (21).

Mechanism of Flavonoid Protection against Cardiovascular Disease

The putative cardioprotective benefits of wine have been largely attributed to its content of flavonoids and their antioxidant activity (22). This, it is suggested, may be important in reducing the tendency of lipoproteins to become oxidised and participate in atherosclerosis. There can be little doubt about the activity of flavonoids as antioxidants in vitro. Many investigators have used a variety of assay systems to study the antioxidant effects of polyphenols derived from wine and other sources. These compounds are able to efficiently scavenge a variety of reactive oxidizing species including superoxide, hydroperoxides and the highly reactive hydroxyl radical (23-30). Flavonoids are not only scavengers of reactive oxygen species but also chelate iron which acts as the template for their formation (31,32).

In relation to atherosclerosis it was of particular relevance that flavonoids were not only free radical scavengers but also potent inhibitors of LDL oxidation. Several investigators have been able to demonstrate in vitro that LDL is significantly more resistant to oxidation in the presence of flavonoids derived from red wine and other sources (33-38). Furthermore, flavonoids are also able to spare alpha-tocopherol (vitamin E) the major endogenous radical-scavenging antioxidant of LDL (35).

Another important antioxidant effect of flavonoids is related to their ability to inhibit the lipoxygenases, a group of enzymes which might also be involved in initiating LDL oxidation (39-41) and reduction in the production of neutrophil derived oxidants (42-44). Flavonoids may also modify a number of other cardiovascular risk factors including cholesterol, blood pressure and thrombosis. However, it is the potent antioxidant properties of wine flavonoids are thought to be the major mechanism underlying their putative protection against cardiovascular disease (45). Nevertheless, it is yet to be resolved whether these well-documented *in vitro* effects can be translated into a meaningful alteration in antioxidant protection *in vivo*.

Impact of Red Wine on Antioxidant Status in vivo

Although there is clearly ample evidence of a powerful antioxidant effect of red wine flavonoids from a variety of in vitro assay systems only three studies have addressed their potential impact *in vivo* following acute ingestion (Table I). All of these studies have used the the enhanced chemiluminescent assay for antioxidant activity developed in our laboratory (*46*). Briefly, a glowing light emission can be produced by mixing the chemiluminescent compound luminol with an oxidant (hydrogen peroxide) and an enhancer phenol (para-iodophenol) in the presence of the enzyme horseradish peroxidase. The light emission can be detected in a conventional luminometer and depends on the constant formation of free radical intermediates of para-iodophenol and luminol (Figure 2). Therefore, serum samples containing radical-scavenging antioxidants interfere with light emission from the glowing chemiluminescent reaction. When all of the added antioxidants are consumed (oxidized) in the reaction light emission resumes (Figure 3). The period of light suppression is then compared with a standard curve created by adding the water-soluble tocopherol analogue trolox (6-hydroxy-2,5,7,8-tetramethylchroman-2-carboxylic acid) to calculate the antioxidant activity of the test sample (μmol trolox Eq./litre). This technique is very reproducible (within- and between-batch coefficient of variation for serum samples are 1.7 and 5.0% respectively), as well as being cheaper and requiring less technical expertise than previously reported antioxidant assays.

In our study (*47*) ten healthy students (5 males, 5 females : mean age - 22.0 years, mean weight - 67.2 kg) attended a clinical investigation unit on two separate afternoons after a four hour fast. Following collection of a basal blood sample each subject consumed a standard meal alone or with red wine (5.7ml French Bordeaux/kg) over 30 minutes. Serial blood samples were taken from an indwelling intravenous cannula for four hours and the serum rapidly separated and cooled. Subjects were given free access to drinking water throughout the study. Following ingestion of red wine there was a rapid increase in serum antioxidant activity to reach a peak after 90 minutes before a gradual decline (Figure 4). The peak antioxidant activity represented a remarkable 14% increase over basal values. Antioxidant activity was still significantly elevated at the end of the study at four hours. No such increase was seen after after the consumption of the meal and water ad libitum.

This study was the first (to our knowledge) to suggest that the ingestion of red wine was associated with a significant increase in the antioxidant activity of a human extracellular fluid. Furthermore, the quantitative increases were of a magnitude that had previously been associated with significant inhibition of LDL oxidation *in vitro* (*36*). This result is perhaps not surprising since the variety of wine used in our study had an antioxidant activity of 11365μmol/l in the chemiluminescent assay compared to normal serum values of only 350-550μmol/l (*46*). Indeed, we had found that antioxidant levels of 10-20mmol/l to be common in red wines as previously mentioned. Such values were far superior to the antioxidant activity seen in white wine and a range of other beverages (Figure 5). Assuming *all* of the antioxidant activity in the red wine given to our volunteers (mean volume 0.38 litres, equivalent to 4353μmol antioxidant activity) had been absorbed the observed mean rise of 66μmol/l suggested a volume of distribution of 66 litres! Clearly, it would require absorption of only a fraction of the available antioxidants in red wine distributed throughout the extracellular fluid compartment to produce the observed increases in serum antioxidant activity. We also concluded from our study that enhanced chemiluminescence offered a simple technique for quantifying antioxidant activity in wines or other beverages and their subsequent impact on body fluids.

Table I. Studies examining the impact of red wine ingestion on antioxidant activity and urate concentration in human serum. All error values are standard deviations. * The percentage contribution of urate to rises in serum antioxidant activity has been calculated assuming a 1:1 stoichiometric equivalence between urate and the assay standard antioxidant trolox (*46*). AOA = antioxidant activity, ECL = enhanced chemiluminescence.

Study	Maxwell et al [1994]	Whitehead et al [1995]	Day & Stansbie [1995]
AOA Assay	ECL	ECL	ECL
Subjects (M/F)	5/5	4/5	6/0
Wine	Bordeaux Red	Bordeaux Red	Port Wine
Volume (ml)	383 (mean)	300	250
Wine AOA (μmol/l)	11365	17000	7079
Control	Water	None	Water + 40g ethanol
Follow-Up (min)	240	120	120
Peak Time (min)	90	60	30
Rise in AOA (μmol/l)	66 (14%)	86 (18%)	109 (24%)
Rise in Urate (μmol/l)	39 (12%)	---	81 (23%)
% rise attributable to Urate *	55%	---	74%

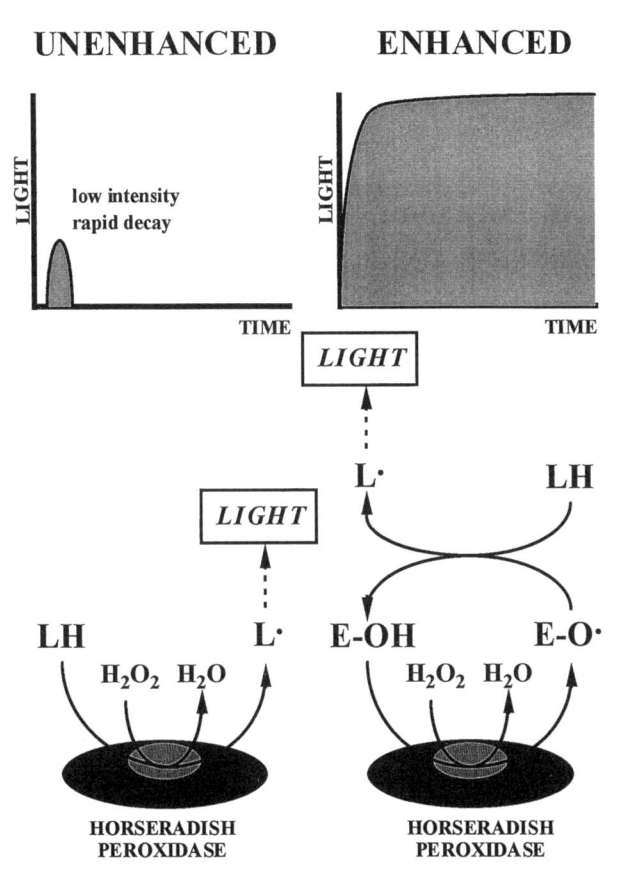

Figure 2. The enhanced chemiluminescent reaction. The chemiluminescent reagent luminol (LH$^-$) is oxidized to its radical form (L$^{-\bullet}$) by the hydrogen peroxide (H$_2$O$_2$)-horseradish peroxidase system. The rate-limiting step of the unenhanced reaction is overcome by the inclusion of enhancer phenols (E-OH) such as para-iodophenol. These are more readily oxidized to their radical form (E-O$^{\bullet}$) than luminol but can subsequently oxidize luminol and in the process are regenerated to their reduced form. In this way the rate of transfer of electrons from luminol to the enzyme is increased with favourable effects on the characteristics of light emission. Radical-scavenging antioxidants will interfere with the reaction sequence and suppress light emission.

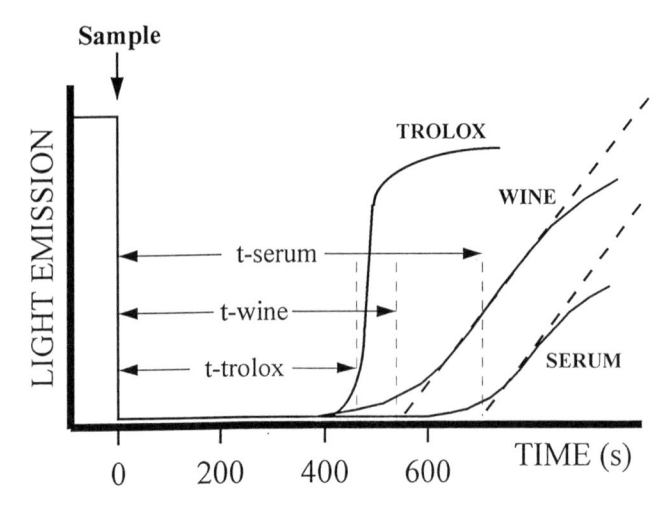

158 WINE: NUTRITIONAL AND THERAPEUTIC BENEFITS

Figure 3. The impact of serum, wine and trolox on light emission from the enhanced chemiluminescent reaction. Antioxidant activity in wine and serum are calculated by comparison of their t-value with that of the trolox standard solution to derive values for antioxidant activity in micromoles of trolox equivalents per litre (μmol/l).

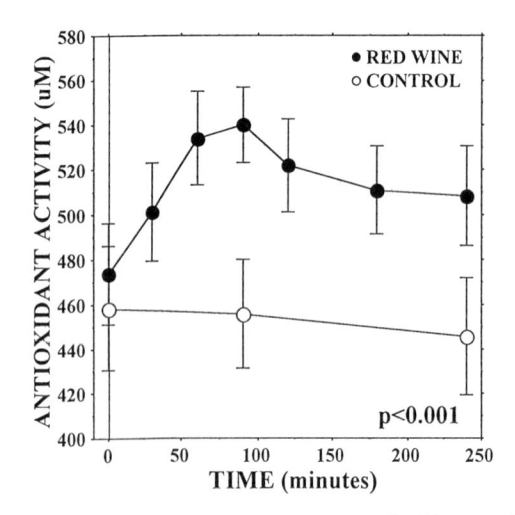

Figure 4. The impact of red wine on serum antioxidant activity in healthy volunteers. Ten healthy volunteers consumed a standard meal alone (control) or together with red wine (5.7ml/kg) over 30 minutes. Water was freely available to subjects throughout both study periods. Antioxidant activity was measured using the enhanced chemiluminescent assay of Whitehead et al (46). Results are expressed as μmol trolox Eq./l and are given as mean ± SE. The interaction of treatment and time has been assessed using analysis of variance. (Reproduced with permission from ref. 47. Copyright 1994 The Lancet.)

A very similar experimental methodology was adopted by Whitehead et al (*48*). Nine subjects (four men, five women) drank 300ml of red wine (1990 Chateau du Juge Bordeaux) over a period of 30 minutes and blood was collected at 1 and 2 hours post ingestion. The red wine itself had an antioxidant activity of 17000µmol/l in relationship to the trolox standard. All subjects showed a rise in serum antioxidant activity after ingestion of red wine with the mean change being from 486µmol/l at baseline to 572µmol/l at one hour and 540µmol/l at 2 hours post-ingestion. No increase in antioxidant activity was observed following ingestion of a similar volume of white wine in three women. Rises in antioxidant activity of a similar magnitude to red wine were seen after ingestion of 1g of ascorbic acid in four women. They also reported the remarkably powerful antioxidant effects of red wine with a selection having mean activity of 15437 $\pm$ 3432µmol/l in comparison to white wine of 1106 $\pm$ 189µmol/l.

Both of these studies appeared to demonstrate that the antioxidants of red wine could have a significant impact on the antioxidant activity of extracellular fluids in vivo. Two obvious potential confounding factors existed. Firstly, since neither study used an alcoholic beverage as a control, could rises in ethanol explain the antioxidant response to red wine? This objection can be safely resisted. Although in some in vitro experiments ethanol has been shown to have weak antioxidant properties it is completely inactive in the chemiluminescent assay. This is in marked contrast to individual flavonoids such as quercetin and other polyphenolic compounds found in wine such as hydroquinone, gallic acid and 1,2,3-trihydroxybenzene were found to be very active antioxidants in the assay by both groups. Secondly, could the apparent increase in antioxidant activity have been a manifestation of alcohol-induced dehydration? The magnitude of the increases (14% and 18%) suggests that this is highly unlikely. In our study the subjects were allowed to drink water ad libitum to try and offset any potential dehydration. Although it remains possible that hydration may have made a *small* contribution we remain confident that the observed increase is genuine.

Although both of the above studies concluded that the powerful *in vitro* antioxidant activity of red wine was being absorbed and detected *in vivo* after its ingestion this assumption has been challenged more recently. In particular, it has been questioned whether these acute increases in antioxidant activity can be simply attributed to the influence of red wine flavonoids. One serum antioxidant that is in high concentration and likely to influence any antioxidant study is urate. Urate may account for as much as 60% of serum total antioxidant activity (*46,49*).

A group from Bristol, UK (*50*) examined the impact of port wine (a blend of red wine and brandy) consumption upon urate concentration as well as total antioxidant activity in serum. Six healthy men consumed 250ml port wine and on a separate occasion 250ml of water containing the equivalent amount of ethanol (40g). Blood samples were taken every 30 minutes for 2 hours. The antioxidant activity of the study port wine was 7079µmol/l. A mean increase in serum antioxidant activity of 109µmol/l (24%) ($p<0.05$) was found after 30 minutes. A similar mean increase in serum urate of 81µmol/l ($p<0.05$) was noted over the same time period. Since urate has previously been shown to hold a 1:1 stoichiometric equivalence with the trolox standard used in the chemiluminescent assay (*46*) it can be inferred that approximately 75% of the antioxidant increase in this study was directly attributable to increases in urate. This belief is supported by the fact that the increase in each parameter was highly correlated

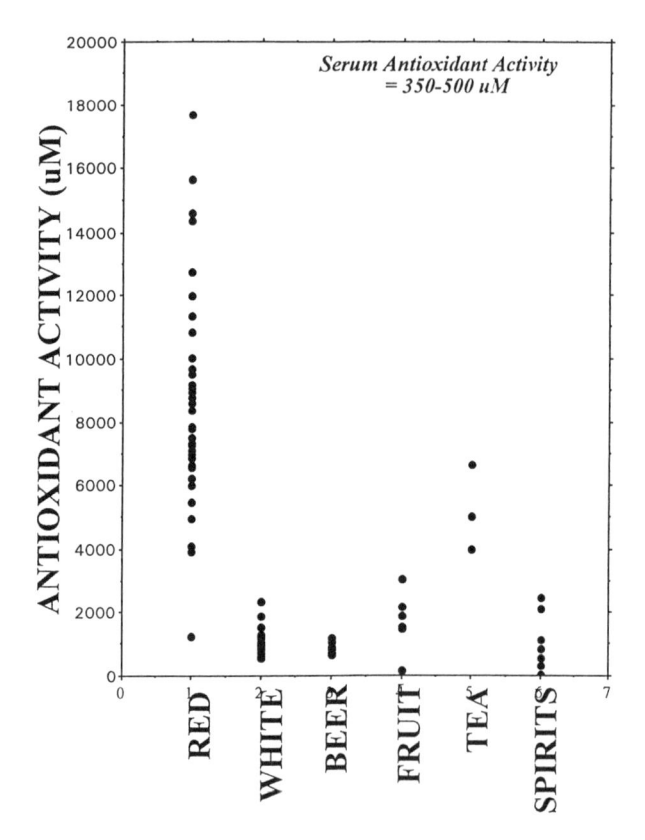

Figure 5. Comparison of the antioxidant activity (µmol/l) measured by enhanced chemiluminescence of a variety of popular beverages.

(r=0.863, p<0.0001). Both measures declined with a half-life of about two and a half hours. No significant increase was seen with either parameter when ethanol was consumed alone. This group also considered the possibility that haemoconcentration may underlie some of the observed effects but discounted this on the basis that there were no changes in urea or protein concentrations during the study period.

This significant increase in urate seen by the Bristol group prompted us to re-examine our own samples for changes in urate. We examined the urate concentrations at baseline and in the 90 minute samples and found the mean increase in serum urate to be 39µmol/l compared to an antioxidant activity increase over the same period of 66µmol/l. Again using the known 1:1 stoichiometric equivalence between urate and trolox this suggested that 55% of the increase could be attributed to urate (Table I). Therefore, we can conclude that even with the most optimistic estimate only half of the antioxidant changes after the acute ingestion of wine can be attributed directly to wine constituents.

The finding that urate may account for much of the antioxidant change itself raises further questions. Why does urate rise in response to wine? Is it specific to wine? Is the rise in urate of any biological significance? Are the antioxidants ingested in wine absorbed at all? The mechanism of the acute rise in urate in response to red wine is unclear. The experiments in Bristol seemed to suggest that the effect must reside in the non-alcoholic component. Whether it is a flavonoid effect and whether it is due to increased production or reduced urinary excretion is unknown. Urate undoubtedly plays an influential role in determining the antioxidant activity of the extracellular fluids but are such increases of any biological relevance? There is evidence to support the belief that urate *does* function as a protective antioxidant in vivo and deserves to be seen as an important antioxidant in human extracellular fluids. Firstly, previous experiments have confirmed that urate directly scavenges free radicals and other oxidants in the aqueous environment in vitro forming oxidation products such as allantoin (*51*). Secondly, urate stabilizes plasma ascorbate not only by direct radical scavenging but also by forming a complex with iron to prevent iron-dependent ascorbate oxidation (*52*). Once urate has been depleted the oxidation of ascorbate is greatly facilitated. This action may be of great importance since ascorbate is often regarded as a pivotal antioxidant of the extracellular fluids. It regenerates alpha-tocopherol in lipoproteins, is itself regenerated intracellularly and is the most efficient plasma antioxidant at preventing peroxyl radical initiated lipid peroxidation (*53*).

It remains to be established that red wine drinking results in an increase in serum flavonoid concentrations significant enough to mediate the antioxidant effects observed in these in vivo studies. Unfortunately, much of the work on flavonoid absorption and bioavailability seems to have been hampered by technical difficulties over their measurement and their chemical diversity. Previous studies have disputed the extent of their uptake following ingestion into the gastrointestinal tract (*54-55*). Unless increases in flavonoid concentrations in the extracellular fluids in the micromolar range are achieved it is hard to believe that bulk scavenging of radicals and protection of lipoproteins against oxidation is a viable proposition. However, lower concentrations might remain active in other ways. Since most of the relevant pathophysiology in atherosclerosis may involve lipoproteins that are trapped in microenvironments of the subendothelial space (*6*) it is possible that local accumulation of flavonoids may have a more profound influence than that suggested by the serum studies described above.

Flavonoids absorbed into lipoproteins themselves where they might have particularly potent antioxidant activities.

This interpretation is suggested by a more recent study comparing the effect of two weeks ingestion of red or white wine (400ml/day) in healthy men (56). Using a different free radical generating system they found that red wine produced a 20% reduction in the propensity of plasma to undergo lipid peroxidation while white wine increased this parameter by 34%. Urate measurements were not reported although other lipid-soluble (lipoprotein-borne) antioxidants such as vitamin E, carotenoids and vitamin A were unchanged. It is then particularly interesting that the resistance of isolated LDL to copper-induced oxidation was significantly increased by red wine consumption but decreased by white wine. This result is of special interest since it points to the possibility that flavonoids may be modifying the antioxidant behaviour of LDL in isolation from any of the other water-soluble antioxidants. It also used a non-specific assay for polyphenols to demonstrate that there was a significant increase in polyphenol content of the LDL isolated after two weeks of red wine ingestion.

Conclusion and Future Studies

The surprising conclusion from these studies is that acute red wine consumption does lead to increases in *serum* antioxidant activity but that, unexpectedly, this appears to have at least as much to do with increases in serum urate as to any increase in red wine flavonoids. The mechanism of the increase in urate is unknown but does not appear to be alcohol-dependent. Urate is undoubtedly an efficient free radical scavenging antioxidant but whether the increase in serum urate is physiologically significant is unknown. These changes in antioxidant activity need to be further confirmed by other groups using alternative techniques for measuring antioxidant status. It is also important that any future studies are matched with measurements of urate and other antioxidants.

Perhaps an even more basic issue that is critical to the putative beneficial effects of red wine is to confirm that there is adequate uptake of flavonoids into the body following their ingestion into the gastrointestinal tract and whether there is indeed accumulation on lipoproteins as suggested above. Three of the studies involved acute wine ingestion. It remains possible that there are other more important long-term antioxidant effects that occur following chronic wine consumption. From the perspective of pathophysiology such studies will be the most valuable. However, the well-recognised impact of regular alcohol consumption on lipoprotein composition and serum urate can be expected to have a major influence on the outcome of such studies. Although some recent epidemiological reviews have been less than enthusiastic about the potential cardiovascular benefits of red wine (20) there remain some very commited protagonists (57). It is certainly true that red wine is the most potent natural antioxidant solution in clinical nutrition. What remains to be discovered is to what extent this activity is translated into meaningful effects in vivo.

References

1. Halliwell, B.; Gutteridge, J.M.C. *Free Radicals in Biology and Medicine;* 2nd Edition; Clarendon Press: Oxford, UK, 1989.
2. Steinberg, D.; Parthasarathy, S.; Carew, T.; Khoo, J.; Witztum, J. Beyond cholesterol. Modifications of low density lipoprotein that increase its atherogenicity. *New England Journal of Medicine* **1989**, *320*, 915-924.
3. Goldstein, J.L.; Brown, M.S. The low-density lipoprotein pathway and its relation to atherosclerosis. *Annual Review of Biochemistry* **1977**, *46*, 897-930.
4. Quinn, M.T.; Parathasarathy, S.; Fong, L.G.; Steinberg, D. Oxidatively modified low-density lipoprotein : a potential role in recruitment and retention of monocyte-macrophages during atherogenesis. *Proceedings of the National Academy of Science USA* **1987**, *664*, 2995-2998.
5. Hessler, J.R.; Robertson, A.L.; Chrisholm, G.M. Low-density lipoprotein-induced cytotoxicity and its inhibition by HDL in human vascular smooth muscle and endothelial cells in culture. *Atherosclerosis* **1979**, *32*, 213-229.
6. Ross, R. Pathogenesis of atherosclerosis : a perspective for the 1990s. *Nature* **1993**, *362*, 801-809.
7. Riemersma, R.A.; Wood, D.A.; MacIntyre, C.C.; Elton, R.; Gey, K.F.; Oliver, M.F. Risk of angina pectoris and plasma concentrations of vitamins A,C, E and carotene. *Lancet* **1991**, *337*, 1-5.
8. Rimm, E.B.; Stampfer, M.J.; Ascherio, A.; Giovannucci, E.; Colditz, G.A.; Willett, W.C. Vitamin E consumption and the risk of coronary heart disease in men. *New England Journal of Medicine* **1993**, *328*, 1450-1456.
9. Stampfer, M.J.; Hennekens, C.H.; Manson, J.E.; Colditz, G.A.; Rosner, B.; Willett, W.C. Vitamin E consumption and risk of coronary disease in women. *New England Journal of Medicine* **1993**, *328*, 1444-1449.
10. Hertog, M.G.; Feskens, E.J.M.; Hollman, P.C.H.; Katan, M.B.; Kromhout, D. Dietary antioxidant flavonoids and risk of coronary artery disease : the Zutphen Elderly Study. *Lancet* **1993**, *342*, 1007-1011.
11. Hertog, M.G.L.; Kromhout, D.; Aravanis, C.; Blackburn, H.; Buzina, R.; Fidanza, F. et al. Flavonoids intake and long-term risk of cornary heart disease and cancer in the seven countries study. *Archives of Internal Medicine* **1995**, *155*, 381-386.
12. Knekt, P.; Jarvinen, R.; Reunanen, A.; Maatela, J. Flavonoid intake and coronary mortality in Finland : a cohort study. *British Medical Journal* **1996**, *312*, 478-481.
13. Waterhouse, A.L.; Frankel, E.N. *Proceedings OIV 73rd General Assembly, San Francisco, August 29-September 3, 1993;* OIV: Paris, France, 1993; Wine antioxidants may reduce heart disease and cancer, pp. 1-15.
14. Rimm, E.B.; Giovannucci, E.L.; Willett, W.C. et al. Prospective study of alcohol consumption and risk of coronary artery disease in men. *Lancet* **1991**, *338*, 464-486.
15. Hein, H.O.; Suadicani, P.; Gyntelberg, F. Alcohol consumption, serum low density lipoprotein cholesterol concentration, and risk of ischaemic heart disease : six year follow up in the Copenhagen male study. *British Medical Journal* **1996**, *312*, 736-741.
16. Lazarus, N.B.; Kaplan, G.A.; Cohen, R.D.; Diing-Jen, L. Change in alcohol consumption and risk of death from all causes and from ischaemic heart disease. *British Medical Journal* **1991**, *303*, 553-556.
17. Friedman, L.A.; Kimball, A.W. Coronary artery disease mortality and alcohol consumption in Framingham. *American Journal of Epidemiology* **1986**, *24*, 481-48.
18. Renaud, S.; de Lorgeril, M. Wine, alcohol, platelets, and the French paradox for coronary artery disease. *Lancet* **1992**, *339*, 1523-1526.
19. Klurfeld, D.M.; Kritchevsky, D. Differential effects of alcoholic beverages on experimental atherosclerosis in rabbits. *Experimental Molecular Pathology* **1981**, *34*, 62-71.

20.   Rimm, E.B.; Klatsky, A.; Grobbee, D.; Stampfer, M.J. Review of moderate alcohol consumption and reduced risk of coronary heart disease : is the effect due to wine, beer or spirits? *British Medical Journal* **1996**, *312*, 731-736.

21.   St Leger, A.S.; Cochrane, A.L.; Moore, F. Factors associated with cardiac mortality in developed countries with particular reference to the consumption of wine. *Lancet* **1979**, *i*, 1017-1020.

22.   Halliwell, B. Antioxidants in wine. *Lancet* **1993**, *341*, 1538.

23.   Troup, G.J.; Hutton, D.R.; Hewitt, D.G.; Hunter, C.R. Free radicals in red wine, but not in white? *Free Radical Research* **1994**, *20*, 63-68.

24.   Laughton, M.J.; Halliwell, B.; Evans, P.J.; Hoult, J.R. Antioxidant and pro-oxidant actions of the plant phenolics quercetin, gossypol and myricetin. Effects on lipid peroxidation, hydroxyl radical generation, and bleomycin-dependent damage to DNA. *Biochemical Pharmacology* **1989**, *38*, 2849-2865.

25.   Husain, S.R.; Cillard, J.; Cillard, P. Hydroxyl radical scavenging activity of flavonoids. *Phytochemistry* **1987**, *26*, 2489-2491.

26.   Robak, J.; Gryglewski, R.J. Flavonoids are scavengers of superoxide anion. *Biochemical Pharmacology* **1988**, *37*, 83-88.

27.   Yuting, C.; Rongliang, Z.; Zhongjian, J.; Yong, J. Flavonoids as superoxide scavengers and antioxidants. *Free Radicals in Biology and Medicine* **1990**, *9*, 19-21.

28.   Hanasaki, Y.; Ogawa, S.; Fukui, S. The correlation between active oxygens scavenging and antioxidative effects of flavonoids. *Free Radicals in Biology and Medicine* **1994**, *16*, 845-850.

29.   Torel, J.; Cillard, J.; Cillard, P. Antioxidant activity of flavonoids and reactivity with peroxyl radicals. *Phytochemistry* **1986**, *25*, 383-385.

30.   Cotelle, N.; Bernier, J.L.; Henichart, J..P; Catteau, J.P. *Free Radicals in Biology and Medicine* **1992**, *13*, 211-219.

31.   Morel, I.; Lescoat, G.; Cillard, P.; Cillard, J. Role of flavonoids and iron chelation in antioxidant action. *Methods in Enzymology* **1994**, *234*, 437-443.

32.   Afanaslev, I.B.; Dorozhko, A.I.; Brodskii, A.V. et al. Chelating and free radical scavenging mechanisms of inhibitory action of rutin and quercetin in lipid peroxidation. *Biochemical Pharmacology* **1989**, *38*, 1763-1769.

33.   Mangipane, H.; Thomson, J; Salter, A.; Brown, S.; Bell, G.D., White, D.A. The inhibition of the oxidation of low-density lipoprotein by (+)-catechin, a naturally occuring flavonoid. *Biochemical Pharmacology* **1992**, *43*, 445-450.

34.   de Whalley, C.V.; Rankin, S.M.; Hoult, J.R.S.; Jessup, W.; Leake, D.S. Flavonoids inhibit the oxidative modification of low-density lipoproteins by macrophages. *Biochemical Pharmacology* **1990**, *39*, 1743-1750.

35.   Jessup, W.; Rankin, S.M.; de Whalley, C.; Hoult, J.R.S.; Scott, J.; Leake, D.S. Alpha-tocopherol consumption during low-density lipoprotein oxidation. *Biochemical Journal* **1990**, *265*, 399-405.

36.   Frankel, E.N.; Kanner, J.; German, G.B.; Parks, E.; Kinsella, J.E. Inhibition of oxidation of human low-density lipoprotein by phenolic sustances in red wine. *Lancet* **1993**, *341*, 454-457.

37.   Frankel, E.N.; Waterhouse, A.L.; Kinsella, J.E. Inhibition of human LDL oxidation by resveratrol. *Lancet* **1993**, *341*, 1103-1104.

38.   Negre-Salvayre, A.; Salvayre, R. Quercetin prevents the cytotoxicity of oxidized low density lipoproteins in lymphoid cell lines. *Free Radicals in Biology and Medicine* **1992**, *12*, 101-106.

39.   Laughton, M.J.; Evans, P.J.; Moroney, M.A.; Hoult, J.R.S.; Halliwell, B. Inhibition of mammalian 5-lipoxygenase and cyclo-oxygenase by flavonoids and phenolic dietary additives : relationship to antioxidant activity and iron ion-reducing ability. *Biochemical Pharmacology* **1991**, *42*, 1673-1681.

40. Moroney, M.-A.; Alcaraz, M.J.; Forder, R.A. et al. Selectivity of 5-lipoxygenase and cyclo-oxygenase inhibition by an anti-inflammatory flavonoid glycoside and related aglycone flavonoids. *Journal of Pharmacy and Pharmacology* **1988**, *40*, 787-792.

41. Takahama, U. Inhibition of lipoxygenase-dependent lipid peroxidation by quercetin : mechanism of antioxidative function. *Phytochemistry* **1985**, *24*, 1443-1446.

42. Busse, W.W.; Kopp, D.E.; Middleton, E. Flavonoid modulation of human neutrophil function. *Journal of Allergy and Clinical Immunology* **1984**, *73*, 810.

43. Hodnick, W.F.; Kung, F.S.; Roettger, W.J.; Bohmont, C.W.; Pardini, R.S. Inhibition of mitochondrial respiration and production of toxic oxygen radicals by flavonoids - a structure-activity study. *Biochemical Pharmacology* **1986**, *35*, 2345-2357.

44. Corvazier, E.; Maclouf, J. Interference of some flavonoids and non-steroidal anti-inflammatory drugs with oxidative metabolism of arachidonic acid by human platelets and neutrophils. *Biochimica et Biophysica Acta* **1985**, *835*, 315-321.

45. Muldoon, M.F.; Kritchevsky, S.B. Flavonoids and heart disease. *British Medical Journal* **1996**, *312*, 458-459.

46. Whitehead, T.P.; Thorpe, G.H.G.; Maxwell, S.R.J. An enhanced chemiluminescent assay for antioxidant capacity in biological fluids. *Analytica Chimica Acta* **1992**, *266*, 265-277.

47. Maxwell, S.R.J.; Cruickshank, A.; Thorpe, G.H.G. Red wine- and antioxidant activity in serum. *Lancet* **1994**, *334*, 193-194.

48. Whitehead, T.P.; Robinson, D.; Allaway, S.; Syms, J.; Hale, A. The effect of red wine ingestion on the antioxidant capacity of serum. *Clinical Chemistry* **1995**, *41*, 32-35.

49. Wayner, D.D.M.; Burton, G.W.; Ingold, K.U.; Barclay, L.R.C.; Locke, S.J. The relative contributions of Vitamin E, urate, ascorbate and proteins to the total peroxyl radical-trapping antioxidant activity of human blood plasma. *Biochimica et Biophysica Acta* **1987**, *924*, 408-419.

50. Day, A.; Stansbie, D. Cardioprotective effect of red wine may be mediated by urate. *Clinical Chemistry* **1995**, *41*, pp.

51. Becker, B.F. Towards the physiological function of uric acid. *Free Radicals in Biology and Medicine* **1993**, *14*, 615-631.

52. Davies, K.J.A.; Sevanian, A.; Muakkassah-Kelly, S.F.; Hochstein, P. Uric acid-iron ion complexes. A new aspect of the antioxidant functions of uric acid. *Biochemical Journal* **1986**, *235*, 747-754.

53. Frei, B.; Stocker, R.; Ames, B.N. Antioxidant defences and lipid peroxidation in human blood plasma. *Proceedings of the National Academy of Science USA* **1988**, *85*, 9748-9752.

54. Das, N.P. Studies on flavonoid metabolism : absorption and metabolism of (+)-catechin in man. *Biochemical Pharmacology* **1971**, *20*, 3435-3445.

55. Gugler, R.; Leschik, M.; Dengler, H.J. Deposition of quercetin in man after single oral and intravenous doses. *European Journal of Clinical Pharmacology* **1975**, *9*, 229-234.

56. Fuhrman, B.; Lavy, A.; Aviram, M. Consumption of red wine with meals reduces the susceptibility of human plasma and low-density lipoprotein to lipid peroxidation. *American Journal of Clinical Nutrition* **1995**, *61*, 549-554.

57. Goldberg, D.M. Does wine work? *Clinical Chemistry* **1995**, *41*, 14-16.

Chapter 13

The Relative Antioxidant Potencies of Some Polyphenols in Grapes and Wines

Alessandro Baldi[1], Annalisa Romani[1], Nadia Mulinacci[1], Franco F. Vincieri[1], and Andrea Ghiselli[2]

[1]Dipartimento di Scienze Farmaceutiche, Università degli Studi di Firenze, via Gino Capponi 9, 50121 Firenze, Italy
[2]Istituto Nazionale della Nutrizione, via Ardeatina 546, Roma, Italy

The antioxidant activities of some polyphenolic fractions of grapes and wines have been tested using *in vitro* and *ex vivo* tests. Polyphenolic fractions were obtained applying a liquid/liquid extraction method and analyzed by using HPLC/DAD, Ion Spray HPLC/MS and Electrospray MS. Some tannin/anthocyan interaction compounds were also extracted and analyzed from wines. EPR spectroscopy, TRAP assay, 2-deoxyribose assay and a platelet aggregation inhibition test were performed to test antioxidant activities of polyphenolic fractions. Results showed that the anthocyans fraction and the fraction containing procyanidins were very effective in antioxidant activity.

Polyphenols are widely spread in plant kingdom (*1*). They are present in most edible fruits and vegetables, and therefore common in the every day diet of many people. It has been calculated that following a mediterranean diet, one can assume up to 2-3 gr of polyphenols a day (*2*). Polyphenols have also a recognized biological activity (*3*). Several pharmaceuticals whose active principles belong to the class of polyphenols are sold in Europe and most of them are extracted from medicinal (or not) plants. Indications include vasoprotection and activities related to their antioxigen effect. There are two different mechanisms to explain the antioxigen effect: the first one is a direct reduction effect on vitamins and fatty acids; the second one is a radical scavenger effect on exogen and endogen free radicals (*4*). Among polyphenols, procyanidins (oligomers of catechin and epicatechin) have been studied for a long time for their biological activities. Michaud and collaborators (*5*) in 1981 isolated several procyanidins and other polyphenols and made comparison among them in order to test their radical scavenging efficiency. In particular, research has been focused on polyphenols contained in grapes and wine for several reasons. First, byproducts from wine production can be an inexpensive source of polyphenols. Second, wine in the mediterranean diet seems to play a very important role for benefits that can bring to the

© 1997 American Chemical Society

human health. Grapes and wine can be a good source of flavonoids (6), even if wine is consumed in amounts that are small enough not to be dangerous for the presence of ethanol. For the above reasons we started a research focused on the study of the antioxidant activities of the polyphenolic fractions of grapes and their relative wines. Several studies have been conducted on this topic using *in vitro* and *ex vivo* tests (7-10). Wine is a good example of a slow evolution of the oxidation process in a quite simple system, thus allowing to study the interaction and the role of some compounds involved in the protection against the oxidative degradation (11). For this reason we chose to analyze two samples of the same wine stored in two different ways and therefore in two different oxidative status. In this way we could check the biological activities of the polyphenolic fractions in the same system but in different moments of the oxidation process. First, we performed a qualitative and quantitative analysis of polyphenols, and after we tested some fractions and some individual compounds for their antioxidant activity, using *in vitro* and *ex vivo* tests.

Materials and Methods

Grapes and Wines. The grapes were grown in an experimental field in the Chianti Classico area (Rocca di Castagnoli, Siena, Italy) and belong to the same cultivar and the same clone (clone Sangiovese R10). The grapes were of the same age and same pruning system, and were harvested at technological ripening. The wine was produced under controlled fermentation conditions. During the following six months, the wine was stored in a stainless steel container. After that, two different samples were prepared for this research: wine A that was stored for the following 12 months in bottle, and wine B stored for six months in barrique (small container in oak wood) and for six months in bottle.

Preparation of teas. Green tea and black tea (from commercial samples) were prepared to compare their radical scavenging efficiency with that of grapes and wines samples. Teas were prepared leaving 2 gr of tea leaves in 100 ml of boiling water for 90 sec.

Low Molecular Weight Polyphenols.
Extraction Methods. Liquid/liquid extraction methods, Figure 1, were performed to obtain several fractions containing single polyphenolic subclasses.

Separation and identification of the compounds. HPLC/DAD analysis were performed on each fraction, applying chromatographic conditions already described in (12). HPLC/MS analysis using an Ion Spray Interface and a triple quadrupole was used to identify the unknown compounds. Negative Ion Spray Mass Spectrometry was applied to the EtOAc extracts analysis, and Positive Ion Spray Mass Spectrometry to the aqueous residues of grapes and wines (13). After the qualitative analysis, a quantitative analysis on the identified compounds was performed, using the external standard method.

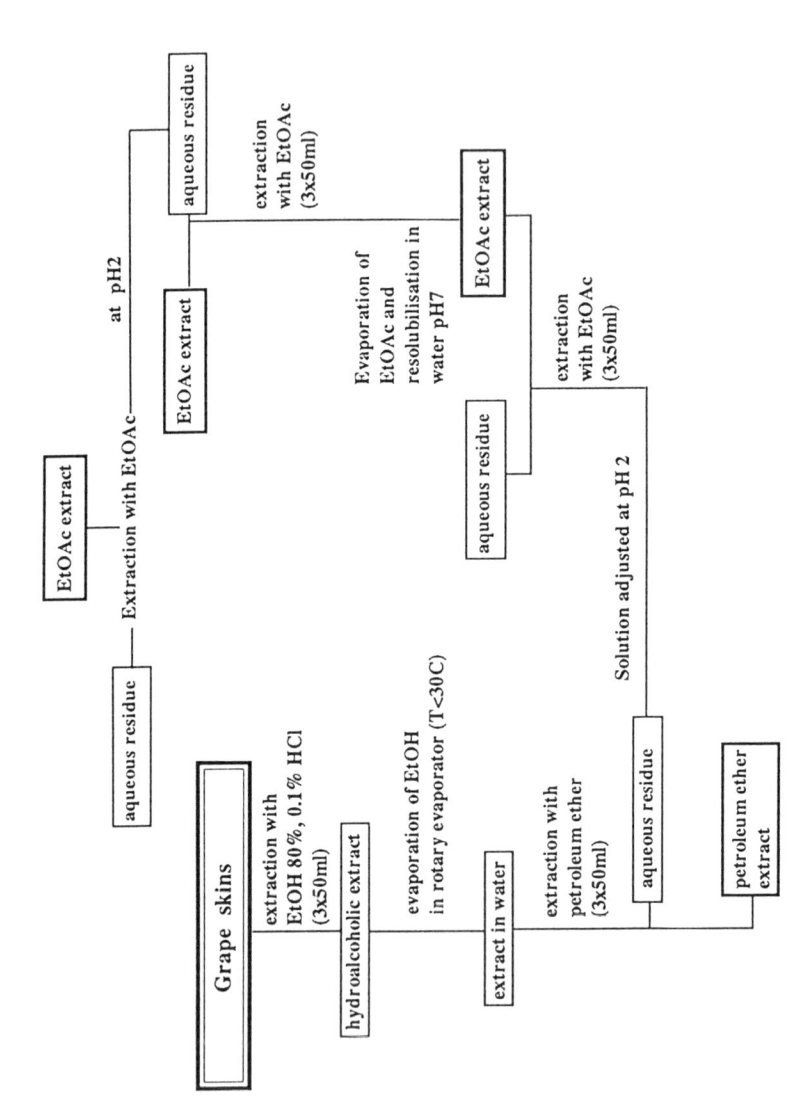

Figure 1. Liquid/liquid extraction method applied on grapes samples.

Tannin-Anthocyan Interaction Compounds.
Extraction and Identification Methods.
Interaction compounds were separated using a Polyvinilpyrrolidon resin (Polyclar AT) LC column and flowing water/ EtOH/ HCl 30/70/0.1, as first eluent, then HCOOH 50% and HCOOH 100% respectively. After neutralization with KOH, a further purification was performed using a short Sephadex LH 20 column, flowing water/ EtOH 50/50 and acetone/ water/ acetic acid 50/50/3 respectively. This allowed to obtain six fractions successively analyzed spectrophotometrically using the method of Glories (14). Further information was obtained using Mass Spectrometry techniques, such as Infusion Electrospray Mass Spectrometry and Negative Ion FAB.

Biological Activity Tests.
EPR Spectroscopy. The samples (water soluble extracts after dilution, lipid soluble extracts after dried) were added to an alkaline solution of hydrogen peroxide. A further addition of acetone to the system generated superoxide ion. A blank was prepared adding KOH instead of the sample. The time of generation of superoxide ion was optimized at 60 sec. and after that the solution was frozen in liquid nitrogen. Then, the frozen blank and the frozen sample solutions were put in the EPR cavity and the $O_2^{\cdot-}$ signal recorded. From the comparison of the two areas associated with the perpendicular features of the EPR spectrum, a reduction index was calculated and converted into a percent scavenger efficiency index.

KOH 40 mM   150µl or KOH 40 mM 100µl + 50 µl of sample
H_2O_2 0.15M   100µl
CH_3COCH_3 50µl
Frozen in liquid nitrogen after 60 sec.
Instrumental setting: υ= 9.459 GHz; modulation frequency = 100 KHz; field modulation amplitude = 6.3 G; gain = 1.6 X 10^{-4}; time constant = 500 ms; microwave power = 2 mW; scan time 500 s.

TRAP assay. A suitable method for measuring TRAP (Total Radical-Trapping Antioxidant Parameter) was applied using the R-Phycoerythrin (R-PE) assay. A 1.5×10^{-8} M R-PE solution in 75 mM phosphate buffer pH 7 was challenged by 4.0 mM of an Azoinitiator (2.2'-azobis-(2-amidinopropane) dihydrochloride, ABAP) with or without a sample (80 µl of a 1:200 dilution to a final pH 7). The decay of R-PE fluorescence was continuosly monitored every 5 min. in a Perkin-Elmer LS-5 Luminescence Spectrometer as described in a previous paper (15). A known amount of Trolox, a water soluble analog of vitamin E was used to quantify the results. ABAP produced a constant flow of peroxyl radicals and TRAP was expressed as µmoles of peroxyl radicals trapped by a liter of sample.

2-Deoxyribose Assay. The reaction mixture was prepared as follows: 100µl of diluted samples (1:10 in appropriate buffers to reach pH 7.4) were added to 690 µl of 10 mM phosphate buffer pH 7.4 containing 2.5 mM 2-deoxyribose. Subsequently, 100 µl of 1.0 mM iron ammonium sulphate premixed with 1.04 mM EDTA were added. Samples were kept in water bath at 37°C and the reaction was started with 100 µl of 1.0 mM ascorbic acid followed by 10 µl of 0.1 M H_2O_2. Samples were mantained at 37°C for 10 min., then 1 ml trichloroacetic acid (2.8%) was added, followed by 0.5 ml thiobarbituric acid (1%) in NaOH 50 mM. Samples were boiled for 8 min., cooled and the absorbance at 532 nm recorded (*16*).

Platelet aggregation assay. Blood samples were obtained from consenting human healthy subjects, fasting from at least 12 hours in B.D. Vacutainer containing 0.129 M Na-citrate as an anticoagulant. Platelet rich plasma (PRP) was prepared by centrifugating blood samples at 150 x g for 10 min. Platelets were washed three times in phosphate buffered saline (PBS) containing 5 mM EDTA, pH 7.4, pooled and resuspended in PBS without EDTA (*17*). 100 ml of lipid soluble extracts (EtOAc extracts or petroleum ether extract) were dried and resolubilized in 50 μl of methanol and dissolved in 1.0 ml (final volume) of PBS. Water soluble extracts (aqueous residues) have been diluted 1:10 in PBS. 10 μl of each samples were then added to 490 μl of PBS containing 3×10^8 platelets and 1.5 mg/ml of fibrinogen. Platelet aggregation was induced by 2 μM ADP and samples were incubated for 5 min. at 37°C. The reaction was stopped by adding 500 μl of trichloroacetic acid (20% w/v). During platelet aggregation, malondialdehyde was produced and detected using the following procedure: 500 ml of 0.8 % thiobarbituric acid were added to the solution and boiled for 8 min. After reaching room temperature, the absorbance at 532 was detected and the results were plotted and compared with a standard curve obtained using tetramethoxypropane. Results were expressed as % of platelets aggregation inhibition.

Results and Discussion.
Grapes.
The application of the liquid/liquid extraction method allowed to prepare fractions containing compounds with similar characteristics. In particular, the application of HPLC/MS techniques like Negative Ion Spray Mass Spectrometry allowed to identify several polyphenolic compounds. Phenolic acids and quercitin-3-glucuronide in the EtOAc extract of the solution adjusted at pH 2 and some procyanidins, catechin, epicatechin and quercitin-3-glucoside as main components of the EtOAc extract of the solution adjusted at pH7, were found. Beside kaempferol-3-glucoside, myricetin-3-glucoside and traces of aglicons quercitin, kaempferol and myricetin, were also found. The aqueous residue after the EtOAc extraction, was analyzed by Positive Ion Spray Mass Spectrometry and several anthocyanins were identified. All the identified compounds are listed in Table I. A quantitative analysis using the external standard method was performed on these compounds.

Wines.
Two different extraction methods were applied to obtain fractions composed by low molecular weight polyphenols and tannin-anthocyan interaction compounds.

Low Molecular Weight Polyphenols. A liquid/liquid extraction method similar to that applied on grapes allowed to obtain EtOAc extracts and aqueous residue similar to that of the grapes extracts. The main differences were the presence of gallic acid and a larger concentration of flavonolic aglycones in wines. Free anthocyanins were present in the aqueous residues even if the relative amounts were different from those found in grapes. Malvidin-3-glucoside was the most represented anthocyanin in wines. Wine A showed a higher content in total polyphenols than wine B. In particular, anthocyanic content was 15% higher in the aqueous residue of wine A than in the aqueous residue of wine B. Same behaviour had the EtOAc extract of the solution at pH 7, containing mainly procyanidins. Probably, during the period spent in barrique, wine B was subject to a faster maturation process, in a higher oxidative status.

Tannin-Anthocyan Interaction Compounds. During the fermentation some interaction compounds between catechins and anthocyans are formed in presence of acetaldehyde. The structures of these compounds were hypotized by Timberlake and Bridle in 1976 (*18*) and further studied by Glories (*14*). The application of the extraction method directly on wine using a Polyvinilpirrolidon resin, allowed to obtain three fractions that were tested by spectrophotometry. Based on their spectral characteristics, the presence of interaction compounds were hypotized on the second and third eluate and a further purification using Sephadex LH 20 was performed. Six fractions were obtained and analyzed by Infusion Electrospray Mass Spectrometry and Negative FAB (Fast Atom Bombardment) Mass Spectrometry. Negative Electrospray Mass Spectrometry showed the presence of signals at 289 m/z and 577 m/z corresponding to the quasimolecular ions of catechin and dimers of catechins in all the six fractions, and Positive Electrospray Mass Spectrometry showed a strong signal at 331 m/z corresponding to the quasimolecular ion of malvidin. Further information was obtained using Negative FAB Mass Spectrometry technique. Mass signals in the range between 600-800 m/z were found in the first three fractions, and 1000-1200 m/z in the second three fractions. These molecular weights could be abscribed to tannin-anthocyan and tannin-anthocyan-tannin interaction compounds as hypotized by Timberlake. A strong signal at 645 m/z corresponding to the quasimolecular ion of malvidin-acetaldehyde-catechin was found. Sufficient amounts of these fractions were prepared to test their biological activity. A part of these fractions was lyophilized to calculate the concentration of each fraction. Biological tests were performed directly on the fractions prior to the lyophilization.

Biological tests.

Biological test *in vitro* and *ex vivo* were applied on the following fractions:
EtOAc extracts of grapes and wines (whole extract and extract of the solution at pH 7 and pH 2 -see fig.1-)
Aqueous residue of grapes and wines
Petroleum ether extract of grapes
Tannin-anthocyan interaction compounds of wines.

EPR Spectroscopy. Initially, the behaviour of grapes and wines fractions as scavenger of free radicals was tested by studying the action of O_2^-. EPR spectrometry was used to allow a direct measurement of the reduction of O_2^- EPR signal intensity. The system generated superoxide ion O_2^- in stable solutions. All samples were treated in the same way of the blank. The reduction of the signal intensity was recorded for each sample and at least three different concentrations were prepared to test the range of linearity. A percent scavenger efficiency index was calculated for each fraction, taking in consideration for all the samples, the same dilution factor. Figure 2 shows the frozen solutions EPR spectra of the blank together with the O_2^- signal of the solution in which the EtOAc extract of wine A was added. A dramatic reduction of the signal intensity can easily be seen. After a mathematical elaboration a percent scavenger efficiency index was calculated for each fraction and they are shown in table II. The dealcoholated wines, A and B, showed the higher values of scavenger efficiency index, but also the EtOAc extracts showed a great inhibition of the O_2^- signal.

Table I. List of identified compounds in grapes and wines

Anthocyans
Delphinidin-3-O-glucoside
Cyanidin-3-O-glucoside
Petunidin-3-O-glucoside
Peonidin-3-O-glucoside
Malvidin-3-O-glucoside
Delphinidin-3-(6-O-acetyl)-glucoside
Cyanidin-3-(6-O-acetyl)-glucoside
Petunidin-3-(6-O-acetyl)-glucoside
Peonidin-3-(6-O-acetyl)-glucoside
Malvidin-3-(6-O-acetyl)-glucoside
Delphinidin-3-(6-O-*p*-coumaroyl)-glucoside
Cyanidin-3-(6-O-*p*-coumaroyl)-glucoside
Petunidin-3-(6-O-*p*-coumaroyl)-glucoside
Peonidin-3-(6-O-*p*-coumaroyl)-glucoside
Malvidin-3-(6-O-*p*-coumaroyl)-glucoside
Flavonols
Quercitin-3-glucoside
Quercitin-3-glucuronide
Quercitin
Myricetin-3-glucoside
Myricetin
Kaempferol-3-glucoside
Kaempferol

Phenolics acids
Caffeic acid
p-Coumaric acid
Ferulic acid
Vanillic acid
p-OH-Benzoic acid
Gallic acid
Protocatechic acid
Hydroxycinnamoyltartaric acids
Caffeoyltartaric acid
p-Coumaroyltartaric acid
Feruloyltartaric acid
Catechins and Procyanidins
(+) Catechin
(-) Epicatechin
Procyanidin B3
Procyanidin B1
Procyanidin B6
Procyanidin B2
Procyanidin B7
Procyanidin C1

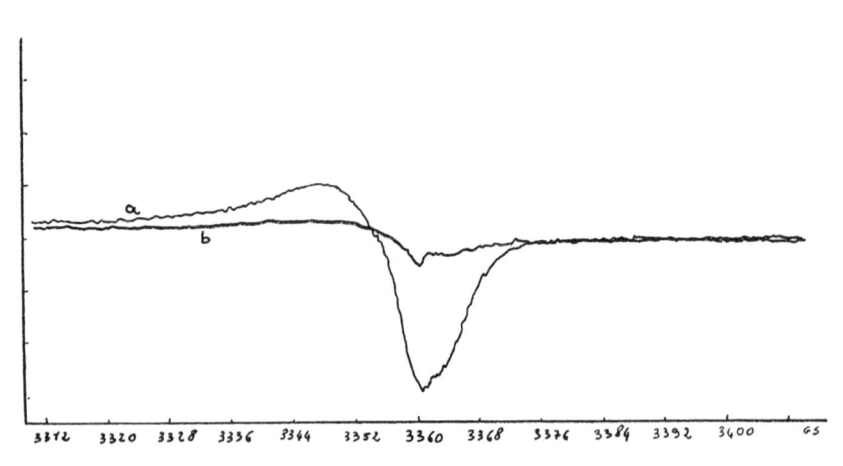

Figure 2. Frozen solution EPR spectra of O_2^- of blank (a) and EtOAc extract of wine (b).

TRAP assay. The Total Radical-Trapping Antioxidant Parameter, whose acronym TRAP well emphasizes its meaning, represents the capacity of a substance, or a mixture, to resist to an artificial induced peroxidation reaction. TRAP value is the result of the efficiency of the system, accounting for the synergism between antioxidants, rather than their single concentrations. This means that the TRAP value includes the effect of unknown and unconsidered compounds, as well as the action of prooxidant factors. This parameter may represent, therefore, a first approach in the study of the supposed antioxidant power of a mixture, deriving from a food, a beverage or something else. The result depends not only on the concentration of the antioxidants in the solution, but also on some eventual sinergistic effects. Figure 3 shows the decay of the R-PE fluorescence in samples at increasing concentrations of wine. The lag-phase of the blank was around 0 min., while increasing amounts of dealcoholated wine gave longer lag-phases. The chart on the top right of Figure 3 shows that lag-phases and increasing concentrations of wine are in linear correlation, demonstrating that the experiment was conducted in the range of linearity. Values of TRAP are shown in Figure 4 and are expressed in μM of peroxyl radicals trapped by the system in a liter of solution. The dealcoholated wines A and B showed a very good activity in radical trapping together with the aqueous residues containing anthocyans. Wine showed the highest values, but the presence of EtOH (12.4%) could give wrong evaluation in this system. All fractions of wine A showed higher activity compared of those of wine B. This could be correlated to the lower amounts in polyphenols of wine B. The activity of black tea and green tea was compared with the activity of the fractions. Dealcoholated wines showed an intermediate activity between those of green and black teas. Tannin-anthocyan interaction compounds were not very active. In particular, Figure 5 shows the comparison of the results of the TRAP test among the six fractions. The first three (composed mainly by tannin-anthocyan interaction compounds) were more active than those showing higher molecular weight (tannin-anthocyan-tannin interaction compounds).

2-Deoxyribose Assay. Next step concerned the study of the antioxidant activity against another and more dangerous species of oxygen radicals, the hydroxyl radical (OH·). A flow of OH· can be generated by using the Fenton reaction summarized below:

$$Fe^{2+} + EDTA + H_2O_2 \longrightarrow Fe^{3+} + EDTA + OH· + OH^-$$

The addition of an electron donor such as ascorbic acid will reduce Fe^{3+} to Fe^{2+}, thus perpetuating the OH· flow. 2-deoxyribose is a suitable substrate for determination of hydroxyl radical production in biological and chemical systems (19). The OH· attack to the 2-deoxyribose molecule gives rise to malondialdehyde which, heated under acid conditions, forms a pink chromogen with TBA, showing a strong absorbance at 532 nm. The use of EDTA as an iron chelator is very important. In fact without EDTA, the inhibition of OH· production can depend not only on the ability of the sample to scavenge OH·, but also on its ability to form complexes with iron (20). This method is simple, inexpensive, and efficient even at low concentrations. Dealcoholated wines A and B showed good ability to inhibit the degradation of 2-deoxyribose. EtOAc extracts of the solution at pH 7 and the aqueous residues gave also good results as shown in Figure 6. So, applying this test, the fractions containing flavonoidic structures (procyanidins and flavonols for EtOAc pH 7, anthocyans for aqueous residues) seem to show the highest activity. Also anthocyans from grapes showed great ability to inhibit

Table II. % of inhibition of the $O_2^{\cdot}$ signal in some wine fractions

Samples	Dilution factor	Values
1. wine A	1:600	84.62
2. wine B	1:600	84.24
3. dealcoholated wine A	1:600	94.03
4. dealcoholated wine B	1:600	96.22
5. EtOAc Tot. (A)	1:600	48.83
6. EtOAc pH 7 (A)	1:600	53.64
7. EtOAc pH 2 (A)	1:600	68.07

Tannin/anthocyan interaction compounds	mg/ml	Values
8. fraction 1	0.01	60.32
9. fraction 2	0.01	63.70
10. fraction 3	0.01	63.90
11. fraction 4	0.01	60.20
12. fraction 5	0.01	56.28

Isolated compounds	Concentration	Values
13. quercitin-3-O-glucoside	8.3×10^{-5}	60.39
14. peonidin-3-O-glucoside	5.7×10^{-5}	69.35

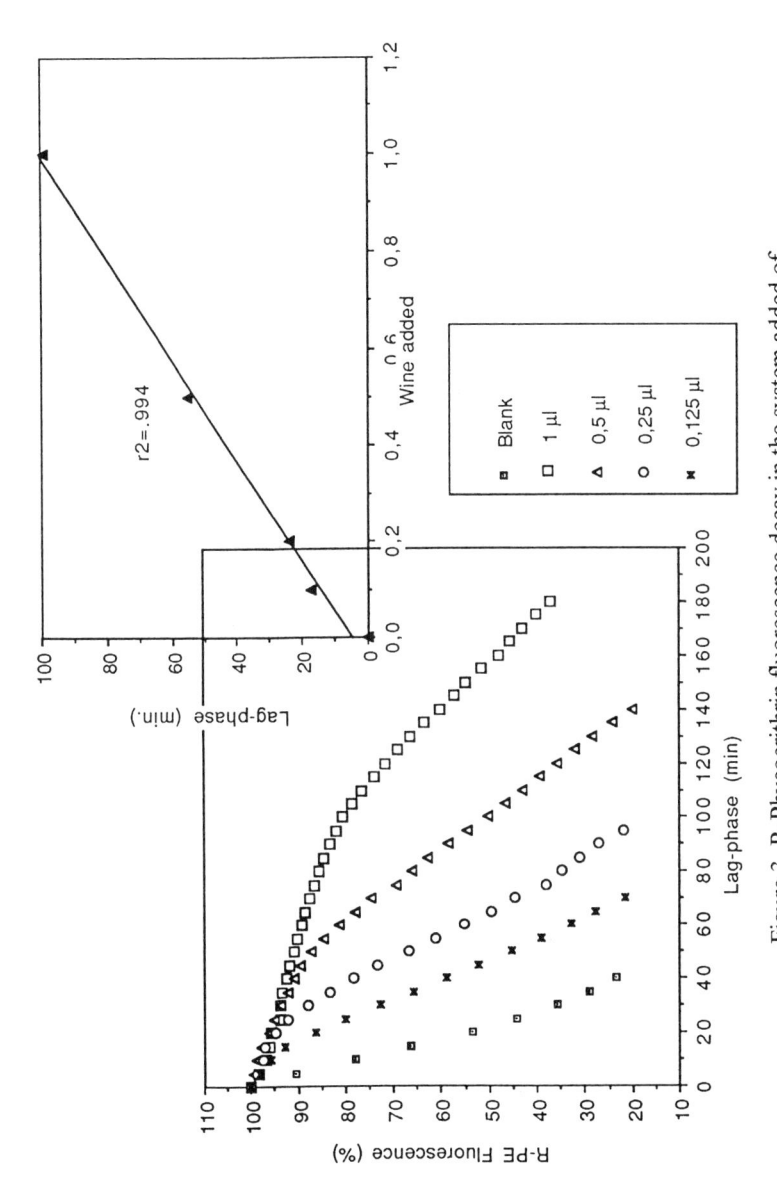

Figure 3. R-Phycoerithrin fluorescence decay in the system added of increasing amounts of wine.

TRAP Test

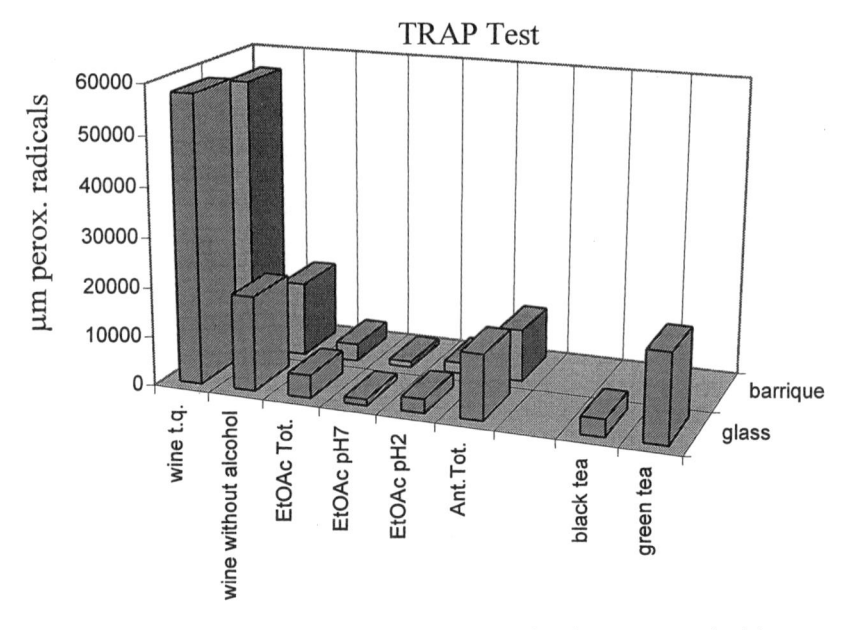

Figure 4. Results of TRAP test on some wine fractions compared with black and green teas.

TRAP test on interaction compounds tannin-anthocyan

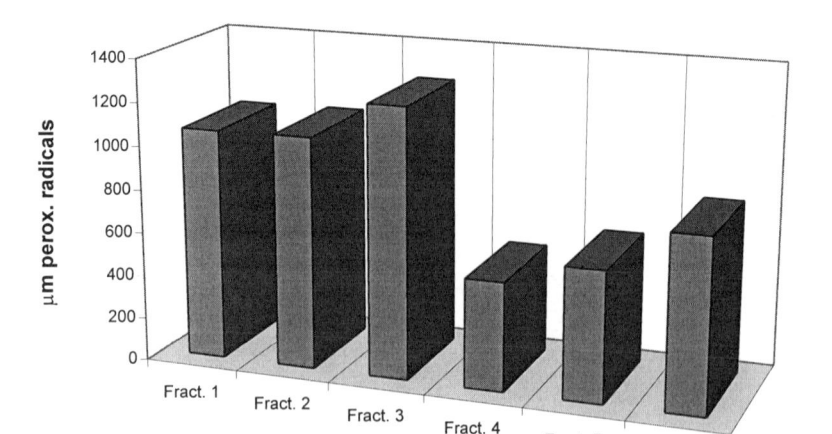

Figure 5. TRAP test values of tannin-anthocyan interaction compounds fractions.

the degradation of 2-deoxyribose, probably due to the higher presence of free anthocyans in grapes respect to wine.
Platelet aggregation assay. Once evaluated the antioxidant effect of wine extracts, their effect on a more complex cellular model was investigated. Human platelets represent an ideal model for this purpose for several reasons:
1- The effect of wine on platelet function is supposed to be a possible explanation of the "French paradox" (*21*)
2- Nutritional antioxidant compounds can influence platelet aggregation (*22-23*)
3- Platelets are a tissue easy to obtain from humans and available in a large number through a simple blood collection followed by centrifugation.
This assay is based on the same principle of the preceding test, with the malondialdehyde (MDA) produced by stimulated platelets instead of the oxidation of the 2-deoxyribose. During platelet aggregation, the cyclooxygenase pathway produces MDA, a reliable marker of the extent of aggregation (*17*). In the platelets, phospholipids of the cellular membrane are involved in the aggregation process, which occurs when a blood vessel is broken. To stop the event, platelets activate the enzyme phospholipase A2 that breaks the fatty acid (usually arachidonic acid) from the phospholipidic molecule. From arachidonic acid, in the cyclooxygenase pathway, cyclic endoperoxides (PGG2, PGH2) are formed, which by means of thromboxanesyntetase, form thromboxane (TXA2). This molecule is an aggregating agent and a vasoconscrictor. For every mole of TXA2, a mole of MDA is produced. The formation of MDA can be detected using the method previously described. This parameter does not represent a measure of the antioxidant power of wine, but a more complex balance in which more than one factor play a role in platelets aggregation (iron chelation, antioxidant activity on free radicals, antienzymatic activity). The results of this test are summarized in Figure 7. Dealcoholated wines A and B showed a great ability to inhibit platelet aggregation in this system. Anthocyans were also very effective to inhibit platelet aggregation, while EtOAc extracts of the solution at pH 7 and pH 2 showed almost the same activity, although lower than the others. Fractions of wine A showed in general higher efficiency than fractions of wine B to inhibit platelet aggregation *in vitro*, findings that could be related to the higher total polyphenolic content.

Conclusion
The application of a liquid/liquid extraction method and the application of some HPLC/MS techniques allowed to separate and identify most of the polyphenols presents in grapes and wines. The different storage conditions allowed to study the same wine in different oxidative status. Particular attention has to be paid to the evolution of the oxidation process. Wine has to be considered as a "living matrix" in which the oxidative status play an important role on organoleptic properties and antioxidant efficiency. On the other side, the application of several *in vitro* and *ex vivo* tests showed that some antioxidant activities could be related to the polyphenolic content. The role of these compounds present in wines has still to be ascertained in living systems, given that *in vitro* experimental conditions are far from physiological conditions. However, results of research indicate that polyphenols in the concentrations present in wines can play an important role in the evolution of the characteristics of wine and can give an antioxidative contribution to the human health.

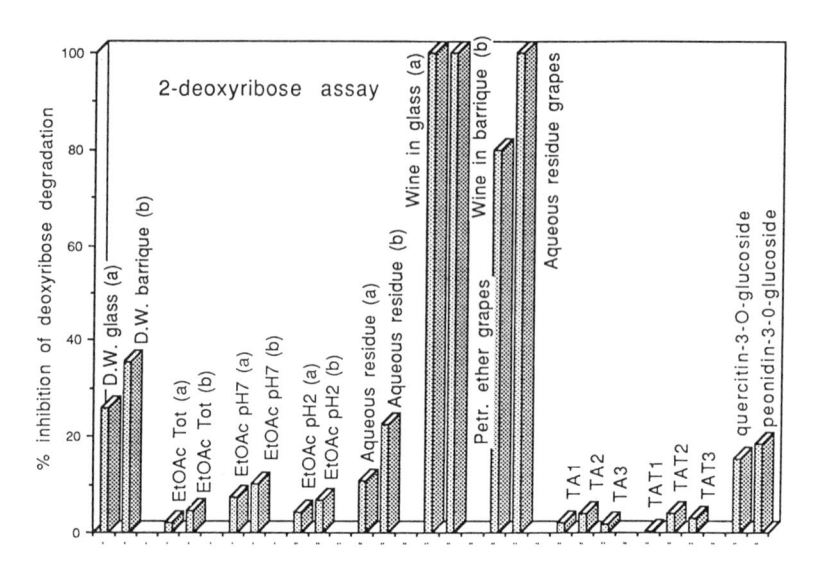

Figure 6. 2-deoxyribose assay results of some grape and wine fractions.

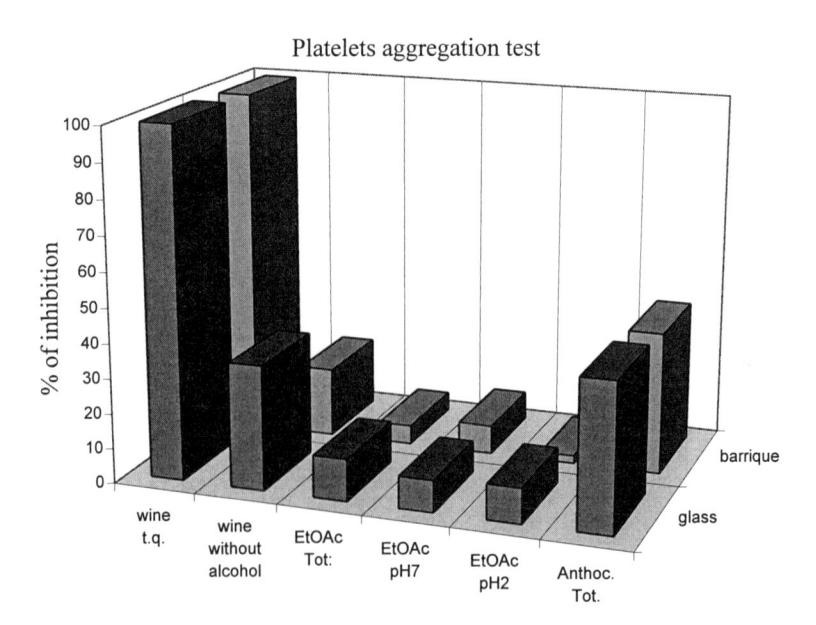

Figure 7. Platelet aggregation assay results of some wine fractions.

Acknowledgment

This work has been supported by grants of CNR (Italian Council of Research). The authors would like to thank the firm "Rocca di Castagnoli" (Gaiole in Chianti, Siena) and in particular Mr. Maurizio Alongi for technical assistance in grape samples collection and wine making.

Literature cited

1. Macheix, J.J.; Billot, J.; Fleuriet, A. In *Fruit Phenolics* C.R.C. Press, Inc. Ed.; I.S.B.N. 0-8493-4969-0; Boca-Raton, FL, USA **1990**; 2-6
2. Kühnau, J. *World Rev. Nutr. Diet* **1976**, *24*, 117-120
3. Okuda, T. In *Polyphenolic Phenomena*; I.N.R.A. Ed.; I.S.B.N./I.S.S.N. 2-7380-0511-X; Paris, France **1994**; 221-235
4. Masquelier, J. *Bulletin O.I.V.* **1991**, 88-93
5. Michaud, J.; Masquelier, J.; Dumon, M.C. *Bull. Soc. Pharm. de Bordeaux* **1981**, *120*, 63-74
6. Bourzeix, M. In *Polyphenolic Phenomena*; I.N.R.A. Ed.; I.S.B.N./I.S.S.N. 2-7380-0511-X; Paris, France **1994**; 157-163
7. Frankel, E.N.; Waterhouse, A.L.; Teissedre, P.L. *J. Agric. Food Chem.* **1995**, *43*, 890-894
8. Frankel, E.N.; Kanner, J.; German, J.B.; Parks, E.; Kinsella, J.E. *The Lancet* **1993**, *341*, 454-457
9. Kanner, J.; Frankel, E.N.; Granit, R.; German, J.B.; Kinsella, J.E. *J. Agric. Food Chem.* **1994** *42*, 64-69
10. Maxwell, S.; Cruickshank, A.; Thorpe, G. *The Lancet* **1994**, *344*, 193-194
11. Mitjavila, S.; Fernandez, Y. *Oenologie* , C.R.A.G. O.I.V. Paris, France **1994**; 13-20
12. Baldi, A.; Romani, A., Mulinacci, N.; Vincieri, F.F. *J. Int. Vigne Vin* **1993**, *27* (3), 201-215
13. Baldi, A.; Romani, A., Mulinacci, N.; Vincieri, F.F.; Casetta, B. *J. Agr. Food Chem.* **1995**, *48*, 2104-2109
14. Riberau-Gayon, P.; Pontallier, P., Glories, Y. *J. Sci. Food Agr.* **1983**, *34*, 505-516
15. Ghiselli, A.; Serafini, M.; Maiani, G.; Azzini, E.; Ferro-Luzzi, A. *Free Rad. Biol. Med.* **1995**, *18*, 29-36
16. Winterbourn, C. *Arch. Biochem. Biophys.* **1986**, *244*, 27-34
17. Violi, F.; Ghiselli, A., Iuliani, L.; Alessandri, C.; Cordova, C.; Balsamo, F. *Haemostasis* **1988**, *18*, 91-98
18. Timberlake, C.F.; Bridle, P. *Am. J. Enol. Vitic..* **1976**, *27*, 97-105
19. Halliwell, B.; Gutteridge, J.M.C.; Aruoma, O.I. *Anal. Biochem.* **1987**, *165*, 215-219
20. Gutteridge, J.M.C. *Biochem. J.* **1984**, *224*, 761-767
21. Renaud, S.; De Lorgeril, M. *The Lancet* **1992**, *339*, 1523-1526
22. Cowan, D.H.; Graham, R.C.; Shook, P.; Griffin R. *Thromb. Haemostas* **1975**, *34*, 50-62
23. Szczeklik, A.; Gryglewski, R.J., Domagala, B.; Dworski, R.; Basista, M. *Thromb. Haemostas.* **1985**, *54*, 425-430

Chapter 14

Metabolic Syndrome X and the French Paradox

Linda F. Bisson

Department of Viticulture and Enology, University of California, Davis, CA 95616-8749

The "French Paradox" is a popularized term referring to the reduction in incidence of coronary heart disease in the French population, in spite of significant fat intake. Since moderate alcohol consumption has also been associated with a reduced risk of coronary heart disease and since the French diet includes wine as a staple, the explanation of the French Paradox has been proposed to be due to moderate daily alcohol consumption. Ethanol increases the level of the so-called "good" HDL cholesterol. However, the effect of ethanol on cholesterol is predicted to account for only a fraction of the impact on cardiovascular health. Increased risk of coronary heart disease has recently been associated with a physiological syndrome called Metabolic Syndrome X. Metabolic Syndrome X is also known as insulin resistance syndrome and is an indicator of increased risk of a cluster of diseases (Reaven, G., 1988, Diabetes 37:1595). Ethanol is a macronutrient energy source in man. It is suggested herein that the effect of ethanol on metabolism of other energy sources may possibly contribute to its effect in reduction of coronary heart disease.

It is well known that diabetic individuals have a dramatically increased risk of development of coronary heart disease. In 1988 Dr. Gerald Reaven and colleagues (19,50-52) reported a correlation between risk for several diseases and impaired glucose tolerance. The failure of the body to properly respond to glucose and insulin signals and clear the bloodstream of this energy source seems to be an early predictor of predisposition to disease. They termed this condition "syndrome X". Since the term "syndrome X" had been previously used to describe another condition, several alternative names have been suggested: Reavan's syndrome, insulin resistance syndrome, Metabolic Syndrome X, metabolic cardiovascular syndrome, and atherothrombogenic syndrome (4,7-10,14,16,19,22,23,29,32,51-53, 62,64, 66). The term "Metabolic Syndrome X" will be used here to refer to this syndrome.

© 1997 American Chemical Society

Metabolic Syndrome X is initially manifested as impaired glucose tolerance and a reduced response of peripheral cells to insulin which leads to high circulatory levels of glucose (51-53) (Figure 1). The failure of peripheral cells to "recognize" that glucose is present leads to a cascading disorder of fuel mobilization and metabolism, eventually leading to even greater insulin resistance and glucose intolerance. In the presence of circulatory glucose, adipose cells impaired in the ability to respond to insulin continue to mobilize lipid for transport to the liver for conversion to ketone bodies. The energy stored in fatty acids can also be used for gluconeogenesis from amino acid carbon. The liver uses a different mechanism for the detection of glucose than the peripheral cells and is still able to recognize that glucose is available. This results in a situation of very high levels of both glucose and lipid circulating in the blood stream and hyperglycemia and dyslipidemia (53). The high levels of these compounds increases the chance of plaque formation in arteries and of overt heart disease. In addition, the impairment of the insulin response may progress to full insulin resistance and diabetes mellitus.

The diseases associated with Metabolic Syndrome X, cardiovascular disease, non-insulin dependent diabetes mellitus, hyperuricemia, certain dietary cancers, obesity and hypertension, can be viewed as consequences of the failure to properly recognize the presence of and respond to fuel sources. This situation will be worsened by excessive caloric intake. The speed with which a pathological condition develops once glucose tolerance has become impaired is dependent upon many factors including diet, lifestyle, and genetic inheritance. Thus, Metabolic Syndrome X appears to define a segment of the population that, while still clinically healthy, is at increased risk for the development of overt disease. The loss of glucorecognition that defines Metabolic Syndrome X disrupts normal macronutrient metabolic interactions. Agents capable of restoring or maintaining normal fuel source regulation may be protective against the development or progression of Metabolic Syndrome X.

Epidemiological studies have suggested that alcohol consumption can reduce risk of both diabetes (50,55) and coronary heart disease (6,15,24,49,54,59,60), two conditions associated with Metabolic Syndrome X. "The French Paradox" is a term that has become equated somewhat erroneously with the epidemiological investigations demonstrating a protective effect of moderate alcohol consumption against coronary heart disease. The French Paradox actually encompasses several dietary and lifestyle differences between American and Mediterranean cultures (54). Ethanol consumption is only one of these differences that may be an important factor in risk of certain diseases. However, the popularization of the French Paradox has resulted in a much needed re-evaluation of the role of ethanol in the human diet.

Ethanol is a macronutrient energy source in man and its presence in the diet affects the metabolism of other fuels as well as the body's response to those fuels. Ethanol enhances both insulin secretion and glucorecognition when present in the bloodstream at the same time as glucose (2,13,20,21,30,35,42,44,46,47,57,65). It also depresses lipid mobilization and fatty acid absorption from the diet (7,11,12,31,38,48,57). These effects of ethanol on overall macronutrient fuel metabolism may explain the reduced incidence of both coronary heart disease and type II diabetes that has been observed in populations of moderate alcohol consumers (50,54,55). The discovery of Metabolic Syndrome X and the possibility of a corrective role played by dietary ethanol clearly warrants further study.

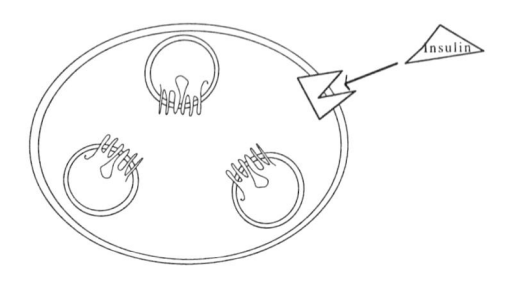

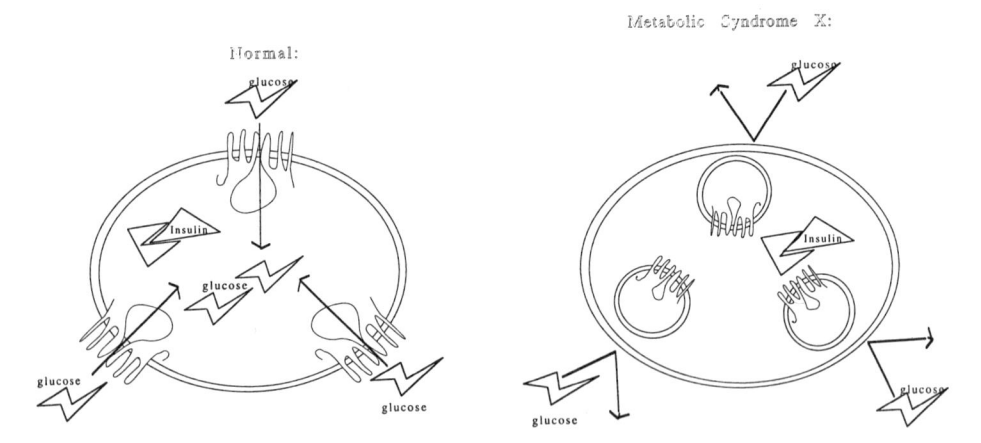

Figure 1. Glucose utilization in normal peripheral cells and in cells from individuals with metabolic syndrome X. In the case of normal cells, insulin stimulates translocation of glucose transporters to the plasma membrane resulting in the uptake of glucose. In the case of metabolic syndrome X, the insulin-mediated stimulation of uptake does not occur.

ACKNOWLEDGMENTS: The author would like to acknowledge George Theodoris for preparation of the figures.

Ethanol as a Macronutrient

Metabolism of ethanol. Three mechanisms for the oxidation of ethanol have been proposed: the alcohol/acetaldehyde dehydrogenase pathway, the microsomal ethanol oxidizing system (MEOS), and catalase (3,39). Since the catalase reaction requires hydrogen peroxide, its physiological significance has been questioned (3). In the first pathway, ethanol is converted to acetaldehyde by alcohol dehydrogenase. Acetaldehyde is then oxidized to acetic acid via aldehyde dehydrogenase. The acetate that is produced from these two reactions is either further metabolized to acetylCoA by acetate thiokinase, an ATP-requiring process, or is released from the liver into the bloodstream for use by the peripheral cells and tissues. The acetylCoA produced from ethanol is then metabolized via the tricarboxylic acid cycle and electron transport chain.

Ethanol can also be metabolized using the microsomal ethanol oxidizing system, also known as the cytochrome P450 system (38,39). In the MEOS system the oxidation of ethanol to acetaldehyde involves molecular oxygen and the reduced cofactor, NADPH. In contrast to the dehydrogenase pathway, this reaction does not generate potentially energy yielding $NADH_2$. The MEOS system is not specific for ethanol and is capable of the oxidation of many other compounds. Also, while alcohol and acetaldehyde dehydrogenase are present constitutively, the MEOS system is only active if ethanol is present. Additional research is needed to determine the exact conditions of MEOS activation in response to dietary ethanol. The variable effects of ethanol on incidence of cancer (17) are likely a consequence of the role of ethanol in activation of the MEOS system and the conversion of other compounds in the diet to potential carcinogens.

Unique aspects of ethanol as an energy source. Ethanol is capable of providing energy for all normal functions of a multicellular organism: cell growth and replication, cell maintenance and function, physical work and thermogenesis. However, in contrast to all other human energy sources, there is no macromolecular storage form of ethanol. Glucose can be stored as glycogen, fats as lipid, and amino acids as protein. While ethanol can be converted to acetylCoA and might be expected to be utilized in lipid biosynthesis, this does not appear to be the case (33,39,56). Rather than be stored for future use, excess ethanol seems to be simply oxidized to carbon dioxide, water and heat by brown adipose tissue (39). How efficient this conversion is depends upon the level and activity of brown adipose tissue in an individual (26). There is some evidence that excessive, chronic alcohol consumption leads to the development of brown adipose tissue in man (26) which is part of the adaptation to ethanol as an energy source. The consequence of the inability to store dietary energy consumed as ethanol means that ethanol will be metabolized in preference to other caloric compounds in a mixture of energy sources. Storage would be preferred for glucose and fatty acids when consumed in the presence of ethanol. Indeed, this is exactly what is observed. In addition, dietary uptake of carbohydrate is enhanced by the presence of ethanol while fatty acid absorption is decreased. The enhancement of utilization of carbohydrate (glucose) is due to the fact that ethanol is not a substrate for gluconeogenesis or lipogenesis and cannot be used to build body mass, therefore glucose must also be consumed. Thus, while ethanol is a source of energy it is not a source of carbon.

A second unique feature of ethanol as an energy source is the fact that the plasma membrane is freely permeable to this compound. Fuel consumption in complex multicellular organisms is a highly coordinated process. Certain cells and tissues, those with a vital function, must have a higher priority for fuel use than the non-vital cells and tissues. For example, the energy needs of the brain must be continually met while muscle and adipose tissue can survive periods of fast. The vital tissues therefore respond directly to the presence of an energy source in the bloodstream. In this case, the energy source functions as a regulatory molecule eliciting a specific cascade of responses from the target cell leading to the consumption of the energy source and the performance of cell function.

When energy sources are in short supply as would occur during a period of fast, the vital tissues utilize the available substrate while non-vital tissues do not. This differential regulation of energy consumption is achieved via hormonal controls. Non-vital tissues do not respond directly to the presence of glucose in the bloodstream, but will only consume glucose if directed to do so by the presence of the hormone insulin. The ultimate target of hormone action is the proteins responsible for the transport of the energy source across the plasma membrane. A cell can be prevented from consuming an energy source if that compound is unable to be transported into the cell. Regulation of transporter protein expression is the primary mechanism utilized by multicellular organisms for the prioritization of fuel use (34). The fact that ethanol freely diffuses across a plasma membrane precludes this type of regulation inoperative.

Multicellular organisms have evolved two mechanisms to regulate ethanol use. First, dietary ethanol is rapidly converted to acetate by the liver which is released into the bloodstream. Between 50 to 100% of dietary ethanol can be converted to acetate by the liver (25,41). Cells of the brain can use acetate as efficiently as glucose (37). Since translocation of acetate across a cell membrane requires a transporter, regulation via transport can be restored. Second, a cell's ability to utilize ethanol can be controlled by adjustment of the level and activity of alcohol dehydrogenase. Cells with reduced total levels of alcohol dehydrogenase will not utilize ethanol as rapidly as those cells containing a high level of activity of this enzyme.

Interactions of Macronutrient Energy Sources and the Coordination of Fuel Consumption

There are two metabolic mechanisms for the generation of energy as ATP in eukaryotic organisms: respiration and fermentation. Only sugars can be fermented. All other energy sources are metabolized via the tricarboxylic acid cycle and the electron transport chain. Of these, most are ultimately converted into acetylCoA, the point of entry to the TCA cycle for respiratory metabolism. Fatty acids, ethanol and amino acids can only yield energy via this pathway in humans, while glucose and fructose can additionally yield energy during glycolysis. Lipid is the most dense chemical form of energy, and is therefore preferred for storage of fuel. As mentioned above, ethanol is unique among the energy sources in not being converted into a macromolecular storage form. The different chemical and biochemical characteristics of energy compounds has led to a specific prioritization of consumption and differentiation of function.

Ethanol and fatty acids. Ethanol and fatty acid oxidation are mutually competitive (48). Both are directly converted to acetylCoA. Both yield circulating energy sources — acetate for ethanol and the ketone bodies for fatty acids, which are converted to acetylCoA post-transport by the recipient cells. The energy derived from fatty acid catabolism can be used to generate glucose for fermentative metabolism and formation of body mass. However, ethanol metabolism does not seem to yield energy that is recaptured in gluconeogenesis. While neither the carbon of ethanol or fatty acids is converted to glucose carbon in gluconeogenesis, energy derived from fatty acid mobilization seems to be able to fuel glucose production in contrast to what is observed with ethanol. The interaction between ethanol and fatty acid metabolism is quite straight forward. Ethanol depresses mobilization of fatty acids from adipose tissue (7,31,38,57), reduces β-oxidation of fatty acids in the liver (11,12), enhances esterification of free fatty acids to triglycerides (12), increases uptake of unesterified fatty acids by the liver (1) and decreases absorption of fatty acids from the diet (7,31,38,57). In short, ethanol blocks fatty acid utilization and directs free fatty acids towards storage as lipid (Figure 2). Ethanol and its metabolite acetate are then utilized as principal energy source.

Ethanol and carbohydrate. The interaction of ethanol and carbohydrate metabolism is more complex but still inherently logical. Since the acetate derived from ethanol does not appear to be utilized in gluconeogenesis (38,39,56), ethanol cannot serve as a source of carbon to build new cell material and body mass in humans. Ethanol stimulates the absorption of carbohydrates from the diet (18,47) (Figure 2). The carbohydrate can then be utilized as carbon source, stored as glycogen or converted to lipid, depending upon the level of carbohydrate consumed and the needs of the body. Ethanol and acetate serve as readily utilizable energy sources for vital tissues, such as the brain (25,37,41). Thus the demand for carbohydrate in the presence of ethanol is restricted to growing or dividing cells, to cells requiring substrate level phosphorylation for efficient function such as muscle, or to cells converting glucose to fatty acids for storage such as adipose tissue. The cells with a higher demand for glucose in the presence of ethanol are the peripheral cells that normally respond to insulin. It is not surprising, therefore, that ethanol results in more efficient usage of glucose by the peripheral cells. The greater efficiency of glucose utilization occurs because ethanol augments the glucose effect on secretion of insulin by the β cells of the pancreas (46). When glucose and ethanol are both present at the same time, a higher concentration of insulin is produced by the β cells, leading to a greater consumption of glucose by the peripheral cells and a lower circulating glucose concentration than would occur with glucose alone. This ethanol-induced hypoglycemia has been observed in numerous studies (28,30,35,44,47,65). In essence, circulating acetate and ethanol substitute for glucose as immediate use energy sources. What is important is the total concentration of circulating energy sources and not the absolute concentration of glucose. Thus, when glucose is the sole energy source the level of glucose in the bloodstream will be set at a higher point than in the presence of ethanol and acetate.

Ethanol (or acetate) also seems to be able to directly stimulate glucose consumption by the peripheral cells in an insulin-independent manner, further reducing blood glucose levels. Ethanol has no effect on the generation of insulin secretion in the absence of glucose (46). It simply augments the glucose signal for insulin secretion but does not generate a signal of its own. Ethanol's protective effect against development of coronary heart disease and adult onset diabetes may be a consequence of its ability to adjust the insulin response to glucose and enhance glucorecognition by peripheral cells. These effects would best be observed if ethanol is consumed simultaneously with other energy sources, that is, only if ethanol accompanies a meal. If ethanol were consumed such that its

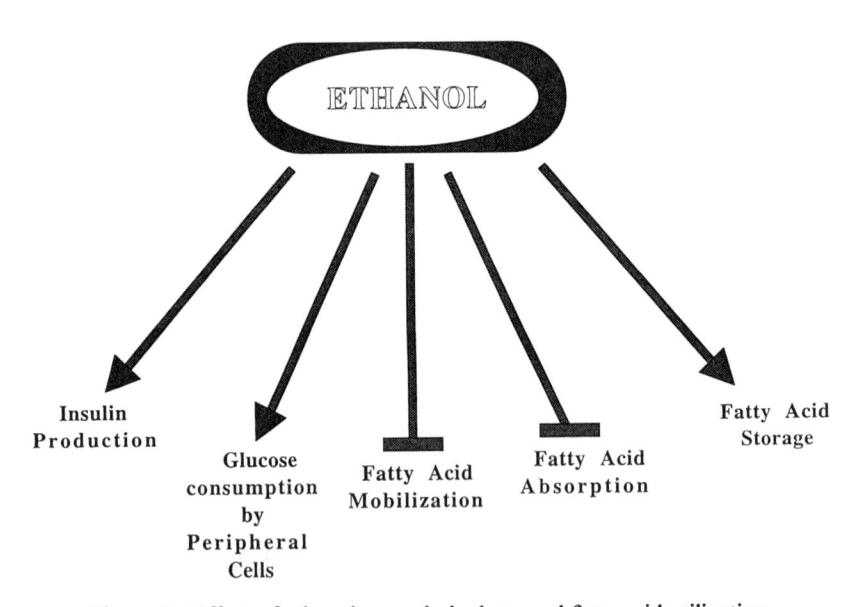

Figure 2. Effect of ethanol on carbohydrate and fatty acid utilization.

metabolism is complete by the time of food intake, it would not be predicted to have the same effects on absorption and metabolism of other macronutrients.

Factors affecting the interplay between ethanol and other macronutrient energy sources. The pattern of energy source consumption is dramatically influenced by other dietary and lifestyle factors. The interactions described above occur in the presence of an overall well-balanced diet of multiple macronutrients and free of micronutrient deficiencies. Efficient consumption of individual energy sources often requires different cofactors or vitamins, the micronutrients. A diet deficient in a particular micronutrient may completely alter the preferences and characteristic pattern of fuel metabolism. Dietary ethanol seems to depress the uptake of certain vitamins like folic acid, thiamin and cobalamin (43,61). With chronic, heavy alcohol consumption, these deficiencies can become acute and negatively impact normal metabolism. Thiamin, as thiamin pyrophosphate, is required for the decarboxylation of pyruvate derived from glucose. If pyruvate decarboxylation is prevented due to a thiamin deficiency, glucose will not be fully metabolized. In this situation, ethanol would block both energy generation and fatty acid biosynthesis from glucose. Similarly, fatty acid and amino acid catabolism requires cobalamin (B12). If cobalamin is deficient because of ethanol depression of uptake, metabolism of these substrates will be much less efficient (6,61). Folic acid is required for biosynthesis, particularly of nucleotide bases used as building blocks for DNA. The inability to produce dTTP for DNA synthesis and repair which accompanies folic acid deficiency will lead to a greater percentage of errors in the DNA and increase the risk of development of certain cancers (27).

Another critical factor influencing the pattern of energy source consumption is the energy demand of the body. Physically active individuals will display a greater requirement for carbohydrate than any other energy source because muscle utilizes fermentation or substrate level phosphorylation for the production of a high level of energy quickly. Respiratory substrates seem unable to confer the same level of performance to muscle tissue as is afforded by glucose. Also, while the physiological mechanisms of this regulation remain obscure, the storage demand will also influence fuel use. There will be more efficient utilization of fatty acids under conditions of expansion of lipid reserves. Lastly, genetic factors and lifestyle influence such things as amount of brown adipose tissue and muscle mass, which will affect energy storage and demand.

Ethanol and Metabolic Syndrome X. With respect to Metabolic Syndrome X and loss of glucose tolerance, dietary ethanol would improve glucose tolerance by generating a higher insulin signal for a given concentration of glucose (Figure 3) and would also stimulate the peripheral cells to respond to insulin and consume glucose (Figure 4). In this case, ethanol might be able to restore proper circulating glucose levels and delay or even prevent the cascading derangement of fatty acid metabolism accompanying the defect in glucorecognition. Ethanol consumed with carbohydrate would behave differently than ethanol consumed independently of carbohydrate. This may also explain some of the discrepancies in the literature on the protective effect of ethanol against coronary heart disease. The results of such studies would be impacted by the manner in which alcohol is consumed. This is true in general of metabolic studies.

Insulin Production by Beta Cells

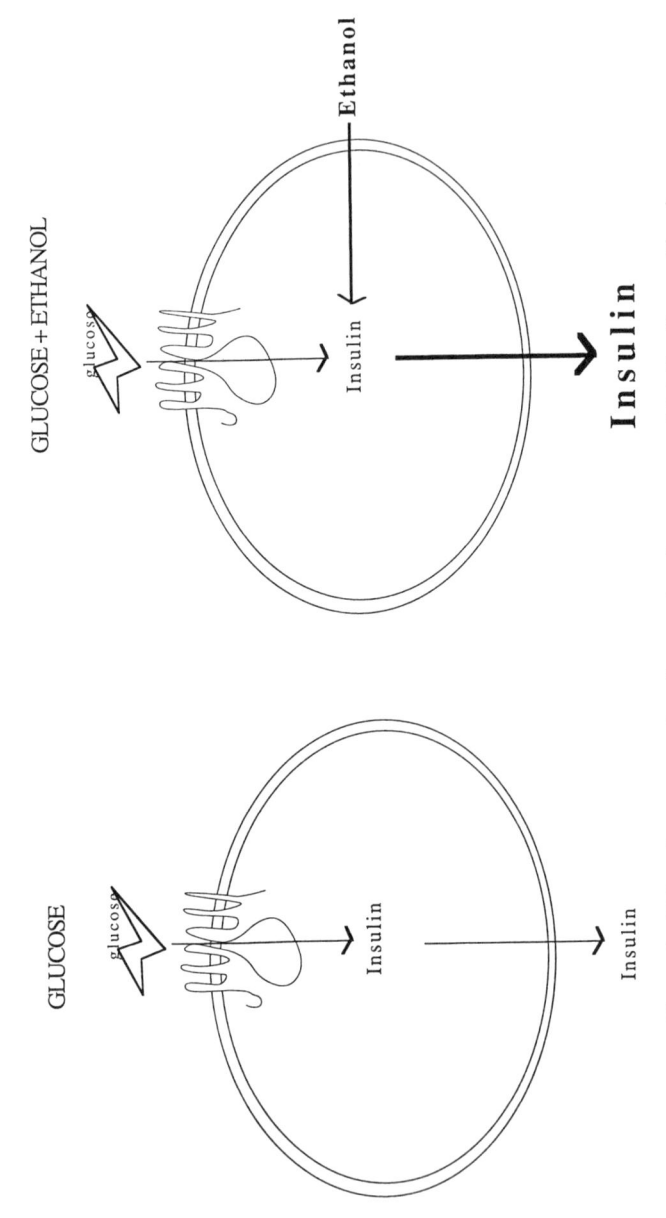

Figure 3. Ethanol augments the glucose signal to pancreas islet β cells resulting in production of elevated levels of insulin.

Effect of Ethanol on Glucose Consumption by Peripheral Cells

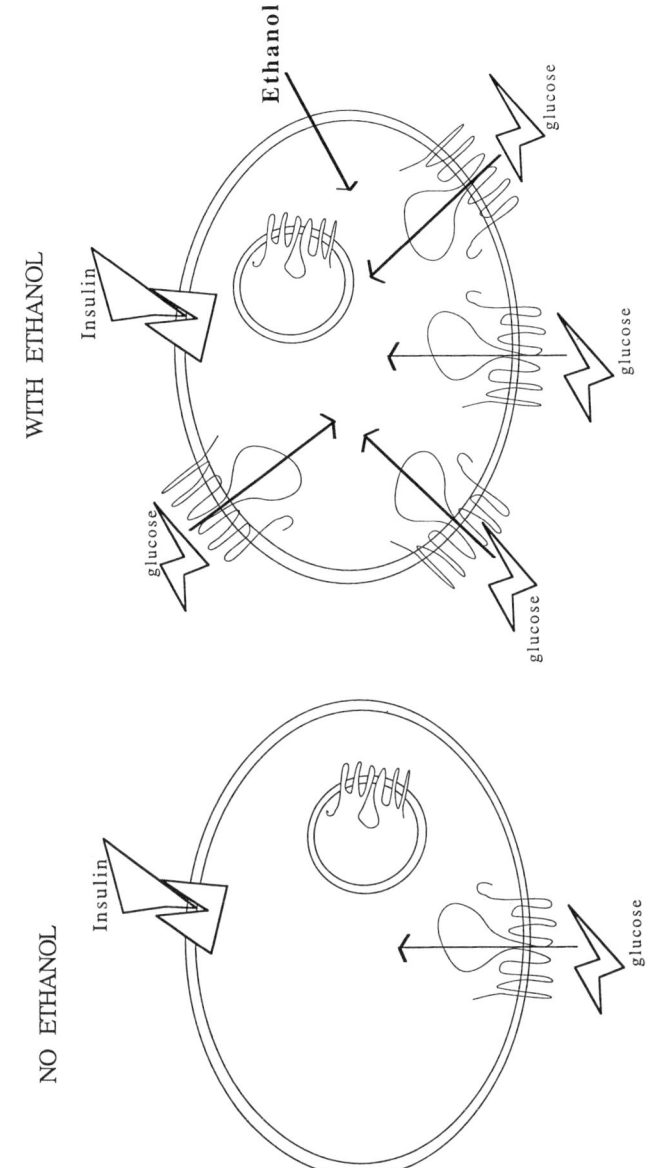

Figure 4. Effect of ethanol on glucose consumption by peripheral cells. Ethanol augments the insulin signal leading to greater uptake of glucose by peripheral cells as compared to insulin alone.

Toward a Definition of Moderate Consumption

While moderate consumption of ethanol may be beneficial for reducing risk of certain diseases, chronic, excessive alcohol consumption clearly leads to disease. The definition of moderate ethanol consumption remains a critical and open question. It is as irresponsible to recommend a given amount of ethanol be consumed by the entire population as it would be to recommend a single level of carbohydrate (glucose) consumption. In the case of glucose, the "safe" level of consumption obviously would differ for individuals with diabetes or a predisposition to diabetes as compared to the rest of the population. The recommended level of carbohydrate consumption would also vary depending upon the amount of physical activity sustained by the individual.

Similar arguments can be made against a blanket recommendation for a generic level of ethanol consumption. As a consequence of genetic background, certain individuals are at high risk of development of physiological disorders from alcohol consumption. The appropriate level of alcohol consumption for these individuals would be lower than that of the rest of the population. This situation is exactly analogous to the negative physiological impact of continued glucose consumption in individuals with type II diabetes. While there are clearly defined tests to determine the level of glucose intolerance in individuals, there is no such equivalent assay for ethanol intolerance. Recommendations for specific patterns of consumption of calorie sources cannot ignore genetic predisposition to adverse effects from that consumption. In the case of alcohol, it is not yet clear what types of biochemical markers should be analyzed to define the segment of the population at high risk from ethanol consumption. However, given the possible protective effect of ethanol against development of the Metabolic Syndrome X diseases, specifically of type II diabetes and coronary heart disease, a blanket recommendation to abstain from alcohol is equally irresponsible. It is imperative that studies be undertaken to refine our understanding of the role of ethanol in macronutrient metabolism and maintenance of health.

With these caveats in mind, it is possible to begin to define moderate ethanol consumption. The level of moderate ethanol consumption that would be considered ideal for the prevention of coronary heart disease or diabetes is clearly dependent upon the composition of the rest of the diet. If ethanol consumption leads to a micronutrient deficiency, then that level of consumption is too high. This of course could be corrected by increasing the content of vitamin-rich foods in the diet as well as by reducing ethanol. Given the potential involvement of the MEOS system in increased risk of certain cancers, moderate ethanol consumption can in addition be defined as that level of ethanol that enhances glucorecognition without sustained induction of the MEOS system. Ethanol consumption becomes excessive when oxidative metabolism becomes so saturated that fatty acids begin to accumulate in the liver leading to fatty liver and cirrhosis. In this case, the optimal level of ethanol will be directly dependent upon the enzymatic composition of the liver and its metabolic capacity for the conversion of ethanol to acetate. Ethanol consumption is also excessive when acetaldehyde accumulates as in the case of saturation of acetaldehyde dehydrogenase. Finally, ethanol consumption is excessive if ethanol exceeds the level of alcohol dehydrogenase activity and the liver's ability to convert ethanol to acetate. In this case, circulating ethanol levels are elevated. If ethanol consumption leads to any one of the above mentioned metabolic scenarios, the level of consumption is too high. It is important to correlate the protective effect of ethanol consumption with these indicators of a potential problem to determine if a level of consumption can be identified that is desirable from an overall health perspective. Because of its solubility properties, ethanol is capable of perturbing plasma membrane function which may lead to a disruption of cellular function and even cell death. Thus, the recommended level of ethanol consumption to reduce risk of disease will differ based upon the metabolic capacity of an individual, genetic predisposition to an alcohol-related disorder, as well as on overall diet and lifestyle. It is unlikely that there will be a single definition of moderate ethanol consumption, but many definitions depending upon genetic and physiological factors.

Conclusion: The Need for Further Research

The observation that coronary heart disease may be correlated with an impairment of glucose tolerance suggests that ethanol's protective effect against the development of this disease may be a consequence of its known impact on carbohydrate metabolism and role as a macronutrient energy source in the human diet. Ethanol is able to augment the glucose-induced secretion of insulin and stimulates glucose consumption by peripheral cells. The mutually competitive nature of ethanol and fatty acid metabolism may also explain the health-promoting effects of ethanol on lipid mobilization and metabolism. The possible effect of dietary ethanol on the development and progression of Metabolic Syndrome X may in part explain the French Paradox and the beneficial effects of the Mediterranean diet. Hopefully the arguments presented above have been provocative enough to stimulate much needed research on the interactions of macronutrient fuels in the diet and on the role of perturbation of the normal pattern of fuel metabolism in health and disease.

Literature Cited

1. Abrams, M. A. and C. Cooper. Mechanism of increased hepatic uptake of unesterified fatty acid from serum of ethanol-treated rats. Biochem. J. 156:47-54 (1976).
2. Adner, N. and A. Nygren. The influence of indomethacin, theophylline, and propranolol on ethanol augmentation of glucose-induced insulin secretion. Metab. 41:1165-1170 (1992).
3. Badaway, A. A.-B. The metabolism of alcohol. Clinics Endocrin. Metab. 7:247-271 (1978).
4. Bain, S. C. and P. M. Dodson. The chronic cardiovascular risk factor syndrome (Syndrome X): mechanisms and implications for atherogenesis. Postgrad. Med. J. 67:922-967 (1991).
5. Baraona, E. Ethanol and lipid metabolism. **In: Alcohol Related Diseases in Gastroenterology.** H. K. Seitz and B. Kommerell, Eds., pp. 65-95. Springer, Verlag, Berlin (1985).
6. Baraona, E. and C. S. Lieber. Effects of ethanol on lipid metabolism. J. Lipid Res. 20:289-315 (1979).
7. Beck-Nielsen, H., O. H. Nielsen, P. Damsbo, A. Vaag, A. Handberg and J. E. Henriksen. Impairment of glucose tolerance: mechanism of action and impact on the cardiovascular system. Am. J. Obstet. Gynecol. 163:292-295 (1990).

8. Beer, S. F., D. A. Heaton, K. G. M. M. Alberti, D. A. Pyke and R. D. G. Leslie. Impaired glucose tolerance precedes, but does not predict insulin-dependent diabetes mellitus. A study of identical twins. Diabetologia 33:497-502 (1990).
9. Bergstrom, R. W., D. L. Leonetti, L. L. Newell-Morris, W. P. Shuman, P. W. Wahl and W. Y. Fujimoto. Association of plasma triglyceride and C-peptide with coronary heart disease in Japanese-American men with a high prevalence of glucose intolerance. Diabetologia 33:489-496 (1990).
10. Bjorntorp, P. Abdominal fat distribution and the metabolic syndrome. J. Cardiov. Pharmacol. 20:S26-S28 (1992).
11. Blomstrand, R. and L. Kager. The combustion of triolein-1-^{14}C and its inhibition by alcohol in man. Life Sci. 13:113-123 (1973).
12. Blomstrand, R., L. Kager and O. Lantto. Studies on the ethanol-induced decrease of fatty acid oxidation in rat and human liver slices. Life Sci. 13:1131-1141 (1973).
13. Boyd, A. E. and L. G. Moss. When sugar is not so sweet: glucose toxicity. J. Clin. Invest. 92:2 (1993).
14. Clauster, E., I. Leconte and C. Auzan. Molecular basis of insulin resistance. Horm. Res. 38:5-12 (1992).
15. Crouse, J. R. and S. M. Grundy. Effects of alcohol on plasma lipoproteins and cholesterol and triglyceride metabolism in man. J. Lipid Res. 25:486-496 (1984).
16. Cusin, I., F. Rohner-Jeanrenaud, J. Terrettaz and B. Jeanrenaud. Hyperinsulinemia and its impact on obesity and insulin resistance. Int. J. Obes. 16:S1-S11 (1992).
17. Doll, R., D. Forman, C. LaVecchia and R. Woutersen. Alcoholic beverages and cancers of the digestive tract and larynx. *In*, Health Issues Related to Alcohol Consumption. P. M. Verschuren (Ed), pp. 125-166 ILSI Europe (1993).
18. Dornhorst, A. and A. Ouyang. Effect of alcohol on glucose tolerance. Lancet 2:957-959 (1971).
19. Ferrannini, E. Syndrome X. Horm. Res. 39:107-111 (1993).
20. Field, J. B., H. E. Williams and G. E. Mortimore. Studies on the mechanism of ethanol-induced hypoglycemia. J. Clin. Invest. 42:497-506 (1963).
21. Freinkel, N., A. K. Cohen, R. A. Arky and A. E. Foster. Alcohol hypoglycemia. J. Clin. Endocrinol. 25:76-94 (1965).
22. Haffner, S. M., R. A. Valdez, H. P. Hazuda, B. D. Mitchell, P. A. Morales and M. P. Stern. Prospective analysis of the insulin-resistance syndrome (Syndrome X). Diabetes 41:715-722 (1992).
23. Hjermann, I. The metabolic cardiovascular syndrome, Syndrome X, Reaven's Syndrome, insulin resistance syndrome, atherothrombogenic syndrome. J. Cardiovasc. Pharmacol. 20:S5-S10 (1992).
24. Hojnacki, J. L., J. E. Cluette-Brown, M. Dawson, R. N. Deschenes and J. J. Mulligan. Alcohol delays clearance of lipoproteins from the circulation. Metab. Clin. Exp. 41:1151-1153 (1992).
25. Huang, M.-T., C.-C. Huang and M.-Y. Chen. *In vivo* uptake of ethanol and release of acetate in rat liver and GI. Life Sci. 53:165-170 (1993).
26. Huttunen, P. and M.-L. Kortelainen. Long-term alcohol consumption and brown adipose tissue in man. Eur. J. Appl. Physiol. 60:418-424 (1990).

27. James, S. J., A. G. Basnakian and b. J. Miller. In vitro folate deficiency induces deoxynucleotide pool imbalance, apoptosis and mutagenesis in Chinese hamster ovary cells. Cancer Res. 54:5075-5080 (1994).
28. Kallner, A. and L. Blomquist. Effect of heavy drinking and alcohol withdrawal on markers of carbohydrate metabolism. Alc. Alcoholism 26:425-429 (1991).
29. Karam, J. H. Type II diabetes and Syndrome X: Pathogenesis and management. Endocrin. Metab. Clin. N. Am. 21:329-350 (1992).
30. Kendrick, Z. V., M. B. Affrime and D. T. Lowenthal. Effect of ethanol on metabolic responses to treadmill running in well-trained men. J. Clin. Pharmacol. 33:136-139 (1993).
31. Kondrup, J., N. Grunnet and J. Dich. Interactions of ethanol and lipid metabolism. **In: Human Metabolism of Alcohol, Volume III. Metabolic and Physiological Effects of Alcohol.** K. E. Crow and R. D. Batt, Eds., pp. 97-113. CRC Press, Boca Raton, FL (1989).
32. Koutis, A. D., C. D. Lionis, A. Isacsson, A. Jackobsson, M. Fioretos and L. H. Lindholm. Characteristics of the "Metabolic Syndrome X" in a cardiovascular low risk population in Crete. Eur. Heart J. 13:865-871 (1992).
33. Koziet, J., P. Gross, G. Debry and M. J. Royer. Evaluation of (^{13}C) ethanol incorporation into very-low density lipoprotein triglycerides using gas chromatography/isotope ratio mass spectrometry coupling. Biolog. Mass. Spec. 20:777-782 (1991).
34. Kraegen, E. W., J. A. Sowden, M. B. Halstead, P. W. Clark, K. J. Rodnick, D. J. Chisholm and D. E. James. Glucose transporters and *in vivo* glucose uptake in skeletal and cardiac muscle: fasting, insulin stimulation and immunoisolation studies of GLUT1 and GLUT4. Biochem. J. 295:287-293 (1993).
35. Larue-Achagiotis, C., A.-M. Poussard and J. Louis-Sylvestre. Does alcohol promote negative hypoglycemia in the rat? Physiol. Behav. 47:819-823 (1990).
36. Leahy, J. L., S. Bonner-Weir and G. C. Weir. Beta cell dysfunction induced by chronic hyperglycemia. Current ideas on mechanism of impaired glucose-induced insulin secretion. Diab. Care 15:442-455 (1992).
37. Lear, J. L. and R. F. Ackermann. Evaluation of radiolabeled acetate and fluoroacetate as potential tracers of cerebral oxidative metabolism. Metab. Brain Dis. 5:45-56 (1990).
38. Liber, C. S. Alcohol, liver and nutrition. J. Am. Coll. Nutr. 10(6):602-632 (1991).
39. Lieber, C. S. Perspectives: Do alcohol calories count? Am. J. Clin. Nutr. 54:976-982 (1991).
40. Lieber, C. S. and R. Schmid. The effect of ethanol on fatty acid metabolism; stimulation of hepatic fatty acid synthesis *in vitro*. J. Clin. Invest. 40:394-399 (1961).
41. Lundquist, F., N. Tygstrup, K. Winkler, K. Mellemgaard and S. Munck-Peterson. Ethanol metabolism and production of free acetate in the human liver. J. Clin. Invest. 41:955-961 (1962).
42. Marks, V. Alcohol and carbohydrate metabolism. Clinics Endrocrinol. Metab. 7:333-349 (1978).

43. Martin, P. R., G. Impeduglia, P. R. Giri and J. Karanian. Acceleration of ethanol metabolism by past thiamin deficiency. Alcohol. Clin. Exp. Res. 13:457-460 (1989).
44. McMonagle, J. and P. Felig. Effects of ethanol ingestion on glucose tolerance and insulin secretion in normal and diabetic subjects. Metab. Clin. Exp. 24:625-632 (1975).
45. McPherson, K., E. Engelsman and D. Conning. Breast cancer. *In:* Health Issues related to Alcohol Consumption. P. M. Verschuren, pp. 221-224. ILSI Europe (1993).
46. Metz, R., S. Berger and M. Mako. Potentiation of plasma insulin response to glucose by prior administration of alcohol. Diabetes 18:517-522 (1969).
47. Nikkila, E. A. and M. R. Taskinen. Ethanol-induced alterations of glucose tolerance, postglucose hypoglycemia and insulin secretion in normal, obese, and diabetic subjects. Diabetes 24-933-943 (1975).
48. Ontko, J. A. Effects of ethanol on the metabolism of free fatty acids in isolated liver cells. J. Lipid Res. 14:78-86 (1973).
49. Parkes, J. G., R. A. Hussain and D. M. Goldberg. Effect of alcohol on lipoprotein metabolism I. High density lipoprotein binding. Clin. Physiol. Biochem. 7:269-277 (1989).
50. Perry, I. J., S. G. Wannamethee, M. K. Walker, A. G. Thompson, P. H. Whincup and A. G. Shaper. Prospective study of risk factors for development of non-insulin dependent diabetes in middle aged British men. Brit. Med. J. 310:560-564 (1995).
51. Reaven, G. M. and Y.-D. I. Chen. Role of insulin in relation of lipoprotein metabolism in diabetes. Diabetes Metab. Rev. 4:639-652 (1988).
52. Reaven, G. M. Role of insulin resistance in human disease. Diabetes 37:1595-1607 (1988).
53. Reaven, G. M. Role of insulin resistance in human disease (Syndrome X): An expanded definition. Ann. Rev. Med. 44:121-131 (1993).
54. Renaud, S., M. H. Criqui, G. Farchi and J. Veenstra. Alcohol drinking and coronary heart disease. *In:* Health Issues Related to Alcohol Consumption. P. M. Verschuren (Ed.). pp. 81-123. ILSI Europe (1993).
55. Rimm, E. B., J. Chan, M. J. Stampfer, G. A. Colditz and W. C. Willett. Prospective study of cigarette smoking, alcohol use, and the risk of diabetes in men. Brit. Med. J. 310:55-559 (1995).
56. Schumann, W. C., I. Magnusson, V. Chandramouli, K. Kumaran, J. Wahren and B. R. Landau. Metabolism of [2-^{14}C] acetate and its use in assessing hepatic Krebs cycle activity and gluconeogenesis. J. Biol. Chem. 266:6985-6990 (1991).
57. Shelmet, J. J., G. A. Reichard, C. L. Skutches, R. D. Hoeldtke, O. E. Owen and G. Boden. Ethanol causes acute inhibition of carbohydrate, fat, and protein oxidation and insulin resistance. J. Clin. Invest. 81:1137-1145 (1988).
58. Taskinen, M.-R., E. A. Nikkilä, M. Välimäki, T. Sane, T. Kuusi, A. Kesäniemi and R. Ylikahri. Alcohol-induced changes in serum lipoproteins and in their metabolism. Am. Heart J. 113:458-464 (1987).
59. Taskinen, M.-R., M. Valimaki, E. A. Nikkila, T. Kuusi, C. Ehnholm and R. Ylikahri. High density lipoprotein subfractions and postheparin plasma lipases in

alcoholic men before and after ethanol withdrawal. Metabolism 31:1168-1174 (1982).
60. Taskinen, M.-R., M. Valimaki, E. A. Nikkila, T. Kuusi and R. Ylikahari. Sequence of alcohol-induced initial changes in plasma lipoproteins (VLDL and HDL) and lipolytic enzymes in humans. Metabolism 34:112-119 (1985).
61. Thompson, A. D. Alcohol and nutrition. Clinics Endocrin. Metab. 7:405-428 (1978).
62. Vague, P. and D. Raccah. The syndrome of insulin resistance. Horm. Res. 38:28-32 (1992).
63. Venkatesan, S., N. W. Y. Leung, and T. J. Peters. Fatty acid synthesis *in vitro* by liver tissue from control subjects and patients with alcohol liver disease. Clin. Sci. 71:723-728 (1986).
64. Winocour, P. H. Coronary heart disease in diabetes mellitus — antecedents and associations. Postgrad. Med. J. 67:917-921 (1991).
65. Yki-Jarvinen, H. and E. A. Nikkila. Ethanol decreases glucose utilization in healthy man. J. Clin Endocrin. Metab. 61:941-945 (1985).
66. Zavaroni, I., S. Mazza, M. Fantuzzi, E. Dall'aglio, E. Bonora, R. Delsignore, M. Passeri and G. M. Reaven. Changes in insulin and lipid metabolism in males with asymptomatic hyperuricemia. J. Int. Med. 234:25-30 (1993).

Chapter 15

Wine Phenolics and Targets of Chronic Disease

J. Bruce German[1], Edwin N. Frankel[1], Andrew L. Waterhouse[2], Robert J. Hansen[3], and Rosemary L. Walzem[3]

Departments of [1]Food Science and Technology, [2]Viticulture and Enology, and [3]Molecular Biosciences, University of California, Davis, CA 95616-8749

The role of oxidative stress in the development of chronic diseases such as atherosclerotic cardiovascular disease, cancer and autoimmunity, and post-ischemia injury, trauma and ultimately in aging is under intensive investigation. As the significance of oxidation in the etiology of disease has been recognized, the ability of certain nutrients - antioxidants - to retard these processes chemically has led to the hypothesis that ingestion of such nutrients may prevent these disease states. Wine is one of the richest natural sources of the flavonoid class of antioxygenic polyphenolics. To understand how wine and plant phenolics in general could affect health status, it is necessary to understand the complexity of oxidation as a chemical process and the biochemistry that has evolved as a response.

Paradoxically, oxidation, the chemical process by which oxygen is added and withdraws energy from reduced carbon-based molecules, is a life-sustaining process. It is the coupled transport of electrons, captured from the oxidation of ingested foodstuffs, in the mitochondria that fuels each of our cells. During a billion-year evolutionary course within an oxygen atmosphere, living organisms have found free radical oxidative reactions to be both highly necessary and potentially disastrous to their highly-reduced constituent macromolecules. The selective pressures of these forces have produced a complex spectrum of biochemical systems that either utilize or detoxify products of free radical chain reactions. We are only now beginning to recognize and understand that these systems interact to control normal growth and development. As our understanding of the interactions between oxidant-generating/utilizing systems and the ancillary protective/repair processes grows, so will our ability to identify points at which normal deviates towards pathological and where intervention by flavonoids may be beneficial.

'Oxidative stress' is a catch phrase that describes a general phenomenon of oxidant exposure or antioxidant depletion. Oxidant exposure and damage are now believed to be caused by many events, both chronic and natural and acute and catastrophic (*1*). Gross tissue damage accrues, for example, following the induction of oxidative stress by chemical intoxication or iron overload (*2-4*). More subtle chronic damage may be caused by production of reactive species during the course of normal metabolism (*5*).

© 1997 American Chemical Society

For example, macrophages release activated oxygen as part of the normal inflammatory response in order to generate the chemically toxic oxygen radicals that kill invading pathogens. In this defensive strategy, the health threat of local tissue damage is balanced against the asset in preventing systemic infection, and further selected for the evolution of repair systems to effectively respond to this transient damage. However, chronic inflammation, as occurs in autoimmune disorders, due primarily to overactive host reactions, creates pathological tissue changes (6,7). That the normally protective processes can create overt tissue pathology underscores the power of oxidative chemistry and the risks associated with the biological generation of oxidative species.

These observations suggest that organisms must tolerate a balance between the benefits and risks of free radical oxidative chemistry. The balance can be shifted in either a detrimental or beneficial direction by changing the predominance of prooxidative processes and antioxygenic protection. Studies that test the implications of this hypothesis are being conducted world wide. Many of these studies are 'natural experiments' in the sense that epidemiology relates disease incidence to genetic and environmental variables in free-living populations. Evidence from such studies suggests that a disparity between basal antioxidant protectants and the oxidative stress experienced by an individual may result in repetitive oxidative damage to sensitive tissue and plasma targets. Imbalance and repetitive oxidative damage also appear to lead to functional deterioration and accumulation of potentially toxic by-products of the oxidant response and repair systems as well.

The concept of balance carries profound implications for the study of oxidation biology and the etiology of chronic disease. Recently, a further conceptual advance was made with the recognition that non-essential components of the diet may actively participate in the oxidative balance of living creatures. The non-essential polyphenolic compounds in wine were identified as antioxidants whose level in plasma of moderate wine consumers was proposed to retard the oxidative modification of low density lipoproteins (LDL), a chemical event causal to atherosclerosis (8).

This review describes the dynamics of oxidative chemistry within biological systems. The multistage nature of the process is emphasized since complexity forms the basis for multiple mechanisms of pathogenesis. Furthermore, it is by virtue of the chronic and pervasive nature of free radical oxidative events that routine dietary consumption of polyphenolic materials is thought to be of broad benefit.

Chemistry of Oxidation

Thermodynamic equilibrium strongly favors the net oxidation of reduced, carbon-based biomolecules. The rather paradoxical (and fortuitous) kinetic stability of all biological molecules in our oxygen-rich atmosphere is due to the unique spin state of the unpaired electrons in ground state molecular oxygen in the atmosphere. Ground state molecular (triplet) oxygen is kinetically stable due to the spin state of its unpaired electrons. This property renders atmospheric oxygen relatively inert to reduced, carbon-based biomolecules. Hence, reactions between oxygen and protein, lipids, polynucleotides, carbohydrates, etc. proceed at vanishingly slow rates unless they are catalyzed. However, once a free radical chain reaction is initiated, the free radicals that it generates rapidly propagate, interacting directly with various targets and also yielding hydroperoxides. These hydroperoxides are readily attacked by reduced metals leading to a host of decomposition products. Some of these products are capable of causing further damage, some, formed through self-propagating reactions, are themselves free radicals; thus, oxidation is re-initiated. A voluminous literature has emerged during the gradual unraveling of this chemistry among biological lipids, and points to several key participants in the reaction course (*9-10*).

Initiators of oxidation eliminate the reactive impediments imposed by the spin restrictions of ground state oxygen by converting stable organic molecules, RH, to free radical-containing molecules, R·. Oxygen reacts immediately with such species to form the peroxy radical, ROO·. Initiators of lipid oxidation are relatively ubiquitous, primarily single electron oxidants, and include trace metals, hydroperoxide cleavage products and light. A risk of evolving biological systems that use polyunsaturated fatty acids (PUFA) is that these molecules are oxidized by the ROO· species to yield another free radical, R·, and a lipid hydroperoxide, ROOH. This effectively sets up a self-propagating free radical chain reaction, $R· + O_2 \rightarrow ROO \rightarrow ROOH + R$, that can lead to the complete consumption of PUFA in a free radical chain reaction (*11*). The ability of the peroxy radical to act as an initiating, single-electron oxidant drives the destructive and self-perpetuating reaction of PUFA oxidation.

Decomposition of hydroperoxides formed during lipid oxidation produces a variety of short-chain aldehydes, ketones and alcohols (*9*). Products such as these, in addition to radicals, can damage functional molecules in a variety of ways (Table I) and compromise the health of the animal. The susceptibility of an individual lipid to oxidation, and therefore its overall rate of oxidation, is controlled by the ease of hydrogen abstraction, which in turn is related to the abundance of double bonds on fatty acids. As the number of double bonds in a molecule increases, the number of methylenic hydrogens increases as well, which increases the rate of oxidation. For example, the fatty acids 18:1, 18:2, 18:3 and 20:4 have relative oxidation rates of 1, 50, 100 and 200. The relative rate of oxidation as a function of number of double bonds may be important to rates of deterioration of biological molecules in vivo. It has now been documented that diets high in PUFA require more antioxidant nutrients such as tocopherols to prevent oxidation and rancidity. Significantly, animals consuming diets high in PUFA also have been suggested to require additional antioxidant protection to prevent tissue damage. Unfortunately, to date the precise molecular nature of this increased requirement is not clear, and many of the studies that purport to show an increase in oxidative damage actually show only an increase in crude measures of lipid oxidation, namely thiobarbituric acid-reactive substances (TBARS). The assay for TBARS is fundamentally unable to distinguish varying oxidative damage between dietary fats since it is differently responsive to the same amount of oxidation from different levels of unsaturation. Although on the basis of chemical reactivity, a diet enriched in highly unsaturated fatty acids would appear to increase the tendency to oxidation and increase the incidence of all chronic degenerative diseases associated with increased oxidation, this has not been observed. To the contrary, in many cases the replacement of more saturated fat diets with highly unsaturated fats, including fish oils, frequently results in a reduction in atherosclerosis, thrombosis and other chronic diseases (*7*). Thus, when considering the myriad effects of dietary fats on tissue oxidation, it is critical to understand all of the various biochemical and metabolic consequences as well. The means by which PUFA actually decrease oxidation in circulating LDL was recently proposed to be due to a significant reduction in circulating age of the lipoproteins (*12*). Similarly, the ability of phenolic phytochemicals from wine to inhibit oxidative biochemical and metabolic pathways may significantly alter their net effect on tissue oxidative damage.

Antioxidants and Biological Containment of Inappropriate Oxidation

The chemistry of free radical oxidations is multistage and complex. Oxidation is not a single catastrophic event. There is no single dangerous or reactive product of oxidation, rather there are classes of products many of which are both selectively and broadly damaging. There is no single initiating oxidant that generates all free radicals, rather there are a great many sources of single electrons. Thus, there is no simple means to prevent them. Free radicals and their products react with virtually all biologically-important molecules, and no single defense will protect all targets of oxidative damage. To counter this diversity of potential devastation, organisms have evolved a variety of strategies and mechanisms to prevent or respond to oxidative stresses and the presence of free radicals and their products (Table II). Thus, the corollary to the inherent complexity of the multistage process of oxidation is that it can be inhibited at one or more of its many steps.

To fully appreciate the potential health effects of wine phenolics in antioxidant protection, they must be placed within the context of the overall response of living organisms to oxidation. Living organisms do not react passively to oxidant stress. This is not surprising given the precarious dependence of living organisms on the kinetic impediment of ground state oxygen to prevent their rapid oxidation. All organisms have evolved highly complex biochemical pathways to deal with oxidation. Pathways range from regenerating oxidized protectants to extra- and intracellular oxidant recognition mechanisms to oxidant-sensing genetic response elements. Among higher animals, these response pathways also extend to wholesale induction of gene families that code for protection and repair proteins up to the recruitment of distant cells to affected tissues. The complexity and interdependence of these systems indicate that oxidative stress could increase requirements for not only direct antioxidants but also those nutrients essential for proper up-regulation of oxidant defense and repair mechanisms.

Antioxidants

Antioxidant is a broad classification for molecules that may act prior to or during a free radical chain reaction, at initiation, propagation, termination, decomposition or during the subsequent reaction of oxidation products with sensitive targets. Antioxygenic compounds can participate in several of the protective strategies described for higher animals (Table II). Differences in point of activity are not trivial, and influence the efficacy of a given compound to act as a net antioxidant or protectant. Distinctions in how different molecules act can also profoundly affect the impact of oxidation, and its inhibition, on normal biological function and damage. The alkyl radical, R·, is considered much too highly reactive in an oxygen-rich environment for any competing species to successfully re-reduce R· to RH before oxygen adds to form the peroxy

Table I. Consequences of Inappropriate Oxidation

Reaction	Examples
Direct oxidation of susceptible molecules with resultant loss of function	Oxidation of membrane lipids alters membrane integrity, promotes RBC fragility and membrane leakage; oxidation of proteins results in loss of enzyme catalytic activity and/or regulation
Adduct formation with loss of native functions	Oxidative modification of the apoB molecule on LDL prevents uptake by the LDL receptor and stimulates uptake by the scavenger receptor
Oxidative cleavage of important molecules that impairs or destroys their functionality	DNA cleavage, point, frame shift, deletion and base damage all translate into altered sequence at replication
Liberation of signal molecules or analogs to signal molecules that elicit specific but inappropriate cellular responses	Leukotoxin and eicosanoid analogs activate cellular responses such as platelet aggregation, and down-regulate vascular relaxation

Table II. Antioxidant Defense Strategies and Systems

Strategy or System	Examples
Prevent oxidant formation	Isolate initiators, oxidants or reactive metabolites: Mitochondria and peroxisomes are specialized cellular organelles that contain the generation and transfer of electrons, and which dispose of toxic intermediates and products of metabolism. Transferrin and ceruloplasmin are plasma proteins that actively sequester iron and copper ions capable of initiating oxidation.
Scavenge activated oxidants	Primary chain-reaction breaking antioxidants include α-tocopherol, ubiquinone, ascorbate, uric acid, polyphenolics, various flavonoids and their polymers, amino acids and protein thiols. Use of amino acids and protein thiols as antioxidants implies functional and energetic compromise.
Reduce reactive intermediates	Higher animals possess enzyme systems that scavenge active oxygen, including superoxides dismutase, catalase and peroxidases. Other enzymes detoxify reactive intermediates, and include catalase (hydrogen peroxide scavenger), glutathione peroxidase (removes hydroperoxides) and superoxide dismutase (reduces superoxide anion). Natural food constituents with antioxidant activity can also act as free radical quenchers, antioxidants and or protectors/regenerators of other antioxidants. Synergistic (13) and antagonistic effects among mixtures of antioxidant compounds are possible based on the nature of redox couples formed by compounds present in tissues. Phenolic antioxidants stabilize some enzymes, enhancing activity, while inhibiting others.
Induce repair systems	Proteases, lipases, RNAases, etc. constantly turn over cellular constituents, and degradative enzymes often have higher affinities for modified molecules. Substrate affinities of synthetic enzymes discriminate against oxidized forms of lipids, proteins and nucleotides. This discriminatory process acts to remove damaged molecules from the cell and it's structures. Oxidation of protein transcription factors such as NF-kappa-B (14) change their binding properties. Oxidized transcription factors bind to what are termed 'oxygen response elements' of promoters for selected genes. This is now recognized as a means for the cell to detect oxidant levels and induce gene families (e.g., genes encoding peroxidases) to properly respond to the stress.
Apoptosis	Cells that are unrepairable are abandoned by the process of 'programmed cell death' or apoptosis. This same process is used by higher organisms to selectively reshape tissues during normal growth and development, and when exposed to other types of subnecrotic stress. Whole-scale activation of oxygen response elements is probably involved. This process disassembles cells in a highly regulated and coordinated fashion. Apoptosis is also a damage containment strategy as it prevents the release of reactive and toxic compounds from lysosomes, peroxisomes, etc.

radical, ROO˙. At this point, however, ROO˙ is a relatively stable free radical that reacts relatively slowly with susceptible targets such as PUFA. This is the most widely accepted point of action for free radical scavenging antioxidants such as the phenolic tocopherol. Tocopherol can reduce ROO˙ to ROOH with such ease that tocopherol is competitive with biologically-sensitive targets such as unsaturated lipids, RH, even at 10,000-fold lower concentration. The tocopheroxyl radical, A˙, is in general a poor oxidant and reacts significantly more slowly than the original oxidant, ROO˙. Conversion of ROO˙ to ROOH and formation of A˙ effectively imparts a kinetic hindrance on the propagating chain reaction. The tocopheroxyl radical can be either re-reduced by reductants such as ascorbate, dimerize with another radical or be further oxidized to a quinone. These free radical scavenging functions of tocopherol are very well documented (15).

Tocopherol has vitamin status, and loss of its free radical scavenging properties is believed to be the basis for its essentialness and the pathologies associated with its deficiency. That the basis for the essentialness of tocopherol lies in its ability to prevent oxidative damage raises an important nutritional question: Are these actions also provided by non-essential polyphenolics present in plants and foods derived from them, and in particular wine? A host of chemical studies implicate many of the phenolics in wine as capable of interfering with and inhibiting free radical chain reactions of lipids. Wine phenolics inhibit lipid hydroperoxide formation catalyzed by metals, radiation and heme compounds (13,16). Polyphenolics from wine and other plants scavenge peroxy, alkoxy and hydroxy radicals and singlet oxygen (16-18). Flavonoids have been shown to spare tocopherol consumption in oxidizing lipid systems (19,20). If α-tocopherol is truly an essential antioxidant and acts in situations that no other compound can, the sparing effect of non-essential antioxidants may be one of their most important actions.

Antioxidant activity is not limited to prevention of hydroperoxides (Table II). Hydroperoxides are relatively easily detected, and indicate that oxidation has occurred, but are not considered to be directly damaging to either to foods or biological molecules. However, the reductive decomposition of hydroperoxides by reduced metals generates even more reactive free radicals, the hydroxyl radical, HO˙, or the alkoxyl radical, RO˙. These strongly electrophilic oxidants react with and oxidize virtually all biological macromolecules. Furthermore, the alkoxy radical typically fragments the parent lipid molecule and liberates electrophilic aldehydes, hydrocarbons, ketones and alcohols. Both the highly reactive hydroxy and alkoxy radicals and the electrophilic aldehydes liberated with their reduction react readily with polypeptides (proteins) and polynucleotides (DNA). Thus, vital additional modes for antioxidant action in protecting biologically-sensitive molecules include either prevention of hydroperoxide decomposition, reduction of the alkoxyl radicals or scavenging the electrophilic aldehydes produced. Different antioxidants vary in their efficacy during this phase of the oxidation progress. Even tocopherol isomers differ with respect to their ability to prevent decomposition of hydroperoxides (21,22). The phenolics found in wine vary in their ability to interrupt a free radical chain reaction with differences detectable among different lipid systems, oxidation initiators and other antioxygenic components.

Biology Uses Risky Oxidation Chemistry

Organisms need to cascade and amplify chemical signals to develop appropriate responses to many stressors, including oxidants. It is notable that many of these signaling systems are themselves oxidant-generating pathways. Among the most familiar examples of such signaling are the enzymatic systems that oxidize specific PUFA moieties to form potent signaling molecules. These molecules, termed oxylipins (prostaglandins, leukotrienes, etc.), all serve to alert adjacent or responsive cells of a state of stress. Enzymatically produced oxidized lipids even act on higher order brain functions such as pain and even sleep. Oxidation of some protein transcription factors allows binding to 'oxidant response elements' within DNA and directly affect its transcription. This cascading proliferation of oxidized molecules does accomplish the tasks of intracellular and multicellular signaling, but also places a burden on oxidant defense systems. These chemical signals clearly co-evolved with the increasingly sophisticated oxidant repair systems. Perhaps the presence of these oxidant defenses (Table II) allowed the non-fatal use of oxidants. The comparative biochemical evidence is consistent with a parallel evolution of both oxidant response and oxidant signaling pathways of ever increasing sophistication.

Net Oxidation: A Balance between Prooxidants and Antioxidants

As now described, oxidation is initiated in cells, tissues and fluids by a host of chemical, and more importantly, enzymatic and protein factors. Many of the oxidation events initiated by organisms are necessary for, or at least valuable to, the success of the organism. Thus, organisms use oxidation, but there is a clear risk-benefit relationship (Table III). Biology seemingly accepts the risk because, at least in the short term, oxidation provides a net benefit. The long-term consequences may only be relevant to aging organisms and poorly defended tissues. Unfortunately, both situations occur in humans.

There is a growing point of view that many chronic diseases develop as a result of unprotected or aberrant oxidation. Repetitive oxidant damage can accrue over a life-time and greatly influence the health of the individual. Developments in the field of oxidant biology emphasize the need to re-evaluate antioxidant requirements in relation to cellular dysfunction. The requirement for oxidant defense will vary with oxidant stress. It is difficult to believe that antioxidant effects defined under conditions of zero stress are in any way meaningful for a system under even brief, acute stress such as viral infections, inflammation, trauma and exposure to environmental pollutants. Even less relevance is discernible during states of chronic and sustained oxidant stress such as autoimmunity, chronic infection, elevated circulating lipoproteins or mild antioxidant deficiency. Thus, estimates of population requirements for antioxidant defense would seem to be best based on individuals exposed to an 'average' or 'typical' amount of oxidant stress. The concept of what constitutes 'typical' oxidant stress is undefined. Definition of such a parameter would be difficult since a variety of insults can elicit an oxidant stress both directly and indirectly in ways heretofore unrecognized.

Diseases Associated with Oxidation

Increasing evidence implicates oxygen free radicals as mediators of numerous degenerative and chronic deteriorative, inflammatory and autoimmune diseases (*23*), including rheumatoid arthritis (*24*), diabetes, vascular disease and hypertension (*25,26*), cancer and hyperplastic diseases (*5,27*), cataract formation (*5,28*), emphysema (*29*), immune system decline and brain dysfunction as well as the aging process (*5*). An imbalance in oxidant-antioxidant activity is involved in free radical-mediated pathologies such as ischemia-reperfusion and asthma (*30*).

As outlined in the preceding sections, a number of cellular and organismal processes are controlled or affected by oxidants or oxidation. Mechanisms for how perturbations of oxidant balance lead to systemic, multifactorial diseases can now be postulated. In fact, multiple mechanisms probably operate simultaneously. One of the best examples of how oxidant imbalance can cause cellular dysfunction and disease is found in the 'French paradox.'

French Paradox - Fat vs. Antioxidant Intake. The association of saturated fatty acid intake with mortality and morbidity from atherosclerotic cardiovascular disease, (ASCVD) does not apply for certain French populations. Whereas the reported coronary mortality per 10,000 people in the USA is 182, the mortality of the French, in general, is 102, while in the Toulouse region, it is 78 (*31*). This discrepancy is referred to as the "French paradox." The French people have similar intakes of saturated fatty acids, similar risk factors and comparable plasma cholesterol as the US population. The only dietary factor that showed a negative correlation with ASCVD was wine consumption. Renaud and de Lorgeril (*31*) pointed out that while there is an association between reduced ASCVD and alcohol consumption generally, the "alcohol" in red wine was superior to that provided in other alcoholic beverages. Thus, it appeared that the beneficial effects of red wine were partly contributed by components other than alcohol. To understand how wine could reduce the incidence of ASCVD, we must understand the pathogenesis of this disease.

LDL Oxidation and ASCVD. The lesions of ASCVD are progressive, that is, they become larger and more severe over time. The first identifiable is the fatty streak, a cluster of lipid-engorged macrophages whose appearance earned the name foam cell. The lipids in these cells were recognized decades ago as largely derived from LDL but how the macrophage, without an LDL receptor, accumulated such high levels of LDL was only reconciled recently by the oxidation hypothesis. Oxidative modification of LDL makes native, and possibly quite benign, LDL a substrate for the macrophage scavenger receptor, and hence more atherogenic (*32,33*). Oxidized cholesteryl esters and other PUFA oxidation products modify LDL and contribute to ASCVD etiology (*33*).

Table III. Endogenous Oxidant Generating Systems with Potentially Pathogenic Consequences

Oxidant Generating System	Pathogenic Potential
Fenton chemistry	The univalent reduction of hydroperoxides by transition metals, especially ferrous and cuprous salts, yields an unpaired electron as either the alkoxyl or hydroxyl radical. Probably the most destructive free radical-initiating system, the presence of free metals and oxidized lipids in atherosclerotic plaque is strong evidence that oxidation of tissues and lipoproteins contributes to lesion progression.
Mitochondrial electron transport	Mitochondria transfer billions of electrons per day into oxygen in single-electron steps that eventually converts metabolizable hydrocarbon into carbon dioxide and water. Even with the fidelity of transfer equal to 99.999% of total electrons transferred, leakage from this system is a significant source of reactive oxygen species. Release of free radicals has been estimated to be in excess of 10^6 free radical species per day. This imperfection of mitochondrial oxidative coupling is the basis of the mitochondrial damage theory of aging.
Respiratory burst	The immune system has evolved a 'leaky' oxygen-reducing system to combat pathogenic organisms. Stimulation of the terminal oxidase in phagocytes produces a literal burst of oxygen consumption that is stoichiometrically converted to superoxide. Superoxide kills cells in the immediate vicinity of the oxidant burst, but is non-specific and can damage host cells as well as invading pathogens. The animate immune response is a good example of the overall cost-benefit equation that is inherent to animal stress responses.
Oxygenating enzymes	Many, and perhaps all, cells respond to various external stimuli by liberating PUFA from cellular membranes. Arachidonic acid is particularly labile, and initiates a signal cascade that depends upon its free radical-catalyzed, enzymatic oxygenation to hydroperoxide derivatives broadly termed eicosanoids. These stereospecific molecules are local signals that activate that cell and its immediate neighbors. In this way, the eicosanoids act as part of the cellular stress response system in higher organisms. Chronic or over-activation of this system constitutes and oxidative stress that can produce inflammation and activate additional systems. Often referred to as 'peroxide tone.'
Reductive cleavage of peroxides	A general class of enzymes called peroxidases eliminate peroxides as a general detoxifying mechanism. Certain of the peroxidases catalyze oxidant production as a result of this reaction. Peroxidase oxidant production generally accompanies a response to pathogen invasion, and so are considered as additional elements in the killing mechanisms of immune cells. Chronic or over-activation of this system constitutes an independent oxidative stress.
Xenobiotic metabolism	The liver of higher animals is the primary tissue involved in the conversion of toxic chemicals into excretable compounds. This conversion is effected by inducible enzymes that are typically oxidases. As a result, toxin metabolism can and does produce free radical species. The poisonous properties of a host of pesticides, etc, are now recognized to result from the secondary by-products produced during the metabolism of xenobiotics.

The increased atherogenicity of LDL following oxidative modification is proposed to result from their uncontrolled uptake into subendothelial macrophages by a receptor specific for damaged (oxidized) particulates, like red blood cells, and LDL (*34*). The result of the accumulation of oxidized LDL by these macrophages is a gradual development of an inflamed and proliferative tissue site that leads ultimately to atheromatous plaque and vascular disease. An actual heart attack occurs when the roughened surface of the vascular tissue that overlies the plaque activates platelets, which form a clot or thrombus and occlude the artery. Platelet activation is also an oxidant-dependent reaction. Prevention of ASCVD by antioxidant protection could result from both prevention of peroxidative lipoprotein modification and the additional effects of antioxidants on cellular or immunological activity (*35*). As such, there are several sites at which interference with oxidant generation and its consequences would slow ASCVD or reduce the incidence of heart attacks. Antioxidants, including those from wine, may reduce peroxidation of PUFA and LDL and thereby decrease macrophage foam cell formation. They could reduce chronic inflammation tendencies by reducing peroxides, down-regulating the arachidonic acid cascade and reducing platelet aggregability and thrombotic tendencies (*36*).

The view of oxidation as the key to ASCVD is somewhat at odds with traditional views of atherosclerotic risk. Elevated LDL is the fundamental correlate of disease incidence and has captured considerable attention due to its ability to predict death from ASCVD in humans. However, until quite recently there was no verifiable explanation for why, if LDL oxidation was causing ASCVD, high levels of LDL should be more readily oxidized. In experiments using lipoproteins during circulation, Walzem et al. (*12*) showed that the susceptibility of lipoproteins to oxidation increases as their age in circulation increases. Since increased intravascular LDL residence time in humans almost invariably accompanies elevated plasma LDL cholesterol, the average LDL of hypercholesterolemics is older. Thus, individuals with high LDL cholesterol are in essence imposing an elevated oxidant stress on LDL by prolonging their exposure to the oxidative environment of the intravascular compartment.

If protection of LDL from oxidant stress prevents or slows the development of ASCVD, it becomes important to determine how and what can protect LDL. Vitamin E has a well-recognized physiological function as a biological antioxidant in scavenging free radicals and preventing oxidant injury to PUFA in cell membranes or within the surface of lipoproteins. Considerable evidence suggests that vitamin E is the major lipid-soluble free radical scavenger in vivo (*37*). LDL is the metabolic end-product of very low density lipoprotein (VLDL) catabolism. The number of tocopherol molecules present in each LDL particle is determined by the activity of tocopherol transfer protein during VLDL synthesis. Once secreted, if the protectors of lipoprotein are consumed, they are not likely to be replenished. Depletion of LDL α-tocopherol precedes LDL oxidation. LDL contain less than ten tocopherol molecules per particle. Whether or not this amount of tocopherol as the sole antioxidant protection available to the LDL particle is adequate or reflective of the conditions that humans evolved with is not known.

Plant Phenolics as Antioxidants

The relative role of different antioxidants in LDL protection is still controversial. Some of the controversy stems from differences in methodologies. When water-soluble oxidants are used in studies of this type, water-soluble plasma antioxidants such as ascorbate appear to elicit the most effective protection (38). However, when LDL are isolated and their susceptibility in vitro is measured, preparation of the LDL via centrifugation and dialysis removes all water-soluble protection; then the lipid-soluble antioxidants, particularly vitamin E, appear to be the sole protection. Tocopherols are quite effective in delimiting propagation of free radical chain reactions, and they may be partially regenerated by other reductants. However, tocopherols do not stop free radical initiation reactions, hence their action as the sole protectant may be limited.

Wine Phenolics and ASCVD. Kinsella et al. (36), Frankel et al. (8) and Kanner et al. (13) proposed that nonalcoholic compounds, the phenolic antioxidants, that are abundant in red wine are responsible for protection of the French from ASCVD via prevention of LDL oxidation and inhibition of platelet aggregation. Consumption by the French of red wine, fruits and vegetables containing phytochemical antioxidants may decrease the peroxidative tendencies and retard interactions involved in atherogenesis and thrombosis. Wine phenolics can effectively participate in several antioxidant defenses (Table II), inhibit platelet aggregation, spare α-tocopherol and may protect sensitive targets like proteins or DNA.

Phenolic Composition of Grapes, Wines and Foods. Among the numerous natural constituents of foods, principally of plant origin, that have antioxidant activity are the polyphenols. The phenolic compounds are primary antioxidants that act as free radical acceptors and chain breakers. Polyphenols include salicylic, cinnamic, coumaric and ferulic derivatives and gallic esters. In grapes alone, the following phenolics have been identified: phenolic acids (hydroxybenzoic, salicylic, cinnamic, coumaric and ferulic derivatives, and gallic esters), flavonols (kaempferol and quercetin glycosides), flavan-3-ols (catechin, epicatechin and derivatives), flavanonols (dihydroquercetin, dihydrokaempferol and hamnoside) and anthocyanins (cyanidin, peronidin, petunidin, malvidin, coumarin and caffein glucosides). In compounds that are derivatives of benzoic and cinnamic acids as well as flavonoids, the degree of hydroxylation and position of hydroxylation are important in determination of the antioxidant efficiency (39). For example, in white mustard, p-hydroxybenzoic acid is the major phenolic present, followed by sinapic acid; together, these represent 36% of the total phenolics (40). Among the antioxidative components of low-pungency mustard flower, the major antioxidants are sinapic acid, p-hydroxybenzoic acid and trihydroxy phenolic compounds, such as flavones or flavones (41).

Evaluation of antioxidative activity of naturally-occurring substances has been of interest; however, there is a lack of knowledge about their molecular composition, the amount of active ingredients in the source material and relevant toxicity data. The proposal that the altered disease risk in specific populations could be explained by a mechanism involving antioxidant polyphenolics in fruits and fruit products focused considerable scientific and public scrutiny on the actions of these compounds in human health. This interest has produced epidemiological studies, mechanistic hypotheses and testing of oxidant/antioxidant effects in the progression of several diseases. These diseases can be classified by the aberration in oxidant balance that is believed to cause them. The breadth of associations between consumption of plant phenolics and improved human health demands scientific investigation. This research group has focused on candidate molecules, their absorption and their mechanisms of action (8,12,13,36). The research community is now developing testable hypotheses to further assess the mechanisms of these associations.

Diseases Associated with Direct Oxidation/Damage

DNA Damage and Cancer. Aside from ASCVD, cancer is the most significant chronic disease associated with direct oxidative damage. In a review of epidemiological literature on vegetable and fruit consumption and human cancer, Steinmetz and Potter (42) found a consistent association between higher levels of fruit and vegetable consumption and a reduced risk of cancer, particularly with epithelial cancers of the alimentary and respiratory tracts. These authors also addressed possible mechanisms by which these foods might alter risk of cancer (43). The authors hypothesized that humans are adapted to a high intake of plant foods that supply crucial substances to maintain the organism. Cancer may result from decreasing the level of intake of foods that are metabolically necessary. Among the potentially anticarcinogenic agents in foods are carotenoids, vitamin C, vitamin E, selenium, dietary fiber, dithiolthiones, glucosinolates, indoles, isothiocyanates, flavonoids, phenols, protease inhibitors, sterols, allium compounds and limonene. The complementary and overlapping mechanisms suggested for these compounds by Steinmetz and Potter (43) include "the induction of detoxification enzymes, inhibition of nitrosamine formation, provision of substrate for formation of antineoplastic agents, dilution and binding of carcinogens in the digestive tract, alteration of hormone metabolism, antioxidant effects, and others."

The biochemical backgrounds for the actions of cancer-protective factors in fruits and vegetables were reviewed in detail (44). The authors based their simplified model on a generalized initiation-promotion-conversion model for carcinogenesis. In this model, initiators are directly or indirectly genotoxic, promoters are substances capable of inferring a growth advantage on initiated cells and converters are genotoxic. The mechanisms of anticarcinogenic substances in fruits and vegetables were related by the authors to the prevention and inhibition of cancer, notably by antioxidant-related activities. Among many other compounds discussed, these authors noted that polyphenols from fruits and vegetables could protect against cancer initiation by scavenging activated mutagens and carcinogens, acting as antioxidants, inhibiting activating enzymes and by shielding sensitive structures (e.g., DNA). Mechanisms acting at the biochemical level towards anti-promotion include the scavenging of activated oxygen, stabilization of membranes and the inhibition of ornithine decarboxylase.

Diseases Associated with Oxidant Signaling

With the recognition that cellular stimulation activates oxidant production systems to generate very potent signal molecules has come the logical possibility that such systems could be inappropriately stimulated (*11,45,46*). Thus, the very systems that respond to stress may be destructive and exacerbate or even initiate distinct pathological states. The best described of the stress response systems are the oxygenated fatty acids or eicosanoids, and several examples of pathologies associated with their excessive production are known.

Prostaglandins and Thrombosis. The processes of thrombosis are ostensibly those of inappropriate blood clotting; however, it is actually the culmination of many factors that produces a clotted artery. The critical principle underlying this pathology, and the practical problem in successful interventions, is that platelet clotting is ultimately an absolutely essential event that prevents an individual from excessive bleeding. The vascular system is basically a plumbing network conducting a relatively viscous fluid at high flow and pressure. The utility of the self-contained hole-plugging response system provided by platelet aggregation is obvious. Platelets are the cell type that act most directly to recognize vessel wall disruptions, to signal a rapid, multicellular response and then to initiate the construction of a physical barrier to prevent further blood loss.

In view of the paradigm developed above, it is not surprising that oxidant signaling systems have evolved in biology to respond rapidly to stress, and that platelets take advantage of this system as well. Platelets are known to oxygenate arachidonic acid via two discrete oxygenating systems: the prostaglandin synthetase-thromboxane synthetase couple that produces thromboxane, the most active platelet aggregating and vasoconstricting of the arachidonic acid metabolites (and one of the most potent yet described), and the 12-lipoxygenase enzyme that produces 12(S)-HPETE, an arachidonic acid hydroperoxide that promotes adherence of platelets to vascular surfaces. Interestingly, these enzymes are not absolutely required elements of the platelet-clotting cascade since in their absence platelets will still clot; nevertheless, these two systems of oxygenating fatty acids act to accelerate and amplify the clotting processes. Thus, platelets, in response to both appropriate (bleeding) and inappropriate (atherosclerosis) conditions, actively produce oxidants as a means to cascade the signaling of clotting. This knowledge has been the basis for developing oxygenase inhibitors as pharmacological agents to prevent thrombosis, and many prostaglandin inhibitors, notably aspirin, are widely recommended as antithrombotic agents. Aspirin is a salicylate phenol originally derived from willow (*Salix*) bark. The therapeutic successes of small doses of aspirin beg the question, do natural polyphenolics consumed in foods that inhibit oxidation inhibit the enzymatic oxygenation of platelets that promote thrombosis? In vitro, the epithelial lipoxygenase is inhibited by the grape phenolic catechin at low micromolar concentrations (47). The platelet enzyme from humans was found to be inhibited by wine phenolics, the most likely candidate of which was catechin, which in pure form showed half-maximal inhibition at 1 µM concentration (Matsuo and German, unpublished).

Leukotrienes and Asthma. Asthma is a prototypical autoimmune condition in which the excessive recruitment of inflammatory immune cells is distinctive. Several immune cell modulators are known to be responsible for the bronchoconstriction associated with allergen challenge to pulmonary mast cells. The most potent bronchoconstricting substances characterized are the 5-lipoxygenase products, the leukotrienes. Again, in direct analogy with several other signaling systems, when these cells are challenged, arachidonic acid is released and is actively oxygenated via a free radical oxidation reaction to a stereospecific hydroperoxide, which in the case of the leukotrienes is converted by an additional free radical reaction to the leukotriene precursor LTA4. In the case of asthma, mast cells are considered the main source of histamine and slow-reacting substances of anaphylaxis, SRS-A, the signal molecules implicated in bronchoconstriction, but neutrophils and eosinophils are also well known to be associated with asthmatic lungs. In each case, the recruitment and activation of these cells is enhanced by the production of oxidized lipids, especially the eicosanoids. Similarly, cell activity and severity of bronchoconstriction are reduced by pharmacological agents that block the production of oxidized signal lipids. Various phytochemicals (plant secondary metabolites), including polyphenolics, have been documented to inhibit these pathways, and have been argued to be of therapeutic benefit for inflammatory lung diseases, including asthma.

Diseases Associated with Oxidant-Induced Cell Activation

Phagocyte Activation and Asbestosis. Although the mechanism of lung fibrosis after asbestos exposure is unknown, observations suggest that neutrophils may play a role in the development of the lung injury. Lung mediators attract macrophages which then phagocytize asbestos fibers. Asbestos also exerts a cytotoxic effect on polymorphonuclear leukocytes, which in response release proteolytic enzymes such as collagenase and elastase. In addition, asbestos causes the production of highly-reactive oxidants in neutrophils that are responsible for additional damage to tissues. While the role of polymorphonuclear leukocytes, such as neutrophils, in pathogenesis of asbestosis still remains controversial (48), the potential for antioxidant phenolics both as protectants from direct oxidant damage and for down-regulating oxidant signaling in recruiting phagocytic cells is evident. The benefits of tocopherol to asbestos-induced oxidant damage vividly poses the question, could other phenolics from plants interfere with the aggressive activation and oxidant generation during phagocytosis of asbestos? Similarly, is this a paradigm of phenolic protection from excessive inflammation?

Viral Latency and AIDS. Since there is clearly an oxidant scale that biological tissues have assembled and respond to (Table II), it is not surprising that pathogenic organisms have adapted to this signaling system as well. Viral genomes have now been demonstrated to contain oxidant response elements that enable the virus to remain dormant, in essence to lie in wait, until conditions within the cell are sufficiently compromised that pathogenic success is more assured. This principle of pathogenic latency is another condition in which the balance of oxidant stress and antioxidant protection is important. Whether non-essential antioxidants such as polyphenolics interfere with such signaling, and if so whether in a positive or net negative direction, remains to be determined.

The role of reactive oxygen and free radicals in the activation of latent HIV in infected individuals has been investigated. In 1993, Greenspan (*49*) hypothesized that the existence of oxidative stress is an important element in HIV progression and that this is the basis for the efficacy of phytopharmaceutical substances. Greenspan and Arouma (*50*) reviewed evidence to support the premise that a pro-oxidant condition exists in HIV-seropositive patients. Plants are protected from oxidation-induced cell death by the synergistic action of primary and secondary metabolites of antioxidants in their cells. Some of these same metabolites can inhibit cell death resulting from HIV. These authors proposed a mechanism by which these synergistic antioxidants from plants can inhibit viral replication and cell killing in HIV infection.

Key Issues

The data are clear: plant antioxidants hold promise for preventing and ameliorating disease. The scientific questions are now, which compounds are effective and what is their mechanism of action? A number of key issues remain and must be addressed to ascertain the contribution of food phenolics to prevention or amelioration of specific disease processes. These issues include: (I) identification and quantitation of phenolics in foodstuffs; (ii) determination of the bioavailability to humans and pharmacokinetics of specific phenolics that exhibit the greatest in vitro activity; (iii) determination of the molecular structure of specific phenolics in relation to antioxidant function; (iv) identification and quantitation of phenolic compounds in clinical samples from humans and in samples from animals; (v) determination of the molecular targets of action and the doses required to achieve and maintain levels that provide the greatest efficacy; and (vi) determination of the molecular mechanisms by which disease intervention occurs.

Although some of the above stated issues have been addressed in the literature, much of the available published data are questionable. The chemistry of oxidation, and the biological response to oxidation are complex. There is a temptation, irresistible to many investigators, to use non-specific 'global' indicators of oxidation to discern mechanism or clinical status. This is a risky approach. The highly interactive nature of oxidant balance is still being revealed, and what constitutes a relevant global tissue biomarker of antioxidant status is unknown. The better approach, one that will be more likely to contribute to our understanding of oxidation and health, is the measurement of specific compounds in tissues and biological fluids. The contribution from such experimental care cannot be overestimated since, until recently, there have been problems related to the fact that composition and quantitation of phenolics in various foods have been based upon measurements of total classes of polyphenols as opposed to specific polyphenols. Other inaccuracies in the literature have resulted from identification and quantitation being determined by unsophisticated methodology that only recently has been replaced by analytical techniques with lower detection levels, which are required for quantitation of minor, but potentially biologically-active compounds. An additional problem that has been recognized as a vital issue is related to appropriate handling of clinical samples to be measured for the appearance or disappearance of polyphenols absorbed following ingestion or other means of administration. To date, no study has determined the proper methods for collection, transport, storage, etc. most appropriate for application to the variety of clinical samples (i.e., plasma vs. serum, temperature, binding of polyphenols to proteins, etc.) prior to measurements of polyphenols. Another issue not yet addressed in animal or human studies relates to the effects of various foods consumed with polyphenol-containing foods on the absorption of these antioxidant compounds.

The future of mechanistic research on phenolics in health is full of promise. Epidemiology has already provided convincing support for the positive outcome. It is now essential to transform population level correlations into specific responsible molecules, their mechanisms of action, biomarkers of their status and functions, the most efficacious methods for delivery and finally to improve the agricultural food supply to realize fully the value of this intensive scientific scrutiny. In this context, wine will likely emerge as an unusual delivery vehicle for plant phenolics whose conspicuous abundance in certain populations has proven to be a key observation in the search for mechanisms of health improvement.

Acknowledgments

The authors acknowledge the support of BARD, United States - Israel Binational Agricultural Research and Development Fund, Dean's Council: College of Agricultural and Environmental Sciences, and Formula Funds for the School of Veterinary Medicine, University of California-Davis.

Literature Cited

1 Halliwell, B.; Gutteridge, J. M. C. *Free Radicals in Biology and Medicine;* Clarendon Press: Oxford, 1989.
2 Stohs, S. J.; Bagchi, D. *Free Radical Biol. Med.* **1995**, *18*, 321-336.
3 Gutteridge, J. M. *Chem.-Biol. Interact.* **1994**, *91*, 133-140.
4 Halliwell, B. *Am. J. Med.* **1991**, *91(3C)*, 14S-22S.
5 Ames, B. N.; Shigenaga, M. K.; Hagen, T. M. *Proc. Natl. Acad. Sci. (USA)* **1993**, *90*, 7915-7922.
6 Bashir, S.; Harris, G.; Denman, M. A.; Blake, D. R.; Winyard, P. G. *Ann. Rheum. Dis.* **1993**, *52, 659-666.*

7. Keen, C. L.; German, J. B.; Mareschi, J. P.; Gershwin, M. E. *Rheum. Dis. Clin. North Am.* **1991**, *17*, 223-234.
8. Frankel, E.; Kanner, J.; German, J. B.; Parks, E.; Kinsella, J. E. *Lancet* **1993**, *341*, 454-457.
9. Frankel, E. N. *J. Sci. Food Ag.* **1991**, *54*, 495-511.
10. Porter, N. A. Caldwell, S. E.; Mills, S. A. *Lipids* **1995**, *30*, 277-290.
11. Kanner, J.; German, J. B.; Kinsella, J. E. *Crit. Rev. Food Sci. Nutr.* **1987**, *25*, 317-364.
12. Walzem, R. L., Watkins, S., Frankel, E. N., Hansen, R. J.; German, J. B. *Proc. Natl. Acad. Sci. USA* **1995**, *92*, 7460-7464.
13. Kanner, J.; Frankel, E.; Granit, R.; German, B.; Kinsella, J. E. *J. Ag. Food Chem.* **1994**, *42*, 64-69.
14. Suzuki, Y. J.; Mizuno, M.; Tritschler, H. J.; Packer, L. *Biochem. Mol. Biol. Internat.* **1995**, *36*, 241-246.
15. Buettner, G. R. *Arch. Biochem. Biophys.* **1993**, *300*, 535-543.
16. Hanasaki, Y.; Ogawa, S.; Fukui, S. *Free Radical Biol. Med.* **1994**, *6*, 845-850.
17. Laughton, M. J.; Evans, P. J.; Moroney, M. A.; Hoult, J. R.; Halliwell, B. *Biochem. Pharmacol.* **1991**, *42*, 1673-1681.
18. Tournaire, C.; Croux, S.; Maurette, M. T.; Beck, I.; Hocquaux, M.; Braun, A. M.; Oliveros, E. J. *Photochem. Photobiol. B Biology* **1993**, *19*, 205-215.
19. Terao, J.; Piskula, M.; Yao, Q. *Arch. Biochem. Biophys.* **1994**, *308*, 278-284.
20. Jessup, W.; Rankin, S. M.; De Whalley, C. V.; Hoult, J. R.; Scott, J.; Leake, D. S. *Biochem. J.* **1990**, *265*, 399-405.
21. Huang, S.-W.; Frankel, E. N.; German, J. B. *J. Agric. Food Chem.* **1994**, *42*, 2108-2114.
22. Huang, S.-W.; Frankel, E. N.; German, J. B. *J. Agric. Food Chem.* **1995**, *43*, 2345-2350.
23. Miesel, R.; Zuber, M. *Inflammation* **1993**, *17*, 283-294.
24. Heliovaara, M.; Knekt, P.; Aho, K.; Aaran, R. K.; Alfthan, G.; Aromaa, A. *Ann. Rheum. Dis.* **1994**, *53*, 51-53.
25. Deucher, G. P. *Exs* **1992**, *62*, 428-437.
26. Harris, W. S. *Clin. Cardiol.* **1992**, *15*, 636-640.
27. Ferguson, L. R. *Mutat. Res.* **1994**, *307*, 395-410.
28. Gershoff, S. N. *Nutr. Rev.* **1993**, *51*, 313-326.
29. Rice-Evans, C. A; Diplock, A. T. *Free Radical Biol. Med.* **1993**, *15*, 77-96.
30. Bast, A.; Haenen, G. R.; Doelman, C. J. *Am. J. Med.* **1991**, *91 (3C)*, 2S-13S.
31. Renaud, S.; de Lorgeril, M. *Lancet* **1992**, *339*, 1523-1526.
32. Steinberg, D. *Circulation* **1992**, *85*, 2337-2344.
33. Steinberg, D., Parthasarathy, S., Carew, T. E., Khoo, J. C.; Witztum, J. L. *New Eng. J. Med.* **1989**, *320*, 915-924.
34. Sambrano, G. R.; Parthasarathy, S.; Steinberg, D. *Proc. Natl. Acad. Sci. USA* **1994**, 3265-3269.

35 Gey, K. F. *Biochem. Soc. Trans.* **1990**, *18*, 1041-1045.
36 Kinsella, J. E.; Frankel, E.; German, B.; Kanner, J. *Food Technol.* **1993**, *47*, 85-90.
37 Burton, G. W.; Ingold, K. *Ann. New York Acad. Sci.* **1989**, *570*, 7-22.
38 Frei, B.; Stocker, R.; Ames, B. N. *Proc. Natl.. Acad. Sci. USA*, **1988**, *85*, 9748-9752.
39 Pratt, D. E.; Hudson, B. J. F. In *Food Antioxidants*, Hudson, B.J.F., Ed.; Elsevier Applied Science: Amsterdam, 1990; pp. 171-192.
40 Kozlowska, H., Rotkiewicz, D. A.; Zadernowski, R. *J. Am. Oil Chem. Soc.* **1983**, *60*, 1191-2223.
41 Shahidi, F.; Wanasundara, U. N.; Amarowicz, R. *Food Res. Internat.* **1994**, *27*, 489-493.
42 Steinmetz, K. A.; Potter, J. D. *Cancer Causes Control* **1991**, *2*, 325-357.
43 Steinmetz, K. A.; Potter, J. D. *Cancer Causes Control* **1991**, *2*, 427-442.
44 Dragsted, L. O.; Strube, M.; Larsen, J. C. *Pharmacol. Toxicol.* **1993**, *72 (Suppl. 1)*, 116-135.
45 German, J. B.; Kinsella, J. E. *Biochem. Biophys. Acta* **1986**, *879*, 378-387.
46 German, J. B.; Hu, M. L. *Free Radical Biol. Med.* **1990**, *8*, 441-448.
47 Hsieh, R. J., German, J. B.; Kinsella, J. E. *Lipids* **1988**, *23*, 322-326.
48 Lewczuk, E.; Owczarek, H.; Staniszewska, G. *Medycyna Pracy* **1994**, *45*, 547-550.
49 Greenspan, H. C. *Med. Hypoth.* **1993**, *40*, 85-92.
50 Greenspan, H. C.; Aruoma, O. I. *Immunol. Today* **1994**, *15*, 209-213.

Chapter 16

An In Vivo Experimental Protocol for Identifying and Evaluating Dietary Factors That Delay Tumor Onset
Effect of Red Wine Solids

Susan E. Ebeler[1], Andrew J. Clifford[2], John D. Ebeler[1], Nathan D. Bills[3], and Steven H. Hinrichs[3]

Departments of [1]Viticulture and Enology and [2]Nutrition, University of California, Davis, CA 95616–8749
[3]Department of Pathology and Microbiology, University of Nebraska Medical Center, Omaha, NE 68198

>Consumption of fruit and vegetable rich diets is protective against cancer, however, the actual dietary factors that may be involved are not known. Recent epidemiologic evidence also indicates that wine may contain non-alcoholic constituents which protect against cancer. We describe a transgenic animal model combined with a chemically defined diet that can be used to identify foods, beverages, and/or their constituents that delay tumor onset in vivo.

Human epidemiologic studies have recently shown that diets rich in fruits and vegetables may reduce the risk of some cancers (1, 2). While a number of potential anticarcinogens have been identified, including vitamins, minerals, and plant phytochemicals, the specific dietary factors or group of factors that are responsible for the observed effects is still an unsettled issue (2, 3).

Animal studies, although varied, have also played an important role in recognizing the role of diet in cancer prevention and have provided important leads for understanding the underlying mechanisms involved. However, some of the variability associated with animal studies has been due to the unavailability of standardized study protocols involving animal models and diets (4). For example, test compounds are often administered by intermittent injection or gavage of individual compounds dissolved in a variety of carrier solvents that may affect their biologic availability or efficacy. These experimental protocols have not always allowed the absorption and metabolism of the test agent to be studied.

Most previous animal studies have also used chemically induced cancer models. These protocols require repeated topical application, intravenous or intraperitoneal injections, or oral administration of the carcinogens, and they induce

© 1997 American Chemical Society

tumors with unpredictable kinetics. In the rat and mouse colon cancer models, the carcinogen is typically injected either in a single large dose or in several smaller doses over a ~6 week period. In this model, colon tumors do not appear until ~38 weeks after dosing and the total tumor incidence (total number of mice with tumors) is ~70% --a protocol and tumor incidence which are typical for most chemically induced animal models (e.g., hamster lung, rat mammary, mouse skin, and mouse bladder) (5). In addition, the carcinogen dose is usually administered at high doses in order to induce a significant incidence of tumors in the target tissue. While some human cancers are induced by chemical carcinogens, the high, genotoxic doses used in many animal studies can result in a cancer etiology that is quite different from that of natural cancers caused by repeated low dose exposures. Finally, there is increasing evidence that many human cancers have a genetic basis and that carcinogen induced animal models do not reflect the pathogenesis of these cancers.

Transgenic mice models provide the opportunity to evaluate the post-initiation tumor prevention activity of natural foods and food constituents without the need for exogenous chemicals. Transgenic mice carrying the human T-lymphotropic virus type-1 (HTLV-1) transactivator (tax1) gene have been recently described (6). These mice develop neoplasms externally (snout, ear, foot and tail) and can be genotyped at an early age, allowing pools of sibling mice with known predisposition for neoplasia to be studied (7,8).

Recently, well defined amino acid based diets and protocols for producing animals with well defined nutritional status were also described (9, 10). Incorporation of individual foods, food fractions, and purified food constituents into these diets at precise concentrations represents a physiologically relevant way to administer specific foods or food constituents and to evaluate their effectiveness in cancer prevention. Using the transgenic mouse model in combination with amino acid based diets, we describe here a protocol that may be useful for identifying dietary factors which may delay tumor onset.

Materials and Methods

HTLV-1 Transgenic Mice. This strain of mice was originally derived via micro injection of the LTR-tax1 gene construct into fertilized eggs from super ovulated CD1 females crossed with C57BL/6 x DBA2F1 males as previously described (6). Tail biopsies (~1 cm) were taken from mouse pups at ten days of age and digested with proteinase K. After extraction, DNA was digested with Bgl II restriction enzymes, electrophoresed in 0.8% agarose, transferred to nylon membranes (11), hybridized with 32P-labeled HTLV-1 tax DNA (6) and labeled via the random primer procedure (12). Membranes were washed and exposed to X-ray film for 24 h. Presence or absence of a band on X-ray film corresponding to HTLV-1 tax1 DNA was used to classify mice as transgenic or control, respectively. After genotyping, the mice were housed in individual stainless steel wire bottom cages in a room with a 12-h light : 12-h dark cycle, a temperature of 20 - 23°C and a relative humidity of 50%.

Table I. Composition Of One Kilogram Of The Amino Acid-Based Diet. (Reprinted with permission [40])

Major Components	g	Minerals	mg	Vitamins	mg
L-Alanine	3.50	$CaCO_3$	14645	Thiamin HCl	6.0
L-Arginine (free base)	11.20	$CaHPO_4 \cdot 2H_2O$	215	Riboflavin	7.0
L-Asparagine·H_2O	6.82	KH_2PO_4	17155	Pyridoxine HCl	7.0
L-Aspartic Acid	3.50	NaCl	12370	Niacin	30.0
L-Cystine	3.50	$MgSO_4 \cdot 7H_2O$	4990	D-Calcium Pantothenate	16.0
L-Glutamic Acid	35.00	$Fe(C_6H_5O_7) \cdot 6H_2O$	623	Biotin	0.20
Glycine	23.30	$CuSO_4$	78	Vit. B_{12} (0.1% titration)	50.0
L-Histidine (free base)	3.30	$MnSO_4 \cdot H_2O$	181.5	Retinyl Palmitate 250,000 U/g	16.0
L-Isoleucine	8.20	$ZnCl_2$	62.5	Alpha Tocopherol 250 U/g	200
L-Leucine	11.10	KI	0.25	Cholecalciferol 400,000 U/g	2.5
L-Lysine·HCl	17.99	$(NH_4)_6Mo_7O_{24} \cdot 4H_2O$	1.25	Menadione $NaSO_3$	48.0
L-Methionine	8.20	$Na_2SeO_3 \cdot 5H_2O$	0.75	Choline Chloride	2000
L-Phenylalanine	11.60	$Crk(SO_4)_2 \cdot 12H_2O$	19.25	Folic Acid	5.0
L-Proline	3.50	NaF	2.25		
L-Serine	3.50	CH_3CO_2Na	8080		
L-Threonine	8.20				
L-Tryptophan	1.74				
L-Tyrosine	3.50				
L-Valine	8.20				
Succinylsulfathiazole	10.00				
Cellulose (Solka Floc 40)	50.00				
Corn Oil (with 0.015% BHT)	100.00				
Dextrin	402.23				
Sucrose	201.12				
Total	939.20g		58.42g		2.38g

The lyophilized residue from one bottle (750 mL) or red table wine was dissolved in 15 mL H_2O and blended into each kg of this amino acid based diet to formulate the wine-solids supplemented diet.

SOURCE: Reprinted with permission from reference 40. Copyright 1996 American Journal of Clinical Nutrition, American Society for Clinical Nutrition.

The use and care of mice was approved by the IACAUC at the University of California, Davis.

The snouts, ears, feet and tails were examined daily for the appearance of the first external tumor. The age of the mouse on the day that the first tumor appeared was used as the age of tumor onset for that mouse. Tumor latency was chosen as the endpoint over the alternative endpoint, tumor multiplicity (number of tumors divided by the number of mice), because tumor multiplicity is typically determined at a predetermined time and some animals may not have a tumor at this time.

When tumor mass approached 1% of body weight, an individual transgenic mouse fed the nonsupplemented diet and a transgenic littermate matched for gender but fed the wine solids supplemented diet were anaesthetized with ether and bled by cardiac puncture. Blood (~50 µL) was drawn into microhematocrit tubes for hematocrit determination. Blood (40 µL) was also transferred into 20 mL of Isoton II (Curtin Matheson, Hilea, FL) for leukocyte and erythrocyte counts. Hematocrit values and leukocyte and erythrocyte counts were used to confirm the general health of the mice. The remaining blood was allowed to clot at 23°C for ~20 min and then cooled on ice. Serum was separated by centrifugation and transferred to small vials and stored at -10°C. A 300 µL aliquot of serum from each of 3 mice fed the nonsupplemented diet and 4 sibling mice fed the supplemented diet were extracted on a solid phase extraction cartridge and the amount of catechin in the extract was analyzed by reverse-phase HPLC as described by Lamuela-Raventos and Waterhouse (13). Identity of the HPLC peak of serum catechin was determined by coelution with an authentic standard, by light spectroscopy, and by negative ion electrospray mass spectrometry of the collected peak.

The Diet. Composition of the diet is indicated in Table I. The solids from 750 mL of red wine (Zinfandel, 1990 harvest, Sonoma Valley, California; wine solids were prepared by lyophilization of the wine to remove water and ethanol), were incorporated into 1 kg of the standard amino acid based diet. This ensured that the wine solids (and the polyphenols contained in the wine solids) were consumed as an integral part of a nutritionally adequate diet of solid consistency. Incorporating wine directly into the diet would have required feeding a liquid diet, which has been shown to alter intestinal microflora and bacterial translocation from the gut (14). We did not incorporate wine into the drinking water because of concerns for the effects this might have on fluid, calorie, and nutrient intake and because of difficulties in controlling and monitoring the polyphenol intake.

Wine solids were added to the diet to yield a measured polyphenol concentration of 0.044%. This represents a dietary concentration approximately one-fourth that of a typical human diet (based on a per unit metabolic size comparison) (15). Small amounts of diet (0.5 - 1 kg) were prepared at a time to ensure that it was fresh when presented to the mice. Mice had free access to the diet and were fed and weighed daily.

Results

Initial body weight, mean growth rates and final body weight of mice fed the wine solids supplemented diet were not statistically different from those of sibling mice fed the same diet but without the wine solids supplement (Figure 1). Mean packed erythrocyte volumes (50 ± 3%) and erythrocyte (5.7 ± 0.1 x 10^{12}/L) and leukocyte (3.1 ± 0.5 x 10^9/L) counts of mice fed the wine solids supplemented diet were normal (16) and did not differ from those of sibling mice fed the same diet but without the wine solids supplement. Mice on the wine solids supplemented diet reproduced normally for three successive generations, indicating that there were no ill health effects associated with consuming the wine solids supplemented diet for prolonged periods.

Time of tumor onset was significantly delayed in mice fed the diet supplemented with wine solids (Figure 2, left panel). Mean ages ± SEM of tumor onset in transgenic mice fed the nonsupplemented and supplemented diets were 71 ± 4 and 102 ± 10 d, respectively, ($p < 0.028$). First tumors appeared at 55 and 74 days of age in nonsupplemented and supplemented mice, respectively. All nonsupplemented mice had a first tumor by 77 d of age, but not until 128 d of age did all supplemented mice exhibit tumors (Figure 2, right panel).

Catechin concentrations in the serum from four mice fed the wine solids supplemented diet were higher (1.36 ± 0.28 μmol/L) than the trace concentrations of catechin (0.26 ± 0.06 μmol/L) found in the three sibling mice fed the nonsupplemented diet. This difference was significant at $p = 0.011$ using an unpaired 1-tailed student t-test.

Discussion

Chemical Carcinogen Models. As previously discussed, there is increasing evidence that many human cancers, including those of the colon, breast, and nerve tissues, have a genetic basis and that carcinogen induced animal models do not accurately reflect the pathogenesis of these cancers, which are among the leading causes of cancer deaths in humans. As reviewed by Steele et al. (5) colon cancer is typically induced in rats and mice with 1,2-Dimethylhydrazine (DMH) or azoxymethane (AOM); DMH requires in vivo activation to AOM, the ultimate carcinogen. The carcinogen produces colon adenomas and adenocarcinomas after ~38 weeks. Breast cancer is typically induced in rats and mice with either the polycyclic aromatic hydrocarbon, 7,12-dimethylbenz(a)anthracene (DMBA) or the direct acting alkylating agent, N-methyl-N-nitrosourea (MNU). Administration of MNU is thought to activate the H-*ras* oncogene (17) resulting in adenocarcinomas which develop within ~20 weeks.

In these models, high carcinogen doses are administered in order to induce a significant incidence of tumors in the target tissue, however, tumor incidences less than 100% are common. These high, genotoxic doses can induce artifactual enzyme and metabolic changes that are not related to the carcinogenic process.

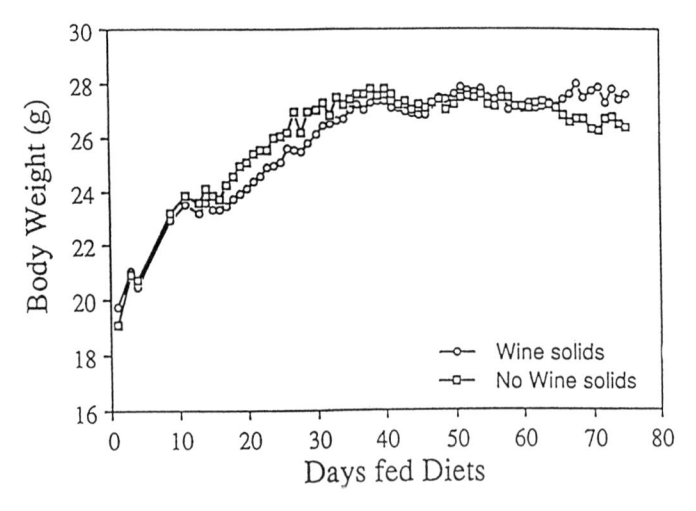

Figure 1. Growth of transgenic mice fed a nutritionally adequate amino acid based diet (no wine solids) or the same diet supplemented with the solids from 750 mL of red table wine per kg diet (wine solids).
Reprinted with permission from reference 40. Copyright 1996 American Journal of Clinical Nutrition, American Society for Clinical Nutrition.

Figure 2. Left Panel: Age at tumor onset in transgenic mice fed an amino acid based diet (no wine solids) or the same diet supplemented with solids from 750 mL red table wine/kg diet (wine solids). Full circles connected with a dashed line represent mean ages when first tumors appeared; vertical solid lines correspond to ± 1 SEM for the wine-solids-supplemented and nonsupplemented diets, respectively.
Right Panel: Tumor free survival curve of transgenic mice fed an amino acid based diet (broken line) or the same diet supplemented with red table wine solids (solid line). Reprinted with permission from reference 40. Copyright 1996 American Journal of Clinical Nutrition, American Society for Clinical Nutrition.

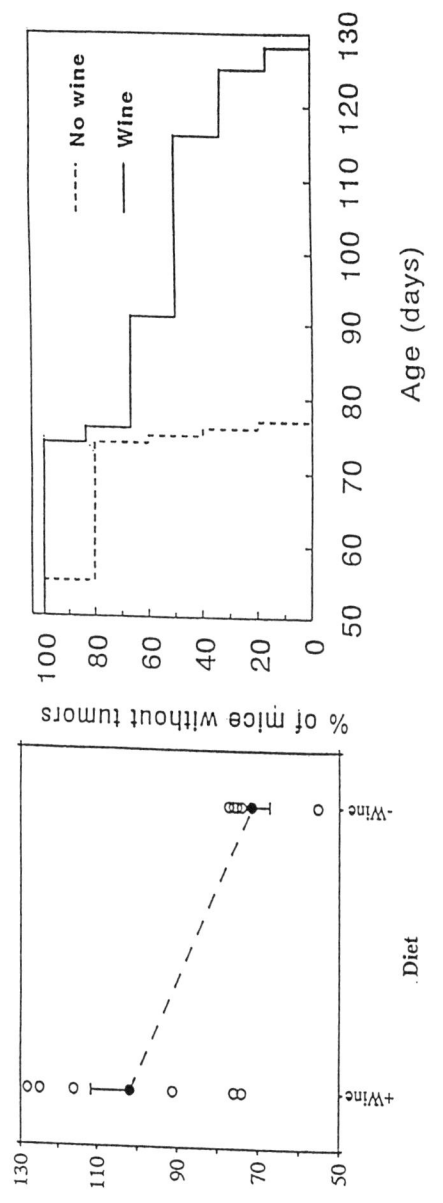

Table II. Mean age of tumor onset for HTLV-1 transgenic mice

Tumor onset Mean age ± S.D. (days)	Fractional Standard Deviation	n	Treatment	Reference
93 ± 6	0.0645	6	Control (amino acid diet)	Bills et al., 1992
83 ± 5	0.0602	20	Control (casein-based diet)	Bills et al., 1993
71 ± 4	0.0563	7	Control (amino acid diet)	Clifford et al., 1996
63 ± 4	0.0635	5	Control (amino acid diet)	Clifford et al., 1996
72 ± 4	0.0556	8	Folate-restricted (amino acid diet)	Bills et al., 1992
93 ± 6	0.0645	20	Calorie-restricted (casein-based diet)	Bills et al., 1993
90 ± 7	0.0778	20	High fat (casein-based diet)	Bills et al., 1993
102 ± 10	0.0980	6	Wine-supplemented (amino acid diet)	Clifford et al., 1996
86 ± 6	0.0698	9	Wine-supplemented (amino acid diet)	Clifford et al., 1996

Transgenic Mouse Models. An animal that gains new genetic information from the addition of foreign DNA, via addition to the egg, is described as transgenic. Cloned fragments of DNA carrying the gene of interest are introduced (via microinjection of DNA or retroviral infection) into the pronucleus of the fertilized egg which is then implanted into a pseudopregnant mouse. The DNA of interest is integrated into chromosomes and copies are inherited by the progeny according to Mendelian genetics. Specific genes can be introduced into the transgenic mice providing animal models for human genetic diseases (18). Whereas transgenic mice have additional genetic material, it is also possible to remove or mutate genes thought to play a role in cancer using embryonic stem cell technology. These mutant mice can also be used for studying the role of nutritional factors in cancer.

Several transgenic animal models have recently been described which are providing valuable insight into the molecular events involved in cancer initiation, promotion, and progression. These models also hold much promise for evaluating the efficacy of dietary and drug interventions therapies without the drawbacks associated with the application of chemical carcinogens previously discussed (e.g., repeated carcinogen application at high doses, unpredictable kinetics, and artifactual metabolic changes). Important features of currently available transgenic models for neurofibromatosis, colon cancer, and breast cancer are summarized in the following paragraphs.

HTLV-1 Transgenic Mouse Model. The transgenic mice used in the present study develop nerve sheath tumors that are similar to those occurring in human neurofibromatosis (7, 8). Neurofibromatosis type-I (NF-1) is the most common dominantly inherited syndrome in humans that predisposes to neoplasia. In this syndrome and the related neurocristopathy, neurofibromatosis type-II, peripheral nerve sheath tumors develop which are initially benign but undergo spontaneous degeneration into highly aggressive malignant tumors known as neurofibrosarcomas (19, 20). The propensity for benign neurofibromas to develop into aggressive malignancies may provide a valuable model to study malignant transformation of premalignant lesions.

The neoplasms develop externally on the snout, ear, foot and tail and are easily viewed and assessed. Because tumor growth can be monitored over several time points, the effects of experimental variables on tumor growth and progression can easily be monitored. The kinetics of tumor development in the HTLV-1 transgenic mice are well defined and consistent. While the absolute age of tumor onset is dependent on experimental conditions, a comparison of the fractional standard deviations for mean ages of tumor onset for 9 different treatment groups in 3 different studies (96 transgenic mice total) ranged from 0.0556 to 0.0980 (Table II). This indicates a small variability in age at tumor onset in this colony.

Min Mouse Model for Colon Carcinoma. Mutations in the *Apc* gene are generally thought to result in colon cancer, one of the leading causes of cancer deaths in humans. Min (multiple intestinal neoplasia) is a mutant allele of the mouse *Apc* (adenomatous polyposis coli) gene and mice carrying this mutation develop intestinal adenomas similar to those of humans with familial adenomatous polyposis as well as those that occur somatically in most sporadic colon neoplasms (21). These mice develop numerous adenomas throughout the intestinal tract which grow to a detectable size in 1-3 months, a small portion of which can go on to become malignant (21, 22). Lesions in other tissue types, consistent with those seen in humans, can also occur: desmoid tumors, epidermoid cysts, and mammary tumors.

Crossing the Min strain with mice of different genetic backgrounds has identified modifier loci which can alter the incidence, tissue involvement, and rate of tumor development (22, 23, 24). These experiments have indicated that mutations to several genes may play a cumulative role in the multi-step processes involved in tumor formation and progression to malignant lesions. This transgenic mouse model has been used to evaluate the chemopreventive effects of nonsteroidal anti-inflammatory drugs (21) and dietary protease inhibitors (25) on the development of intestinal tumors.

Since tumors develop internally, and the animals must be killed in order to observe tumor incidence, tumor multiplicity (the number of tumors counted at one point in time divided by the total number of mice) is used as the normal endpoint for this model. While this endpoint can indicate the relative efficacy of experimental treatments in increasing or decreasing tumor development, the effects on tumor establishment and maintenance or growth and progression cannot be readily evaluated with this model, further complicating these types of studies. (21).

Mouse Models for Breast Cancer. Transgenic animal models have also been used as model systems for studying human breast cancer, one of the major causes of cancer deaths in women. These models involve mutations to a number of genes including *neu*, TGFα, *myc*, *ras*, *src*, and hGH (26, 27, 28, 29). Two promoter regions, the whey acidic protein (Wap) gene and the mouse mammary tumor virus (MMTV) long terminal repeat (LTR) are commonly used. The phenotypic expression and histopathology of each of these genes have been reviewed (27, 28, 30, 31). Combinations of one or more of these genes can alter the phenotype displayed, suggesting that several oncogenes may be involved in the full malignant transformation (27, 28, 30).

Another transgenic mammary tumor model has recently been described using the murine Polyomavirus (MPyV) middle T antigen under the control of the MMTV promoter/enhancer (32). These mice develop rapid neoplasias of the mammary gland which rapidly metastasize to the lung and provide a model for the metastatic process.

As with the Min mouse model, tumor multiplicity is the common endpoint for the transgenic breast cancer models. The mammary tumors develop internally and must be observed antemortem or they require repeated palpation to detect and monitor tumor onset, a time-consuming and difficult procedure requiring a skilled technician (33, 34).

The Chemically Defined Diet and Administration of Test Compounds. Studies on the nutritional effects, metabolism, and biological activity of various nutrients and drugs have been complicated by difficulties in obtaining a standardized diet (4). This is especially true for micronutrients that may be critical in cancer prevention. Many studies have used casein-based diets (e.g., AIN76-A), however, casein is not a pure substance; it is typically 87.3% protein, 1.8% ash, 1.2% fat, 0.1% lactose, and 9.6% moisture, and this composition can vary depending on source, processing and storage conditions (New Zealand Milk Products, Inc., Santa Rosa, CA). Other proteins, such as soy, which are isolated from natural sources also have variable compositions dependent on the isolation procedures. The dietary protein source (e.g., casein vs soy protein) can have important systemic effects, modulating LDL turnover, sterol excretion, and rate of senescence, and protein turnover (35, 36, 37, 38), further complicating dietary studies and emphasizing the need for standardized diets.

Unlike protein based diets, the composition of the amino acid based diet presented in this study can be rigorously defined and controlled, therefore the effects of one or more dietary factors on tumor onset can be evaluated. Mice fed the standard amino acid based diet grow normally and exhibit normal hematologic parameters (9, 10, 39, 40). This amino acid diet also allows the bioavailability of a food, a food fraction, a specific nutrient, or a drug to be readily determined. For example, Bills et al. (39) monitored tissue folate levels following consumption of an amino acid based diet with varying folate levels. They observed changes in tissue folate levels similar to those observed by other investigators using "standard" diets, indicating that nutrient absorption and metabolism by mice consuming the amino acid based diet was normal.

In order to evaluate the potential for toxic effects on growth and reproduction as a result of consuming the wine solids supplemented diet, we monitored initial body weights, mean growth rates, and final body weights of the mice in this study (Figure 1). Mice consuming the wine solids supplemented diet were healthy, grew well, and reproduced normally for 3 successive generations. These results indicate that there were no adverse effects associated with long term consumption of the wine solids in the diet. Finally, when wine was consumed as part of a healthy diet, serum catechin levels increased indicating that catechin, the major phenol of red wine, was absorbed intact by the mice.

Application of protocol for studying tumor onset: Effects of red wine solids. Wine has attracted much attention because of its purported health benefits, particularly with respect to cardiovascular disease (41, 42, 43, 44). However, a number of recent studies indicate that the nonalcoholic constituents of wine may also lower the risk of certain cancer types. For example, Longnecker et al. (45) showed that consumption of beer and liquor, but not wine, was positively related to breast cancer risk. Freudenheim et al. (46), in a case-control study of breast cancer in western New York, also found an indication of a decrease in risk associated with wine intake but a slightly elevated risk associated with increased beer intake (more than 1 drink per day). Macfarlane et al. (47) showed a lowered risk of oral cancer in wine drinkers compared to beer or spirits drinkers in selected populations in US, Italy, and China. Therefore, we used the HTLV-1 transgenic mouse/chemically defined diet protocol described above to specifically evaluate the effects that the non-alcohol components of red wine may have on tumor onset.

We observed that transgenic mice consuming wine solids were significantly older (p = 0.028; Figure 2) when a first tumor appeared, suggesting that red wine contains compounds which may have beneficial tumor preventive properties. First tumors appeared at 55 and 74 days of age in nonsupplemented and supplemented mice, respectively. All nonsupplemented mice had a first tumor by 77 days of age, while only 30% of supplemented mice had tumors at this time. Not until 128 days of age did all supplemented mice exhibit tumors.

A delay in tumor onset of ~1 month is biologically significant in terms of the total lifespan of a mouse (~24 months). In addition, consumption of red wine solids resulted in a more pronounced effect than observed in the same animal model when caloric intake was restricted (48), even though restricting caloric intake is well known to be protective against certain cancer types (49). Because of the genetic nature of the HTLV-1 mouse model, it is not possible to completely inhibit the tumor development; however, since tumor development or onset is an early step in the cancer process, if onset can be delayed and/or prevented, the cancer itself will be delayed and/or prevented.

The actual wine components which may be responsible for the delay in tumor onset are unknown. Red wine contains high concentrations of polyphenolic compounds which are extracted from the grape skins, seeds, and stems during the winemaking process. While total phenol concentrations of 1200 mg/L (expressed as gallic acid equivalents) are common in red wines, much lower levels (~200 mg/L) are found in grape juice and white wines. Grape juice and white wine also contain predominantly nonflavonoid phenols (e.g., hydroxycinnamates) while red wines contain predominantly flavonoids, including catechin and epicatechin. Singleton (50) has reviewed the occurrence, chemistry, and importance of grape and wine phenolics.

As discussed previously, elevated serum catechin levels were observed in mice consuming the wine supplemented diet. This does not identify catechin as the active component, however. Further studies are necessary to identify the specific grape and or wine component(s) which may be responsible for this effect. The dynamics of polyphenol metabolism as well as dose response studies are also necessary to establish the amount of wine solids or individual components that result in a maximum delay in tumor onset.

The biological mechanism(s) by which red wine and/or polyphenols may delay tumor onset are currently unknown. The wine polyphenols may delay tumor onset by acting as in vivo antioxidants, by inhibiting mutagenicity and damage to DNA, by altering eicosanoid synthesis, and by preventing or halting the spread of nascent tumors via alterations in platelet aggregation and angiogenesis (51, 52, 53, 54, 55, 56).

Using the HTLV-1 animal model, Ebeler et al. (57, 58) have shown that levels of some lipid peroxidation products are elevated in the tissues and expired air of tumor-bearing mice compared to non-tumor-bearing controls. Measurement of lipid peroxidation markers in the breath is a non-invasive procedure and may be valuable for monitoring in vivo lipid peroxidation status (57, 59). The highly standardized protocol described here, in which tumors develop externally, provides a sensitive model for characterizing small changes in these lipid peroxidation markers as a function of tumor growth and progression. Application of this standardized protocol will now allow us to evaluate the in vivo antioxidative activity of wine and dietary phenols. This type of mechanistic information is critical for understanding the overall relationships between diet, lipid peroxidation, and cancer.

Conclusions

Understanding the role of diet in preventing cancer has been delayed because of the unavailability of reliable study protocols for creating animal models of known and reproducible nutritional status. We present a transgenic animal model of human disease, combined with chemically defined diets that can be rigorously controlled and supplemented with natural foods, food fractions, and purified food constituents. The protocol is straight forward, uses sibling mice to minimize error, and requires no sophisticated technical help to monitor and detect a first tumor appearance. Because tumors in the HTLV-1 mice develop externally, the effects of dietary interventions on tumor establishment, maintenance, growth, and progression can be readily evaluated.

Using this model we showed that red wine solids, when consumed as part of a healthy diet, significantly delayed tumor onset. Further studies identifying the wine component(s) that may be responsible for this effect as well as their biologic mechanism are currently underway. Application of the protocol described here is a promising way to identify foods, food fractions, extracts, nutrients, and anhedreonpeic chemicals which may protect against cancer in vivo.

Acknowledgments

This research was supported by USDA Regional Research W-143, Hatch 2850 from the California Agricultural Experiment Station; the UC Davis Clinical Nutrition Research Unit (NIH P30 DK 35747); and an Institutional Research Grant (IRG-205) awarded to UC Davis by the American Cancer Society.

Literature Cited

1. Bailey, G. S.; Williams, D. E. *Food Tech.*. **1993**, *47*, 105-118.
2. Willet, W. C. *Science*. **1994**, *254*, 532-537.
3. Ritenbaugh, C. *Prev. Med.* **1993**, *22*, 667-675.
4. Reeves, P. G.; Nielsen, F. H.; Fahey, G. C., Jr. *J. Nutr.* **1993**, *123*, 1939-1951.
5. Steele, V. E.; Moon, R. C.; Lubet, R. A.; Grubbs, C. J.; Reddy, B. S.; Wargovich, M.; McCormick, D. L.; Pereira, M. A.; Crowell, J. A.; Bagheri, D.; Sigman, C. C.; Boone, C. W.; Kelloff, G. J. *J. Cell. Biochem., Suppl.* **1994**, *20*, 32-54.
6. Nerenberg, M.; Hinrichs, S. H.; Reynolds, R. K.; Khoury, G.; Jay, G. *Science*. **1987**, *237*, 1324-1329.
7. Hinrichs, S. H.; Nerenberg, M.; Reynolds, R. K.; Khoury, G.; Jay, G.*Science*. **1987**, *237*, 1340-1343.

8. Baird, A. M.; Green, J. E.; Hinrichs, S. H. *Compar. Path. Bull..* **1992**, *24*, 3-4.
9. Walzem, R. L.; Clifford, A. J. *J. Nutr.* **1988,** *118*, 1089-1096.
10. Clifford, A. J.; Heid, M. K.; Muller, H. G.; Bills, N. D. *J. Nutr.* **1990**, *120*, 1633-1639.
11. Southern, E. M. *J Mol Biol.* **1975**, *98*, 503-517.
12. Feinberg, A. P.; Fogelstein, B. *Anal. Biochem.* **1984**, *137*, 266-267.
13. Lamuela-Raventos, R. M.; Waterhouse, A. L. *Am. J. Enol. Viticul.* **1994**, *45*, 1-5.
14. Alverdy, J. C.; Aoys, E.; Moss, G. S. *JPEN.* **1990**, *14*, 1-6.
15. Kühnau, J. *Wld Rev Nutr Diet.* **1976**, *24*, 117-191.
16. Sanderson, J. H.; Phillips, C. E. *An Atlas of Laboratory Animal Haematology*; Clarendon Press: Oxford, 1981.
17. Gould, M. N. *Seminars in Cancer Biology.* **1995**, *6*, 147-152.
18. Jaenisch, R. *Science.* **1988**, *240*, 1468-1474.
19. Morioka, N.; Tsuchida, T.; Etoh, T.; Ishibashi, Y.; Otsuka, F. *J. Dermatol.* **1990**, *17*, 312-316.
20. Tam, A. W.; Darby, J. K.; Riccardi, V. M. *Neurofibromatosis.* **1988**, *1*, 69-84.
21. Jacoby, R. F.; Marshall, D. J.; Newton, M. A.; Novakovic, K.; Tutsch, K.; Cole, C. E.; Lubet, R. A.; Kelloff, G. J.; Verma, A.; Moser, A. R.; Dove, W. F. *Cancer Res.* **1996**, *56*, 710-714.
22. Moser, A. R.; Luongo, C.; Gould, K. A.; McNeley, M. K.; Shoemaker, A. R.; Dove, W. F. *Eur. J. Cancer.* **1995**, *31A(7/8)*, 1061-1064.
23. Kim, S. H.; Roth, K. A.; Moser, A. R.; Gordon, J. I. *J. Cell. Biol.* **1993**, *123(4)*, 877-893.
24. Clarke, A. R.; Cummings, M. C.; Harrison, D. J. *Oncogene.* **1995**, *11*, 1913-1920.
25. Kennedy, A. R.; Beazer-Barclay, Y.; Kinzler, K. W.; Newberne, P. M. *Cancer Res.* **1996**, *56*, 679-682.
26. Bouchard, L.; Lamarre, L.; Tremblay, P. J.; Jolicoeur, P. *Cell.* **1989**, *57*, 931-936.
27. Dickson, R. B.; Gottardis, M. M.; Merlino, G. T. *BioEssays.* **1991**, *13(11)*, 591-596.
28. Robinson, A. *Can. Med. Assoc. J.* **1995**, *153(8)*, 1123-1124.
29. Smith, G. H.; Sharp, R.; Kordon, E. C.; Jhappan, C.; Merlino, G. *AJP.* **1995**, *147(4)*, 1081-1096.
30. Groner, B. *J. Cell Biochem.* **1992**, *49*, 128-136.
31. Munn, R. J.; Webster, M.; Muller, W. J.; Cardiff, R. D. *Sem Cancer Biol.* **1995**, *6*, 153-158.
32. Fluck, M. M.; Haslam, S. Z. *Breast Cancer Res. Treat.* **1996**, *39*, 45-56.
33. Dexter, D. L.; Diamond, M.; Creveling, J.; Chen, S. F. *Invest. New Drugs.* **1993**, *11*, 161-168.
34. DeWille, J. W.; Waddell, K.; Steinmeyer, C.; Farmer, S. J. *Cancer Lett.* **1993**, *69*, 59-66.
35. Khosla, P.; Samman, S; Carroll, K. K.; Huff, M. W. *Biochim. Biophys. Acta.* **1989**, *1002*(2), 157-163.
36. DeSchrijver, R. *J. Nutr.* **1990**, *120*(12), 1624-1632.

37. Umezawa, M.; Hosokawa, M.; Kohno, A.; Ishikawa, S.; Kitagawa, K.; Takeda, T. *J. Nutr.* **1993**, *123*(11), 1905-1912.
38. Nielsen, K.; Kondrup, J.; Elsner, P.; Juul, A.; Jensen, E.S. *Br. J. Nutr.* **1994**, *72*, 69-81.
39. Bills, N. D.; Hinrichs, S. H.; Morgan, R.; Clifford, A. J.*J. Natl. Cancer Inst.* **1992**, *84*, 332-337.
40. Clifford, A. J.; Ebeler, S. E.; Ebeler, J. D.; Bills, N. D.; Hinrichs, S. H.; Teissedre, P.-L.; Waterhouse, A. L. *Am. J. Clin. Nutr.* **1996**, in press.
41. Renaud, S.; de Lorgeril, M. *Lancet.* **1992**, *339*, 1523-1526.
42. St. Leger, A. S.; Cochrane, A. L.; Moore, F. *Lancet.* **1979**, *May 12*, 1017-1029.
43. Frankel, E.; Kanner, J.; German, J. B.; Parks, E.; Kinsella, J. E. *Lancet.* **1993**, *341*, 454-457.
44. Kinsella, J. E.; Frankel, E.; German, J. B.; Kanner, J. *Food Technol.* **1993**, *47*, 85-90.
45. Longnecker, M. P.; Newcomb, P. A.; Mittendorf, R.; Greenberg, E. R.; Clapp, R. W.; Bogdan, Baron, J.; MacMahon, B.; Willet, C. *J. Natl. Cancer Inst.* **1995**, *87*(12), 923-929.
46. Freudenheim, J. L.; Marshall, J. R.; Graham, S.; Laughlin, R.; Vena, J. E.; Swanson, M.; Ambrosone, C.; Nemoto, T. *Nutr. Cancer.* **1995**, *23*(1), 1-11.
47. Macfarlane, G. J.; Zheng, T.; Marshall, J. R.; Boffetta, P.; Niu, S.; Brasure, J.; Merletti, F.; Boyle, P. *Oral Oncol, Eur. J. Cancer.* **1995**, *31B*(3), 181-187.
48. Bills, N. D.; Hinrichs, S. H.; Birt, D. D. *Federation Proceedings.* **1993**, *7*, 865A.
49. Klurfeld, D. M.; Weber, M. M.; Kritchevsky, D. *Cancer Res.* **1987**, *47*, 2759-2762.
50. Singleton, V. In: *Grape and Wine Centennial Symposium Proceedings*, A. D. Webb, ed.; University of California, Davis, 1982; pp 215-227.
51. Osawa, T. In: *Phenolic Compounds in Food and their Effects on Health;* H. T. Huang; C. T. Ho; C. Y. Lee, eds.; Am. Chem. Soc.: Washington, DC, 1992, Vol. 2; pp 135-149.
52. Ito, N.; Hirose, M.; Shirai, T. In: *Phenolic Compounds in Food and their Effects on Health;* H. T. Huang; C. T. Ho; C. Y. Lee, eds.; Am. Chem. Soc.: Washington, DC, 1992, Vol. 2; pp 269-283.
53. Yoshizawa, S.; Horiuchi, T.; Suganuma, M.; Nishiwaki, S.; Yatsunami, J.; Okabe, S.; Okuda, T.; Muto, Y.; Frankel, K.; Troll, W.; Fujiki, H. In: *Phenolic Compounds in Food and their Effects on Health.*; H. T. Huang; C. T. Ho; C. Y. Lee, eds.; Am. Chem. Soc.: Washington, DC, 1992, Vol. 2; pp 316-325.
54. Kelloff, G. J.; Boone, C. W.; Steele, V. E.; Fay, J. R.; Lubet, R. A.; Crowell, J. A.; Sigman, C. C. *J. Cell Biochem. Suppl.* **1994**, *20*, 1-24.
55. Pace-Asciak, C. R.; Hahn, S.; Diamandis, E. P.; Soleus, G.; Goldberg, D. M. *Clin. Chim. Acta.* **1995**, *235*, 207-219.
56. Stavric, B. *Clin. Biochem.* **1994**, *27*, 245-248.
57. Ebeler, S. E.; Hinrichs, S. H.; Clifford, A. J.; T. Shibamoto. *Anal. Biochem.* **1992**, *205*, 183-186.
58. Ebeler, S. E.; Hinrich, S. H.; A. J. Clifford; T. Shibamoto. *J. Chromatogr B.* **1994**, *654*, 9-18.
59. Lin, Y.; Dueker, S. R.; Jones, A. D.; Ebeler, S. E.; Clifford, A. J. *Clin. Chem.* **1995**, *41*(7), 1028-1032.

Chapter 17

The Role of Wine in Ethyl Carbamate Induced Carcinogenesis Inhibition

Gilbert S. Stoewsand[1], J. L. Anderson[1], and L. Munson[2]

[1]Department of Food Science and Technology, Cornell University, Geneva, NY 14456
[2]Department of Pathobiology, College of Veterinary Medicine, University of Tennessee, Knoxville, TN 37901

A 12% (v/v) ethanol solution and, to a greater extent, wine fed to C3H male mice inhibited tumorigenesis in their liver and lungs induced by the carcinogen, ethyl carbamate. Ethyl carbamate (urethane), a water soluble carcinogen originally used for numerous commercial processes, is a contaminant of fermentation. Wine phenols used in these studies, i.e. caffeic acid, catechin hydrate, and gallic acid, without the presence of ethanol, appeared to enhance liver, but not lung, tumor incidence and frequency. Thus, outside of the presence of ethanol in wine, no other wine constituents have been identified that affords protection against cancer development of ethyl carbamate. Any cancer risk assessment of ethyl carbamate in wine should take into account this ethanol interaction.

Ethyl carbamate (EC), also known as urethane, urethan, or carbamic acid ethyl ester, was formerly used in producing amino resins, as a solvent in the manufacture of pesticides, fumigants and cosmetics and as an antineoplastic drug. These commercial purposes have ceased and the main public exposure to EC is from its presence as a natural contaminant present in alcoholic beverages and other fermented products such as soy sauce (1-3). In one of the largest surveys on wines, EC present in 261 wine samples ranged from undetected to 102 µg/L (4). The U. S. Food and Drug Administration reached an agreement in 1988 with the American Association of Vintners and the Wine Institute that the weighted average of EC in table wines, containing 14 percent or less alcohol by volume, "is not to exceed 15 parts per billion (µg/L) starting with wines produced from the 1988 harvest crush" (5). Guidelines in Canada were established in 1985 limiting the content of EC to 30 µg/L (6).

Carcinogenesis by EC Exposure

EC, the first water soluble carcinogen discovered, can induce many types of tumors in the lungs, liver, thymus, skin and mammary tissue of laboratory animals (7). Distribution of EC after dosing, whether by oral or dermal routes (8) or intraperitoneal injection (9), is widely distributed in tissues and organs. A review of metabolism, carcinogenic effects and risks from EC exposure has been published (10). Carcinogenesis is initiated by the oxidation of EC that is probably accomplished by the

© 1997 American Chemical Society

specific co-factor, cytochrome P-450 IIE1 to a vinyl carbamate, and then epoxidation to an epoxyethyl species forming etheno adducts with nucleic acids in DNA and RNA of various tissues (11-14).These studies on carcinogenesis mechanisms have been accomplished with rodents, but malignant tumors have been observed in nonhuman primates dosed over a long period with EC (15).

Ethanol Interaction with EC

Waddell, et al (16) discovered that radioactive EC administered to mice in a 12% ethanol solution showed an inhibition of radioactivity in tissues as compared to the localization of radioactivity in liver, bone marrow, pancreas and other tissues when EC was administered in water. Further studies in this laboratory (17) showed that ethanol delayed EC metabolism with an inhibition of active metabolites. Ethanol inhibits micronuclei induction by EC in mouse bone marrow erythrocytes (18).
The microsomal ethanol oxidizing system (MEOS) plays a significant role in ethanol oxidation at high ethanol intake or chronic use of alcohol. Cytochrome P-450IIE1 is a necessary co-factor in this MEOS pathway (19). Strain A female mice drinking 10 or 20% ethanol solutions for 12 weeks exhibited significantly reduced incidences of EC-induced pulmonary tumors (20). Studies in our laboratory showed that a 12% ethanol solution, or white or red wines containing this same level of ethanol, fed to C3H mice inhibited EC induced hepatocellular adenomas, hepatocellular carcinomas. as well as pulmonary tumors (21).
Ethanol inhibition of EC induced carcinogenesis may be due, in part, to competitive inhibition for cytochrome P-450IIE1. Metabolism of ethanol, especially under continuous intake, requires this co-factor with the MEOS. The limitation of cytochrome P-450IIE1 for concomitant EC metabolism to effectively form the ultimate carcinogen, namely the EC epoxide metabolite, could play a role in this interactive mechanism.

Wine Interaction with EC

Our initial studies showed that an EC level of 20mg/kg/day in wine given to C3H male mice for 41 weeks resulted in a decreased incidence and frequency of hepatocellular adenomas and other liver tumors as compared to mice drinking water, and even somewhat to a greater extent than ethanol fed mice (21). After alcohol, acids, residual sugars, and perhaps proline, phenols are the constituents major in amount in many wines (22). The wine phenol known as caffeic acid, a nonflavonoid, is found in both red and white wines in appreciable amounts (22). Since caffeic acid has been shown to inhibit tumor development in mice (23,24), we conducted a study to determine if caffeic acid, together with either water or a 12% ethanol solution, could inhibit lung and/or liver tumorigenesis in C3H male mice induced by EC (10 mg/kg body wt/day) with *ad libitum* drinking. Caffeic acid was mixed into a semi-purified diet at 0, 200 or 400 mg/kg of diet and the mice were treated via a similar experimental protocol described in our initial investigation (21). The results of this study, as mean adenoma frequency (number of tumors/tumor bearing mice) in both liver and lung, are presented in Fig. 1. Tumor frequency in both mouse tissues were lower with ethanol treatments as repeated from our earlier work (21). Dietary caffeic acid at 200 mg/kg slightly lowered tumor frequency in the liver of ethanol treated animals but this lowered frequency did not continue at the highest caffeic acid level. Indeed, the highest caffeic acid dietary level with water treatment produced the highest frequency of liver tumors. About 75% of the total number of mice in this study exhibiting liver tumors were on this caffeic acid/water treatment. Caffeic acid produced no changes, in either ethanol or water treatments, on the frequency of lung tumors (Fig.1). It appeared clear that caffeic acid did not enhance EC induced tumor inhibition and may even be responsible, at high dietary levels without ethanol, for liver tumor development.

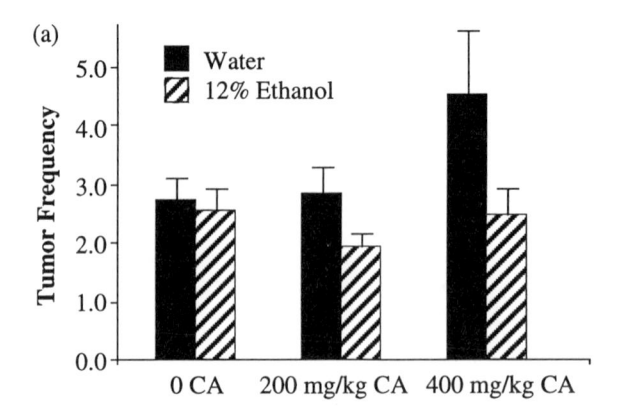

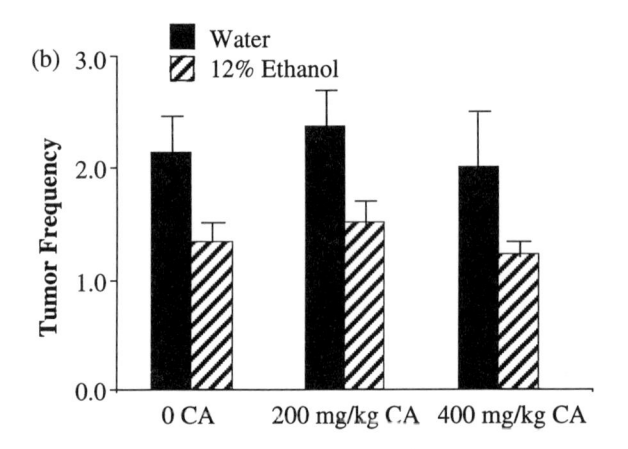

Figure 1. Mean tumor frequency (number of tumors/tumor bearing mice) of EC fed mice.
a) Liver   b) Lung
CA = Caffeic acid
EC = Ethyl carbamate

Wine Phenols. We conducted a more complete study of wine phenolics using the averaged amounts of three major phenolics (P) estimated content in red and white wines (22). P was added to either a 12% ethanol (v/v) solution or water as: caffeic acid, catechin hydrate, and gallic acid at 140, 50, and 25 mg/L, respectively. The wine (Cayuga White/Seyval 50:50 blend), was adjusted to 12% ethanol. In addition, a commercial non-alcoholic (N/A) wine, actually a dealcoholized Chardonnay (.05% ethanol), and water control completed the five treatments used in this 41 week feeding study. The purified diet used in the past (21) was again fed to the mice, but only for 12 hrs during the night (~7:30 pm to 7:30 am) in order to attempt to stop diet wastage and excess body weights. The liquids were fed *ad libitum* with either 0 or 20 mg/kg body wt/day of EC. The incidence and frequency of the two tumor types observed in the liver by detailed pathology, hepatocellular adenomas and hemangioendotheliomas, are presented in Table I. The incidence of spontaneous adenomas, as seen in the 0 EC

Table I. Incidence and Frequency of Hepatocellular Adenomas and Hemangioendotheliomas in C3H Mice Fed Wine, 12% Ethanol or Water with Added Ethyl Carbamate (EC) for 41 Weeks

Treatment	EC mg/kg/day	Incidence (%)[a] Hepatocellular Adenoma	Incidence (%)[a] Hemangio-endothelioma	Frequency[b] Hepatocellular Adenoma	Frequency[b] Hemangio-endothelioma
Wine	0	17.4	0	1.0 ± 0.7^{1}	0
Ethanol + P[c]	0	31.8	0	$1.4 \pm 0.5^{1,2}$	0
N/A[d] Wine	0	70.8	0	$1.5 \pm 0.3^{1,2}$	0
Water + P	0	66.7	0	$1.6 \pm 0.4^{1,2}$	0
Water	0	45.8	0	$1.6 \pm 0.4^{1,2}$	0
Wine	20	47.8	17.4	$1.6 \pm 0.4^{1,2}$	2.2 ± 0.7^{4}
Ethanol + P	20	56.5	17.4	$1.5 \pm 0.4^{1,2}$	1.5 ± 0.7^{4}
N/A Wine	20	83.3	37.5	3.5 ± 0.3^{3}	1.6 ± 0.5^{4}
Water + P	20	77.7	31.8	3.1 ± 0.3^{3}	1.9 ± 0.5^{4}
Water	20	58.3	33.3	$2.4 \pm 0.4^{2,3}$	1.2 ± 0.5^{4}

[a] Percentage of mice with tumors (n= 21-24). Significant (p<0.05) χ^2 measurement of hepatocellular adenoma development dependent on treatments.
[b] Number of specific tumors/ number of tumor bearing mice. Values are means ± SEM. Different superscripts within columns indicate significant differences (p<0.05).
[c] Phenolics added: Caffeic acid - 140 mg/L; Catechin hydrate - 50 mg/L; Gallic acid - 25 mg/L.
[d] Non-alcoholic wine.

Table II Incidence and frequency of alveolar adenomas in C3H mice fed wine, 12% ethanol or water with added ethyl carbamate (EC) for 41 weeks

	EC mg/kg/day	Incidence (%)[a]	Frequency[b]
Treatment		Alveolar adenomas	
Wine	0	0	0
Ethanol + P[c]	0	0	0
N/A Wine	0	8.3	1.0
Water + P	0	0	0
Water	0	4.2	1.0
Wine	20	43.5	1.1 ± 0.3
Ethanol + P	20	43.5	1.2 ± 0.3
N/A Wine	20	58.3	1.8 ± 0.2
Water + P	20	68.2	1.5 ± 0.2
Water	20	87.5	1.8 ± 0.2

[a] Percentage of mice with tumors (n= 21-24). Highly significant (p<0.01) χ^2 measurement of EC induced tumor development dependent on treatments.

[b] Number of adenomas/ number of adenoma bearing mice. Values are means ± SEM. No significant differences in treatment frequencies.

[c] Phenolics added. See Table I.

treatments, seem to occur in a lesser but similar pattern as occured in the EC treated groups. The wine treatments had the smallest incidence of tumors, then the following treatments showed increased tumor incidence: ethanol + P, water, water + phenolics, and N/A wine. Further pathology results indicated that there were no spontaneous hemangioendotheliomas, but mice from the EC treated groups of wine and ethanol + P showed about a 50% less incidence than mice from the other 3 treatments. Additionally, the frequency of hepatocellular adenomas in mice from both the wine and ethanol + P groups were significantly lower as compared to water + P and N/A wine treatments. This data suggests that phenolic intake without the presence of ethanol, either with the natural phenolics present in a N/A white wine or with 3 major wine phenolics, does not inhibit EC-induced liver tumors but seems to actually enhance their incidence and frequency as compared to liver tumor numbers of control mice.

Table II presents the incidence and frequency of lung alveolar adenomas. Very few tumors occurred spontaneously in the lung as seen in the 0 EC treated groups. The mice fed either wine or ethanol + P had the lowest incidence and frequency of alveolar adenomas. However, again it was shown that natural phenolics (N/A wine treatment) or added P to water produced mice with a somewhat larger incidence of alveolar adenomas as compared to mice on treatments containing ethanol. The water drinking, control mice had the highest incidence of EC-induced alveolar adenomas. The trend of tumor frequency was lowest in the wine and water + P treatments. Although these values were not signicantly reduced, the lowered frequency appears correlated with the lowered frequency of hepatocellular adenomas in mice on these treatments (Table I).

Conclusions

EC intake causing tumor induction in liver and lung of C3H mice is inhibited by the accompanying intake of a 12% ethanol solution or wine. The mechanism of this interaction are probably the competitive inhibition of the co-factor cytochrome P-450IIE1 needed for metabolism of ethanol in the MEOS, thus suppressing EC metabolism to its ultimate carcinogen.Wine may have other constituents present that causes somewhat greater protection than ethanol alone against EC carcinogenesis but does not appear to be the wine phenolics. Indeed, there is some indication from these data that wine phenolics in water or non-alcoholic wine increases tumorigenesis in the mouse liver. Any risk assessment of EC should take into consideration this ethanol/wine protective interaction, especially since the major exposure of the public to EC now is from alcoholic beverages.

Acknowledgements

Partial support for this study was granted by the New York Wine and Grape Foundation. The authors thank Widmer's Winery, Naples, New York for donating the wine used in this study.

Literature Cited

1. Ough, C.S. *J. Agr. Food Chem.* **1976**, *24*, 323-328.
2. Canas, B.J.; Havery, D.C.; Robinson, L.R.; Sullivan, M.P.; Joe, F.L.; Diachenko, G.N. *J. A.O.A.C.* **1989**, *72*, 873-876.
3. Matsudo, T.; Aoki, T.; Abe, K.; Fukuta, N.; Higuchi, T.; Sasaki, M.; Uchida, K. *J. Agr. Food Chem.* **1993**, *41*, 352-356.
4. Battaglia, R.; Conacher, H.B.S.; Page, B.D. *Food Additives Contam.* **1990**, *7*, 477-496.
5. Food and Drug Administration. FDA No. T88-7 Talk Paper: Urethane Reduction Plan for Wines. **1988**.

6. Conacher, H.B.S.; Page, B.D. *Proceedings of Euro Food Tox II, Interdiscipllinary Conference on Natural Toxicants in Food, Zurich.* **1986,** Swiss Federal Institute of Technology & University of Zurich, Zurich. 237-242.
7. Mirvish, S.S. *Advances in Cancer Res.* **1968,** *11,* 1-42.
8. Fossa, A.A.; Baird, W.M.; Carlson, G.P. *J. Toxicol. Environ. Health.* **1985,** *15,* 635-654.
9. Berenblum, I.; Haran-Ghera, N.; Winnick, R.; Winnick, T. *Cancer Res.* **1958,** *18,* 181-185.
10. Salmon, A.G.; Zeise, L. Eds. *Risks of Carcinogenesis from Urethane Exposure.* CRC Press/Boca Raton: FL, **1991**.
11. Miller, J.A.; Miller, E.C. *Brit. J. Cancer.* **1983,** *48,* 1-15.
12. Ribovich, M.L.; Miller, J.A.; Miller, E.C.; Timmins, L.G. *Carcinogenesis* **1982,** *3,* 539-546.
13. Svensson, K. *Carcinogenesis.* **1988,** *9,* 2197-2201.
14. Guengerich, F.P.; Kim, D.H. *Chem. Res. Toxicol.* **1991,** *4* , 413-421.
15. Thorgeirsson, U.P.; Dalgard, D.W.; Reeves, J.; Adamson, R.H. *Regul. Toxicol. Pharmacol.* **1994,** *19* , 130-151.
16. Waddell, W.J.; Marlowe, C.; Pierce, W.M. *Food Chem. Toxic.* **1987,** *25,* 527-531.
17. Yamamoto, T.; Pierce, W.M.; Hurst, H.E.; Chen, D.; Waddell, W.J. *Drug Metab. Disposit.* **1988,** *16,* 355-358.
18. Choy, W.N.; Black, W.; Mandakas, G.; Mirro, E.J.; Black, H.E. *Mutat. Res.* **1995,** *341,* 255-263.
19. Lieber, C.S. *Seminars in Liver Disease* **1988,** *8* , 47-68.
20. Kristiansen, E.; Clemmensen, S.; Meyer, O. *Food Chem. Toxic.* **1990,** *28,* 35-38.
21. Stoewsand, G.S.; Anderson, J.L.; Munson, L. *Food Chem. Toxic.* **1991,** *29,* 291-295.
22. Singleton, V.L. In *Wine Analysis*   Linskens, H.F.; Jackson, J.F. Eds. Springer-Verlag, New York. **1988.**
23. Wattenberg, L.W.; Coccia, J.B.; Lam, L.K.T. *Cancer Res.* **1980,** *40,* 2820-2823.
24. Huang, M.-T.; Smart, R.L.; Wong, C.-Q.; Conney, A.H. *Cancer Res.* **1988,** *48,* 5941-5946.

Chapter 18

Endothelium-Dependent Vasorelaxing Activity of Wine, Grapes, and Other Plant Products

David F. Fitzpatrick, Ronald G. Coffey, and Paul T. Jantzen

Department of Pharmacology and Therapeutics, College of Medicine, University of South Florida, Tampa, FL 33612

> This study demonstrates that certain wines and extracts of grape skins and various other fruits, vegetables, nuts, teas and spices stimulate nitric oxide (NO) generation and secretion by endothelial cells of the blood vessel wall *in vitro*, resulting in cyclic GMP-mediated relaxation of vascular smooth muscle (vasodilation). The compounds responsible for this activity appear to be of the catechin type. Since NO is known to decrease platelet aggregation and adhesion, and to diminish oxidation of low density lipoprotein (LDL), as well as relax blood vessels, this mechanism could contribute to the beneficial effects of wine, as well as of plant food products in general.

Over the past few years, several hypotheses have been advanced to explain the beneficial effects of wine in prevention of cardiovascular disease, in particular, atherosclerosis and the subsequent development of coronary heart disease. Several groups have focused on the antioxidant properties of polyphenolic compounds present in wine. The antioxidant effect presumably would either prevent formation of oxygen-derived free radicals such as superoxide, hydroxyl, and peroxyl radicals, or would act by scavenging and neutralizing these deleterious free radicals. There is evidence that such steps could lead to decreased oxidation of LDL and subsequently to diminished or retarded vascular plaque formation in atherogenesis ([1,2]).

Another means by which wine components could exert their beneficial effects is via antithrombotic mechanisms, either by preventing platelet aggregation or causing disaggregation of platelets in established thrombi, or decreasing adhesion of platelets to blood vessel walls. There is evidence to support such an anti-platelet role of wine ([2,3]).

A third potential mechanism of the beneficial effects of wine components relates to one of the hallmarks of hypercholesterolemia and developing atherosclerosis in humans and in experimental atherosclerosis: impairment of endothelium-dependent vasodilation in arteries affected by atherosclerosis (e.g. aorta, coronaries).

The lumen of all blood vessels is lined with a single layer of endothelial cells. These cells are now known to produce and secrete a variety of vasoactive substances, one of the most important of these vasodilating, vasoprotective substance being nitric oxide (NO) (4,5). Nitric oxide is produced in endothelial cells by activation of the enzyme, NO synthase (NOS), the activity of which is dependent on increases in free calcium inside these cells. The substrate for NOS is the amino acid L-arginine, one of whose terminal guanidino groups is converted to NO. The other product of the reaction is L-citrulline. This reaction is inhibited by arginine analogs such as nitroarginine. The NO thus formed (as such or as a nitrosothiol) easily traverses the endothelial cell membrane and enters the smooth muscle cell, where it interacts with the enzyme guanylate cyclase to stimulate formation of cyclic GMP, a second messenger mediating a variety of physiological responses, included vascular relaxation.

Research over the past few years has shown that an adequate level of NO production by endothelial cells is extremely important for maintaining a healthy cardiovascular system. NO exhibits several cardiovascular protective effects in addition to vasodilation, including a reductions in platelet aggregation and adhesion, and oxidation of LDL, as well as inactivation of reactive oxygen species (6). Thus it follows that if too little NO is produced by the endothelium, or if the response to NO by the effector target (vascular smooth muscle, platelets, LDL) is impaired, then protection against atherogenesis is diminished. Evidence is mounting that this is, indeed, the case; there is impairment of endothelium-dependent vasodilation, increased adhesion of platelets to endothelium, and enhanced LDL oxidation during development of atherosclerosis. Therefore, if it were possible to somehow boost NO production by endothelial cells, it might be possible to prevent or delay progression of atherosclerosis.

Our interest in vascular physiology and pharmacology prompted us to test to see whether or not wine or grape products might have some effect on endothelium-dependent blood vessel responsiveness *in vitro*.

Methods

The system we used to study vascular activity of wines and extracts was the isolated rat aortic ring preparation (with or without intact endothelium) suspended in a tissue bath in a physiological salt solution, rigged to measure mechanical responses to various agents (7,8). Cyclic GMP was assayed by the immunoassay method of Coffey et al. (9). Grape skin extracts (GSE) were prepared simply by mincing skins in distilled, de-ionized room temperature water (typically 2 ml water/gm of skins), then filtering 10 min later. Other extracts were prepared in a similar fashion. Pure compounds were dissolved in water or other suitable solvent to give a concentration of 10 mg/ml. Non-aqueous solvent controls were run in parallel.

Results

Endothelium-dependent Relaxation of Aortic rings by Grape Skin Extract (GSE). Initial experiments tested the ability of GSE to cause EDR (Figure 1). The aortic ring is first contracted with phenylephrine (PE, 1μM), then relaxed with acetylcholine (ACh), the classical endothelium-dependent relaxing compound, which is used routinely to test for intactness of the endothelium of the rings. The tissues are then washed (W) to remove drugs in preparation for testing of GSE.

Upon addition of diluted GSE to a ring of intact rat aorta, a rapid relaxation of the contracted ring occurs. The mechanism of the relaxation is also indicated in the figure: The competitive NOS inhibitor N-methyl-L-arginine (L-NMMA) can be seen to inhibit the relaxation induced by GSE. Furthermore, this inhibition is reversed by the normal NOS substrate, L-arginine. The ring which had been denuded of endothelium failed to respond to ACh or GSE. This sequence clearly shows that GSE causes endothelium-dependent vasorelaxations, and that they are mediated by NO. (In a limited number of experiments, GSE caused EDR of canine coronary arteries.)

EDR of Various Grape Products. What about other grape products? Table I shows the EDR activity of various extracts, wines and some compounds present in wines. GSE's prepared from both red and white seedless grapes are capable of virtually 100% relaxation, although the red GSE was more potent. Pulp extracts had no activity. Concord grape juice is an effective relaxer of the rings.

Wines showed great variability in their ability to cause EDR. In addition to the wines listed in the table, several others have been tested, and it appears that of the red wines tested, the cabernet sauvignon samples are consistently more potent and efficacious vasorelaxers than the others. Occasional samples of others such as pinot noir or merlot have activity equivalent to the cabernets, but they are quite variable from sample to sample. Some white wines have some EDR activity, but again it is variable.

Several polyphenolics present in wine have been tested for EDR. Malvidin, the flavonoid largely responsible for the color of red wines, is inactive, as is resveratrol, a natural antifungal compound found in grape skins. Quercetin produces a very slowly developing vasorelaxation, which is partially (about 50%) endothelium-dependent, but the relaxation is not reversed by NOS inhibitors. Other compounds exhibiting at least 50% EDR activity (data not shown) include: chlorogenic acid, diosmin, flavone, kaempherol, myricetin, and rutin (however, unlike active compounds extracted from grape skins, none of these compounds are very water-soluble). Other compounds exhibiting little or no EDR activity include: apigenin, caffeic acid, (+/-) catechin, p-coumaric acid, ellagic acid, esculetin, gallic acid (contracts), gentisic acid, lycopene, morin, naringen, phloridzin, vanillin.

Effect of GSE on Cyclic GMP Levels in Rat Aortic Rings. An elevation of cyclic GMP levels in vascular tissue is considered evidence for involvement of the NO-cyclic GMP pathway in muscle relaxation. Figure 2a shows the effect of GSE

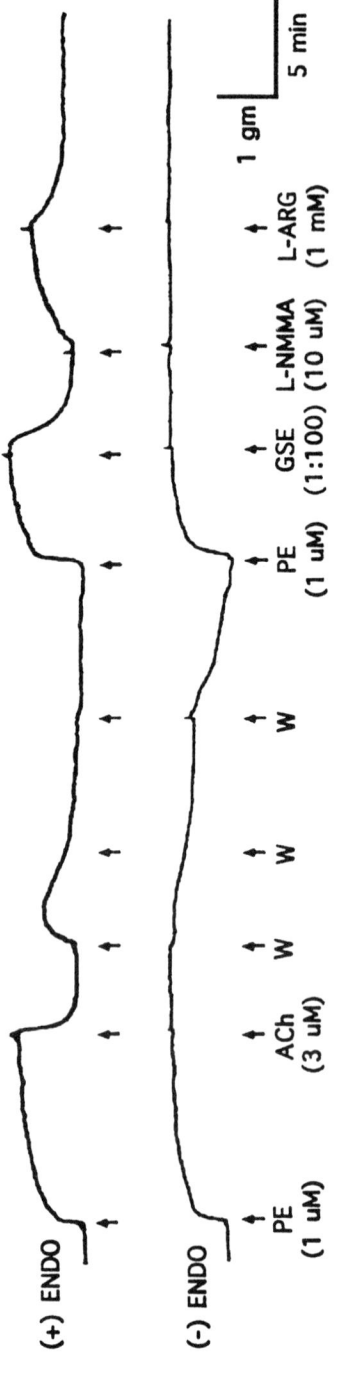

Figure 1. Tracing showing endothelium-dependent relaxing (EDR) activity of grape skin extract (GSE), and effects of an NO synthase inhibitor, N-monomethyl-L-arginine (L-NMMA) and L-arginine (L-ARG). (+) ENDO, ring with endothelium; (-) ENDO. PE, phenylephrine; ACh, acetylcholine; W, wash. Arrows indicate times of application. (Reproduced with permission from ref. 7. Copyright 1993 the American Physiological Society.)

Table I. Endothelium-dependent Vasorelaxing Activity of Various Grape Products

Product	n	EC_{50}	Max. Relaxation (%)
Grape skin extract			
red grape	4	-3.12 ± 0.01	100
white grape	3	-2.85 ± 0.03	96 ± 4
Grape pulp extract			
red grape		indeterminable	0
white grape		indeterminable	0
Grape juice (Concord)	3	-3.08 ± 0.01	97 ± 5
Red wines			
Cabernet Sauv. (Fr '90)	3	-3.22 ± 0.16	86 ± 3
Cabernet Sauv. (CA '91)	4	-3.17 ± 0.01	89 ± 8
Burgundy (CA)	4	-2.14 ± 0.05	53 ± 11
Ethanol		indeterminable	0
White wines			
White Bordeaux (Fr '90)		indeterminable	0
Chardonnay (CA '89)	4	-2.45 ± 0.03	20 ± 4
Malvidin		indeterminable	0
Resveratrol		indeterminable	0
Quercetin	4	-4.00 ± 0.02	97 ± 2

Values are means ± SEM; n: no. of batches tested (for extracts) or no. of replicate samples drawn from the same bottle (wines and pure compounds). EC_{50} values are log dilutions (for extracts and wines) or log of molar concentration for pure compounds) giving 50% relaxation.

Fr and CA: French and California wines, respectively.

SOURCE: Adapted from ref. 7.

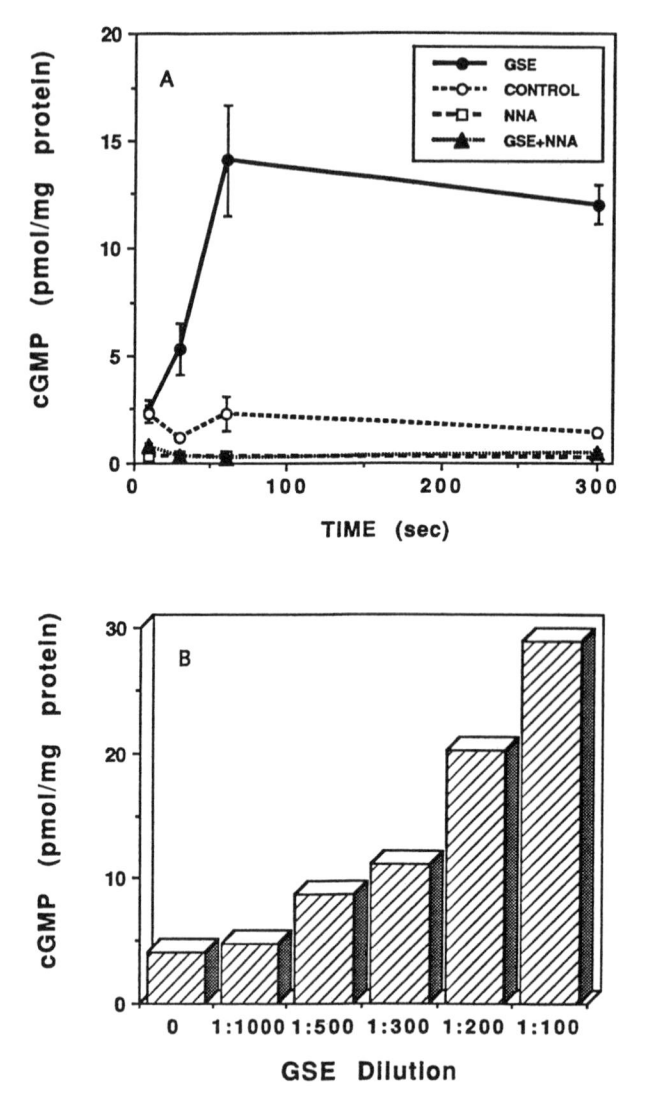

Figure 2. Effects of GSE on cyclic GMP levels in rat aortic rings. *A*: time-dependence experiments; *B*: representative concentration-dependence experiment. (Reproduced with permission from ref. 7. Copyright 1993 the American Physiological Society.)

on cyclic GMP levels in rat aortic rings. GSE augments cyclic GMP accumulation in the rings within the first minute, and the effect is maintained over the 5 min. of the experiment (in the presence of a phosphodiesterase inhibitor). The NOS inhibitor N-nitro-L-arginine (NNA) completely blocks this rise. The cyclic GMP-stimulating effect of GSE is seen at dilutions as low as 1:500 (Figure 2b), and a "dose-response" relationship is evident.

EDR Activity of Extracts of Other Plant Products. Several extracts of commonly consumed vegetables, fruits, teas, and spices have been screened for EDR activity, and many do indeed possess this type of activity (Table II). Among the vegetables tested the variability is considerable; corn, cranberry, and eggplant skin exhibiting the greatest activity. Potato skin and pulp actually enhanced the phenylephrine-induced contraction (about half of which is endothelium-independent, and is inhibited by the alpha-adrenergic blocker prazosin in KCl-contracted aortic rings, data not shown).

In general, the various nut extracts possess high EDR activity, with the skin usually having greater activity than the "meat". Apples (especially the skin) exhibit a great deal of activity, as do guava and plum. Strawberry and watermelon exhibit no activity. Among the teas, green tea showed the greatest activity, and cinnamon was the best of the spices tested.

Effects of Plant Extracts on Cyclic GMP Levels in Aortic Tissue. As in the case of grape skin extracts, some plant extracts which caused EDR, also increased cyclic GMP production, including apple skin extract (ASE) and peanut skin extract (PSE) (Figure 3). However, strawberry extract (SBE), which had no effect on EDR, did not affect cyclic GMP levels.

Discussion

Up until 15 years ago most workers in the cardiovascular field considered the endothelium to be merely a passive barrier which regulated entry and exit of various blood components into and out of the interstitium. In 1980, Furchgott and Zawadzki (10) reported that endothelial cells, upon stimulation by certain vasodilating compounds such as acetylcholine, produced a substance which caused relaxation of blood vessels - an endothelium-derived relaxing factor (EDRF). In 1988 the identity of EDRF was reported to be either nitric oxide or an NO-containing compound (11).

We have shown that grape products as well as other commonly consumed plant foods contain compounds which cause vasorelaxation *in vitro* by an endothelium-dependent process involving the NO/cyclic GMP second messenger system. This demonstrates one possible way in which these foods and beverages could be cardioprotective. Additionally, as pointed out above, NO is involved in other potentially cardioprotective mechanisms including prevention of LDL oxidation and inhibition of platelet stickiness. It would thus appear that this phenomenon is worthy of further investigation, particularly with regard to identification of the

Table II. Vascular Relaxing Activity of Aqueous Extracts of Vegetables, Fruits, Nuts, Teas, Herbs, and Spices

Vegetables	% Relaxation	Fruits	% Relaxation
Bean		Apple	
lima	56.5 ± 10.5	red, skin	92.0 ± 0.9
garbanzo	40.9 ± 8.5	red, pulp	81.2 ± 15.4
green	39.2 ± 6.0	yellow, skin	69.3 ± 18.9
Broccoli	49.2 ± 12.3	yellow, pulp	23.7 ± 7.4
Cabbage		Banana	-21.0 ± 8.6*
green	26.8 ± 3.1	Guava pulp	93.0 ± 2.2
red	42.6 ± 5.1	Orange juice	49.0 ± 4.6
Carrot	5.0 ± 3.0	Plum	
Cauliflower	43.0 ± 14.8	skin	88.1 ± 4.3
Celery	1.4 ± 1.4	pulp	92.6 ± 2.0
Corn	72.2 ± 2.0	Strawberry	0.0 ± 0.0
Cranberry	87.4 ± 6.7	Tomato	
Eggplant skin	77.7 ± 6.2	skin	10.1 ± 2.5
Lentil	48.2 ± 9.7	pulp	5.0 ± 2.6
Mushroom	-21.5 ± 15.8*	Watermelon	0.0 ± 0.0
Pea			
blackeye	53.3 ± 4.1	Teas	
green	35.6 ± 9.5	Black	66.0 ± 6.4
Potato	-52.0 ± 7.0*	Green	91.0 ± 0.7
Rice		Sassafras	69.0 ± 2.6
brown	12.1 ± 4.2		
white	17.7 ± 3.5		
		Herbs, Spices	
Nuts		Bilberry	79.9 ± 4.5
Almond		Cinnamon	98.1 ± 1.9
skin	49.4 ± 11.0	Dill	20.2 ± 4.3
meat	48.1 ± 15.6	Garlic	
Peanut		fresh extract	64.8 ± 8.5
skin	97.0 ± 3.0	Kwai extract	58.0 ± 8.6
meat	60.1 ± 10.3	Onion	43.1 ± 9.7
Pecan		Pepper	
skin	74.0 ± 17.4	red	18.2 ± 4.8
meat	14.4 ± 2.8	white	17.0 ± 2.2
Walnut meat	76.1 ± 13.7	black	0.0 ± 0.0

Results are expressed as percent relaxation ± SEM, caused by a 1:100 dilution of extract, in relation to 3 µM ACh-induced relaxation of same tissue in a given experiment (3-5 experiments).
* Extract caused contraction.
SOURCE: Adapted from ref. 8.

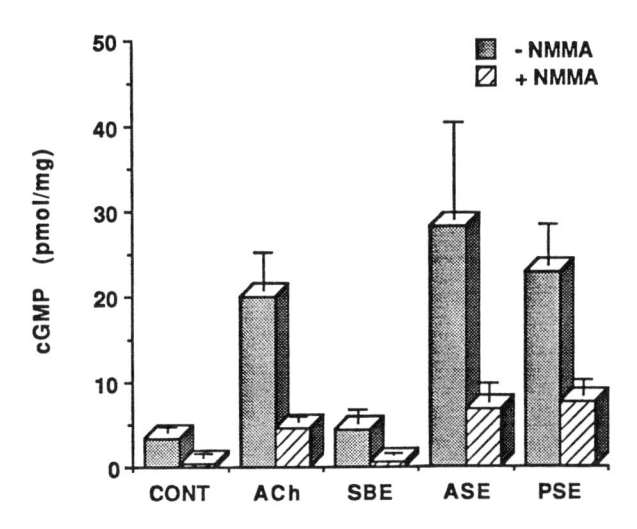

Figure 3. Effects of extracts of food plant products on cyclic GMP levels in rat aortic rings. CONT, control; ACh, acetylcholine (3 µM); SBE, strawberry extract; ASE, apple skin extract; PSE, peanut skin extract; NMMA, N-monomethyl-L-arginine. All extracts were tested at a dilution of 1:100. Other details are presented in Methods. (Reproduced with permission from ref. 8. Copyright 1995 Raven Press Limited.)

EDR-active compounds, and investigation of possible *in vivo* effects. With regard to identification of the compounds, preliminary solvent extraction procedures and HPLC and mass spectrometry analyses indicates that the compounds are of the catechin type (i.e. flavan-3-ols), possibly galloylated catechins.

The question of whether or not the EDR-active compounds are absorbed orally has not been answered. However, work by others suggest that these or similar compounds are indeed absorbed. Absorption of a number of flavonoids from the gastrointestinal tract into the circulation has been demonstrated, including quercetin (*12*) and epigallocatechin gallate (*13*). A potentially important study was reported recently by the Folts group (*3*) showing that both red wine and grape juice (but not white wine), administered orally or intravenously to dogs inhibited cyclic flow reductions (CFRs) in coronary blood flow caused by platelet-mediated thrombus formation. This indicates that: 1) components other than ethanol are responsible for the effect, and 2) these compounds are absorbed intact (or in some active form) in sufficient amounts to produce a biological effect. Experiments to determine possible *in vivo* effects of wine are underway in our laboratory, using the hypercholesterolemic rabbit model. We are also beginning to look at various components of the NO generation pathway in an attempt to determine the biochemical site of action of the phenolics.

Acknowledgments

We wish to thank Stephen Hirschfield, Tessa Ricci, and David Maggi for their technical assistance. This work was supported by a Grant-In-Aid from the American Heart Association, Florida Affiliate, Inc.

Literature Cited

1. Frankel, E.N., Kanner, J., German, J.B., Parks, E., Kinsella, J.E. *Lancet* **1993**, *341*, 454-457.
2. Bierenbaum, M.L., Reichstein, R.P., Bhagavan, H.M., Watkins, T. *Biochem. Intl.* **1992**, *28*, 57-66.
3. Demrow, H.S., Slane, P.R., Folts, J.D. *Circulation*, **1995**, *1182-1199*.
4. Moncada, S., Palmer, R.M.J., Higgs, E.A. *Pharmacol. Rev.* **1991**, *43*, 109-142.
5. Radomski, M.W. *Annals Med.* **1995**, *27*, 321-329.
6. Warren, J.B., Pons, F., Brady, A.J.B. *Cardiovasc. Res.* **1994**, *28*, 25-30.
7. Fitzpatrick, D.F., Hirschfield, S.L., Coffey, R.G. *Am. J. Physiol.* **1993**, *265*, H774-H778.
8. Fitzpatrick, D.F., Hirschfield, S.L., Ricci, T., Jantzen, P., Coffey, R.G. *J. Cardiovasc. Pharmacol.* **1995**, *26*, 90-95.
9. Coffey, R.G., David, J.S., Djeu, J. *J. Immunol.* **1988**, *140*, 2695-2701.
10. Furchgott, R.F., Zawadzki, J.V. *Nature* **1980**, *288*, 373-376.
11. Palmer, R.M.J., Ferrige, A.G., Moncada, S. *Nature* **1987**, *327*, 524,526.
12. Hollman, P., DeVries, J., VanLeeuwen, S., Mengelers, M., Katan, M. *Am. J. Clin. Nutr.* **1995**, *62*, 1276-1282.
13. Unno, T., Takeo, T. *Biosci. Biotech. Biochem.* **1995**, *59*, 1558-1559.

Chapter 19

Antithrombotic Effect of Flavonoids in Red Wine

N. Maalej, H. S. Demrow, P. R. Slane, and John D. Folts[1]

Department of Cardiology, School of Medicine, University of Wisconsin, 600 Highland Avenue, Madison, WI 53792–3248

Moderate daily consumption of alcoholic beverages is a negative risk factor for the development of atherosclerosis and coronary artery disease (CAD), especially in France and other Mediterranean areas where red wine is regularly consumed with meals. The anti-thrombotic activity of red wine was suspected to be due to the alcoholic component. Pure ethanol has been shown to inhibit platelet aggregation in vitro, ex vivo, and in vivo although a blood alcohol content (BAC) of 0.2 g/dl or more is required. However, red wine inhibited platelet activity at a much lower BAC of 0.028 g/dl. We found that red wine and grape juice, but not white wine, inhibited platelet activity. Red wine and grape juice contain a wide variety of naturally occurring compounds including fungicides, tannins, anthocyanins, and phenolic flavonoids (including flavonols and flavones). The antithrombotic effect of red wine and grape juice may be due to the flavonoids common in some vegetable, fruits, and herbs such as tea. Besides having anti-thrombotic properties, flavonoids are also anti-oxidants that prevent lipid oxidization known to contribute to atherosclerosis. Future studies may demonstrate that the consumption of flavonoid rich foods and beverages may have protective effects against the development of coronary artery disease and may decrease the risk of myocardial infarction due to their platelet inhibitory and antioxidant effects.

"The French Paradox", as it has been publicized by both the scientific and popular news media, deals with interesting yet confusing statistics regarding the life-style and the rate of myocardial infarction of the French people. The French eat 3.8 times as much butter as Americans and 2.8 times as much lard (*1*). They have higher serum cholesterol levels and higher blood pressure than Americans (*2*). Other risk factors for cardiovascular disease such as body mass index and cigarette smoking are comparable in both countries (*2*). Yet, Americans have a 2 1/2 times greater rate of death due to coronary heart disease than the French (*2*).

A number of hypotheses have been proposed to account for this paradox. The "Mediterranean diet" may play a role in explaining this paradox. The French

[1]Corresponding author

© 1997 American Chemical Society

drink very little milk and eat a large amount of fresh vegetables, fruits, and drink wine with meals (*3-4*). The reduction in the incidence of coronary artery disease (CAD) with the consumption of alcoholic beverages was first noted by Cabot in 1904 (*5*). Since that time, autopsy, geographic, case-control, cohort, clinical, and epidemiological studies have been conducted to study the effect of alcohol consumption on CAD. The majority of these studies show an inverse relationship between alcohol consumption and CAD (*6*). This protective effect has been attributed in part to the ethanol related increase in HDL cholesterol and the reduced platelet activity.

In the past twenty years, it has become apparent that platelets contribute to the rate of development of atherosclerosis and coronary artery disease by several mechanisms (*7*). In addition, platelet-mediated thrombus formation plays a key role in unstable angina, myocardial infarction and restenosis after angioplasty or atherectomy (*7-9*). One way to study the platelet inhibitory effects of various compounds in vivo is by using an in vivo model such as the "Folts coronary thrombosis model" of platelet aggregation and thrombus formation (*10-11*). Platelet-mediated thrombi periodically form in the stenosed coronary artery followed by embolization distally. This produces cyclical reductions in measured coronary blood flow that is called cyclic flow reductions (CFRs). We have shown that the CFRs in mechanically stenosed canine arteries can be eliminated by platelet inhibitors such as aspirin (*11*), prostacyclin (*11,12*), and the nitric oxide donor sodium nitroprusside (*13*). We have also shown that 1.0 ml/kg of pure ethanol, producing an average blood alcohol content (BAC) of 0.24 g/dl, inhibits platelet activity in this model (*14-15*). Preliminary studies suggested that red wine inhibited platelet activity and coronary thrombosis *in vivo*. (*16*). To ascertain the anti-thrombotic activity of wine, we decided to study the effectiveness of red and white wine in the Folts in vivo model. We also sought to determine if grape juice, a similar beverage yet without the alcohol content, would have a platelet-inhibitory effect. This would help to clarify the platelet inhibitory importance of the ethanol content of wine.

Cardio-Protective Effect of Wine

Wine Consumption and Coronary Heart Disease (CHD). Many studies found an inverse relationship between mortality and moderate consumption of wine. Gronbaek, examined the association between intake of wine, spirits, and beer and the mortality in the Copenhagen city heart study of 13285 subjects. The results showed that the relative risk of dying decreased from 1 for non drinkers to 0.51 for subjects who drank 3 to 5 glasses of red wine per day. Neither beer or spirit consumption was associated with reduced risk (*17*). Gronbaek also observed a U shape relationship between alcohol intake and mortality with the lowest risk for 1 to 6 drinks per week (*18*). Doll assessed the risk of death associated with alcoholic beverage consumption in 1900 British physicians between the age of 50 and 90. He also found a U shape relationship between all causes of mortality and alcohol consumption with a minimum mortality for those consuming 1 to 2 drinks a day (*19*). Fuchs studied the risk of death in 85709 women of 34-59 years of age. The relative risk of death in drinkers, as compared to non drinkers, was 0.83-0.88 for women with light to moderate consumption of alcohol (1.5-29.9 g/day equivalent to 1 to 3 drinks per week). The risk increased to 1.19 for women who consumed more than 30 g/day (*20*).

Many epidemiological studies have investigated the relative cardio-protective benefits of different types of alcoholic beverages. Since 1986, the Framingham Study (*21*), the American Cancer Society Study (*22*), the CORALI Study (*23*), the Kaiser-Permenente Study (*24*), the Health Professionals Study (*25*), the Nurses

Health Study (26), and a recent Boston area study (27,28) have all corroborated the theory of decreased CAD risk with moderate alcohol consumption. Renaud (29), Nanji (30), and St. Leger (31) have suggested that wine consumption is responsible for the low levels of CAD mortality in countries with high wine consumption. Both Nanji and St. Leger found an inverse association between CAD mortality and wine consumption (r = -0.75 and -0.65 respectively). In case-control studies, Hennekens gives the relative risk of CAD mortality for light to moderate drinkers (≤2 oz of ethanol/day) as 0.3 for those consuming beer or wine and 0.2 for those consuming liquor (32). Klatsky gives the relative risk at 0.7 for those preferring beer or wine but calculates the relative risk for those preferring liquor at 1.0-1.1 (33). Moore and Pearson reviewed case-control studies and cohort studies showing that moderate alcohol consumption reduces the risk of CAD to 0.4-0.7 compared to non-drinkers (6). Criqui explored the effect of wine, beer and spirits consumption on CHD and mortality in 21 developed countries. He concluded that moderate wine consumption, particularly wine ethanol, is inversely related to CHD but not to longevity (34). Other studies have also reported the protective effect of moderate alcohol consumption against CHD (35-38). Moderate drinking was also associated with reduced risk of peripheral arterial disease (39,40). Klastky concluded from his study that the risk for CHD and death is minimal for subjects drinking light to moderate amounts (up to 2 drinks/day). The consumption of 3 or more drinks per day has detrimental social, personal, and medical effects that may outweigh any potential benefits (41,42). Camargo reported that moderate alcohol consumption reduces the risk of CHD by increasing HDL. In the physicians health study of 22 071 men age between 40 and 48, they observed a synergistic platelet inhibitory effect when both alcohol and low dose aspirin were taken regularly (43). Anderson reviewed the risk of alcohol consumption and concluded that there is a protective effect of alcohol consumption against CHD. However, there is also evidence for a dose-response relationship between level of alcohol consumption and risk of developing liver cirrhosis, cancers of oropharynx, larynx, esophagus, liver and breast, and blood pressure and stroke (44).

Alcohol Effect on Lipids. Numerous studies have attributed the observed cardio-protective effects of alcohol consumption to an increase in plasma high density lipoprotein (HDL) cholesterol levels (45-49). Lavy studied the effect of a two week dietary supplementation of red and white wine on Human Blood Chemistry, Hematology and Coagulation. He observed that red wine but not white wine increased the plasma HDL cholesterol by 26 % (45). Clevidence studied the effect of moderate alcohol consumption (31.5 ml of alcohol mixed with fruit juice), equivalent to 2 drinks/day, on the lipoprotein profiles of 34 premenopausal women. With alcohol consumption, HDL cholesterol level increased 10%, LDL levels decreased 8%, and levels of lipoprotein (a) were unchanged (46). Gaziano observed that the level of high density lipoproteins cholesterol (HDL) and its HDL2 and HDL3 subfraction were strongly associated with alcohol (beer, wine, and spirit) consumption and are suggested to play a part in the reduced risk of MI (28). Langer observed that the protection of moderate alcohol consumption against CHD is mediated by the increase of HDL and decrease of LDL (47,48). Razay studied 1048 British women aged 25-69 to examine the relationship between alcohol consumption (beer, wine, and spirits) and CHD. He found a reduced risk for women who drank moderately (up to 2 glasses of wine) compared to non-drinkers and heavy drinkers. He observed that women consuming a moderate amount of alcohol had a lower plasma concentration of triglycerides, cholesterol, and insulin. They also had a higher concentration of HDL, HDL2 and HDL3. He attributed the reduced risk of CHD to lower plasma concentration of triglycerides and insulin, as well as higher concentration of HDL as well as HDL2 and HDL3 cholesterol (49).

Effect of Alcohol on the Platelets. Since wine (*50*) and alcohol consumption (*51-53*) has been shown to decrease platelet aggregation, the cardioprotective effects of alcohol may, in part, be related to platelet activity. Many scientists feel that a higher HDL cholesterol level does not fully explain the cardioprotective effects of moderate alcohol consumption (*47-48,54-55*). Seigneur studied platelet aggregation and lipid levels of human volunteers who consumed red wine or white wine for a fifteen day study period. The consumption of both red and white wine increased HDL levels and the consumption of red wine decreased ADP induced platelet aggregation (*50*). Struck compared the effects of red versus white wine consumption upon serum lipids, clotting factors, oxidation products and antioxidant levels in 20 adult hypercholesterolemics, over a three-month period. He observed a reduced thrombin-initiated platelet aggregation from 0.91 to 0.75 U/ml. Additionally, low density lipoprotein cholesterol (LDL) decreased from 167 to 158 mg/dl. The data suggests that wine possesses both antithrombotic and antioxidant effects (*56*).

Renaud studied the effect of alcohol on CHD in industrialized countries. He observed that serum concentration of HDL in the French population is not higher than other industrialized countries. However, platelet reactivity in the French population is lower. He concluded that moderate alcohol consumption does not prevent CHD through its action on high density lipoproteins and atherosclerosis, but rather through a hemostatic mechanism. The data showed that platelet aggregation, which is related to CHD, is significantly inhibited by alcohol at levels of intake associated with reduced CHD (*29,53,57*). McGarry evaluated primary homeostasis in 50 adult patients with idiopathic epistaxis. He observed that the prolongation of the bleeding time was significantly associated with alcohol use even at the low consumption of 1 to 10 units per week (*58*). However, chronic alcoholics are reported to have higher incidence of cardiovascular, endocrine and hematological diseases.

Rubin reviewed the acute effects of ethanol on platelet function both in vivo and ex vivo. Ethanol was observed to inhibit platelet response to specific physiological agonists (*59*). Renaud studied the effect of alcohol consumption on platelet aggregation in 1600 men (aged 49-66). He found that the platelet response to ADP and collagen but not to thrombin were significantly reduced (*60*). Mehta studied the effect of ethanol on human platelet aggregation in vitro. He found that ethanol in concentrations as low as 10 mg% potentiated the platelet aggregation inhibitory response of prostacyclin, at 20 mg% it decreased the formation of thromboxane A2 in whole blood by 41%, and stimulated the formation of neutrophil prostacyclin by 160% (*61*). Ridker found a direct association between alcohol consumption and plasma level of t-PA antigen. This observation supports the hypothesis that changes in the fibrinolytic potential may be an important mechanism whereby moderate alcohol consumption decreases the risk of CHD (*62*).

Animal studies have also confirmed the platelet inhibitory effect of alcohol (*63-66*). Chabielska demonstrated that ethanol (1, 2, and 4 g/kg) in rats significantly decreased blood platelet aggregation in a dose dependent manner. The chronic administration of ethanol (6 g/kg daily for 4 weeks) also altered the sensitivity of rat platelets to ADP (4 ml/l) (*63*). Latta found that chronic short term administration of a moderate amount of ethanol inhibited the enhanced response of platelets from rabbits with diet-induced hypercholesterolemia, via a thrombin-induced, thromboxane A2-independent pathway (*64*). Kitagawa studied the effect of alcohol on bovine platelet membrane fluidity and platelet adenylate cyclase activity. He observed that that alcohol increased the platelet fluidity in the central region of lipid bylayer and the increased the intercellular cAMP concentrations and thus inhibited platelet aggregation (65). Smith observed that moderate alcohol consumption for 4 weeks was associated with reduced platelet count and size in guinea pigs (66).

In Vivo Studies of the Antithrombotic Effect of Wine

Methods. Adult mongrel dogs of either sex were anesthetized. A left thoracotomy was performed and the left circumflex coronary artery was dissected out. An electromagnetic flow probe was placed around the artery to measure blood flow. The coronary artery was squeezed distal to the flow probe with a special surgical clamp to produce intimal and medial damage. A plastic constricting cylinder was then placed around the outside of the injured portion of the artery to produce a 60%-80% stenosis (Figure. 1). Blood pressure and the electrocardiogram of each animal were also monitored. Each animal was observed until cyclic flow reductions (CFRs), due to platelet mediated thrombus formation, were occurring at regular intervals. In order to permit intragastric administration, an abdominal incision over the spleen was made and the stomach was exposed. A 15 French Foley catheter was inserted into the stomach through a small incision in the stomach wall and secured with a purse string suture. After confirming the position of the catheter, the corresponding layers and incision were closed and sutured. In parallel to the in vivo studies, ex vivo whole blood aggregation studies were performed in some experiments to confirm the in vivo results.

Red Wine Study. Five dogs were prepared as described above and given a 4 ml/kg intragastric infusion of red wine. The red wine, 1987 Chateauneuf-du-Pape, is 13% alcohol by volume. Cyclic flow reductions (CFRs) were observed during the initial observation period for all the dogs. In the five dogs, the CFRs were abolished at an average time of 113±32 minutes after wine administration (Figure 2, (67)). The slopes of the CFRs during this time period decreased gradually. The average ethanol content of the red wine given was 0.52 ml/kg producing an average blood alcohol content (BAC) of 0.036±0.013 g/dl.

White Wine Study. Five dogs were prepared as described and given 4ml/kg of white wine intragastrically. The white wine, 1990 Chateau Villotte Bordeaux, is 12% alcohol by volume. Cyclic flow reductions (CFRs) were observed during the initial observation period for all the dogs. The CFRs were not eliminated in any of the animals (Figure 3, (67)). The average ethanol concentration of the wine was 0.48 ml/kg producing an average BAC of 0.024±0.015 g/dl after the administration. The slopes of the CFRs were not significantly different after the intragastric administration of the white wine. The average slope of the CFRs was -18.47±3.56 ml/min^2 before the wine and was -14.85±5.35 ml/min^2 ($p = 0.09$) after the administration of white wine.

Grape Juice Study. Ten dogs were prepared as described above. After observation of CFRs, grape juice was given intragastrically. The grape juice used was Welch's 100% natural grape juice with no sugar, artificial flavors, or colors added. Three doses of grape juice were given: two dogs were given 6 ml/kg, three dogs were given 8 ml/kg, and five dogs were given 10 ml/kg. The dogs given 6 or 8 ml/kg of grape juice intragastrically showed platelet inhibition by a decrease in the slopes of the CFRs and spontaneous embolizations of thrombi, yet the CFRs were not completely eliminated. The CFRs in the five dogs given 10 ml/kg were completely abolished after an average time of 95 ± 33 minutes (Figure 4, (67)). The amount of intragastric grape juice necessary to abolish the CFRs was 2.5 times greater than the amount of intragastric red wine given. The aggregation response to

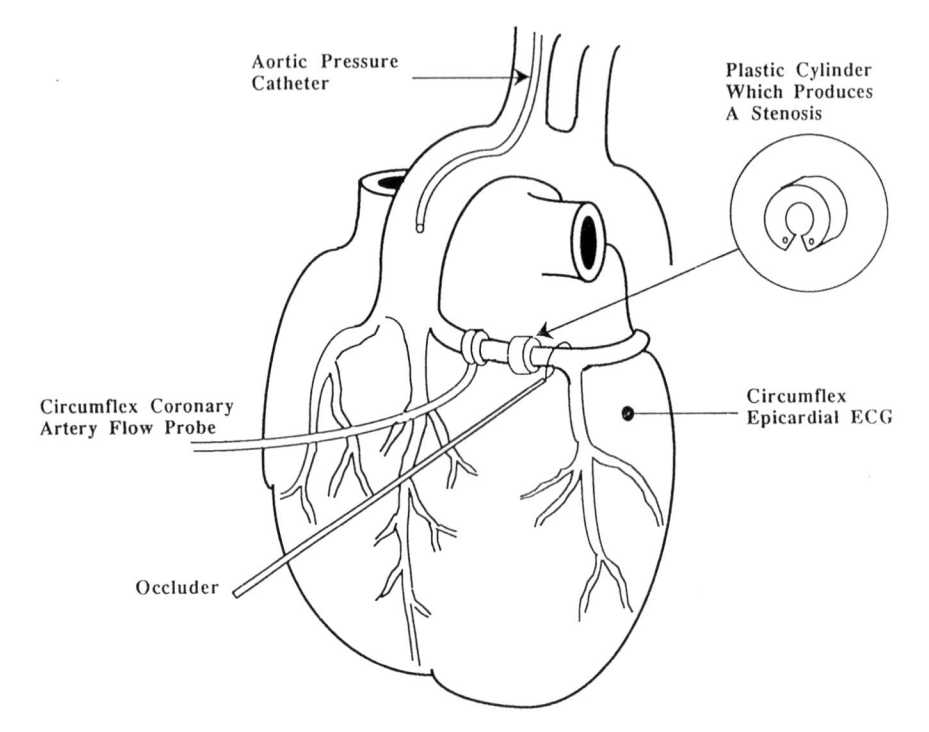

Figure 1. Schematic diagram of the Folts animal model for studying conditions similar to humans with coronary artery disease. The circumflex coronary artery is exposed and clamped to produce vessel wall damage. A plastic cylinder 4 mm in length is placed to encircle and constrict the circumflex coronary artery, producing a 60% to 80% reduction in diameter. An electromagnetic flow probe measures the blood volume flow in the stenosed artery. Platelet mediated thrombus formation in the stenosed artery cause cyclic flow reduction in blood flow (CFRs).

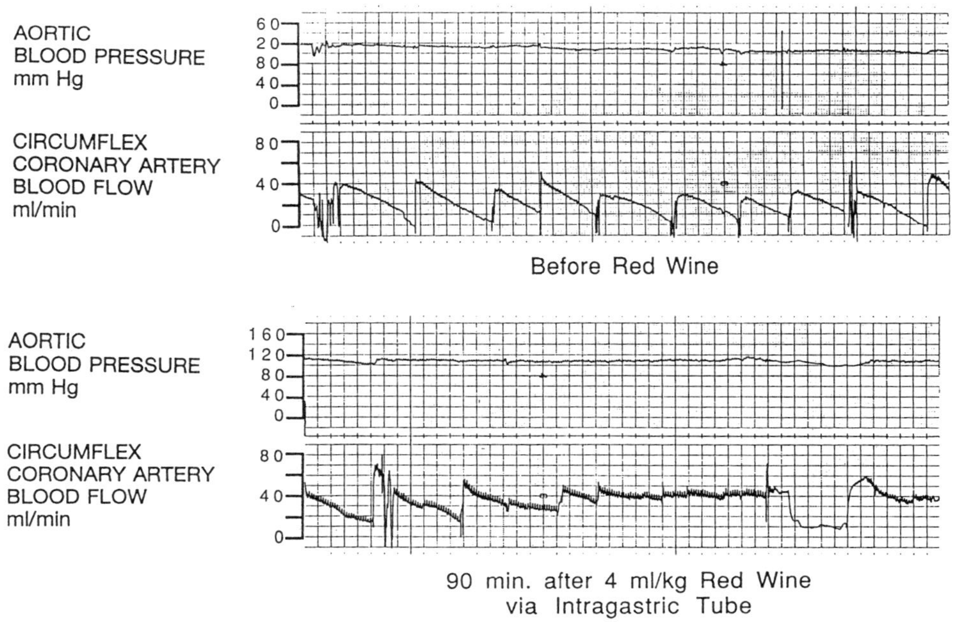

Figure 2. Representative tracing of the hemodynamic effect of intragastric red wine: Top tracing shows mean aortic blood pressure and blood flow in the stenosed left circumflex artery. Cyclic flow reductions were observed before the red wine was given. Bottom tracing shows elimination of the cyclic flow reductions, 90 minutes after 4 ml/kg red wine was given (Reproduced with permission from ref. 67. Copy-right 1995 Am. Heart Assoc.).

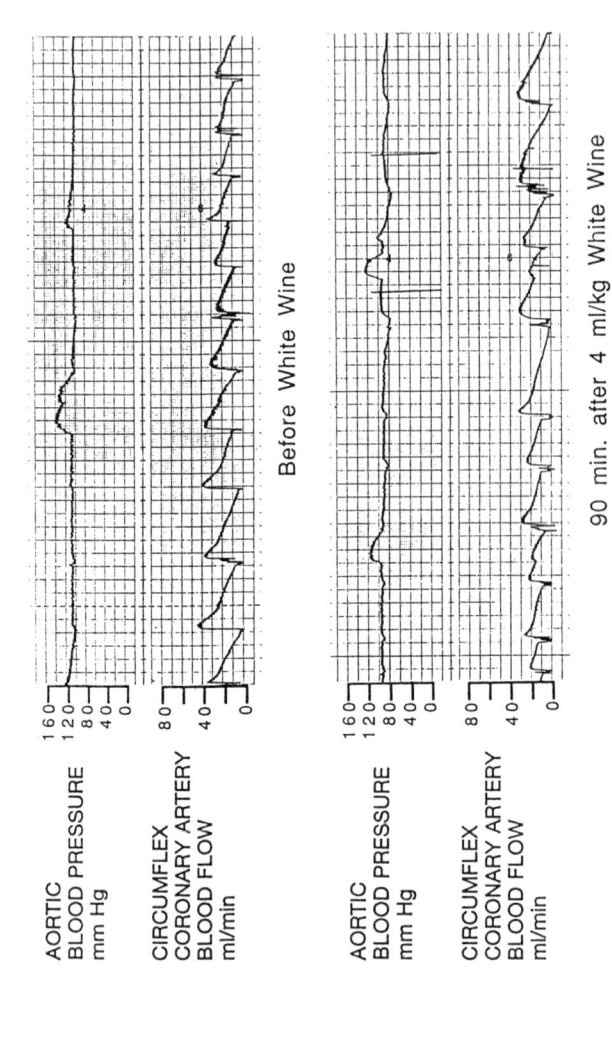

254 WINE: NUTRITIONAL AND THERAPEUTIC BENEFITS

Figure 3. Representative tracing of the hemodynamic effect of intragastric white wine: Top tracing shows cyclic flow reductions before the white wine was given. Bottom tracing shows continuation of the cyclic flow reductions 90 minutes after 4 ml/kg of white wine was given (Reproduced with permission from ref. 67. Copyright 1995 Am. Heart Assoc.).

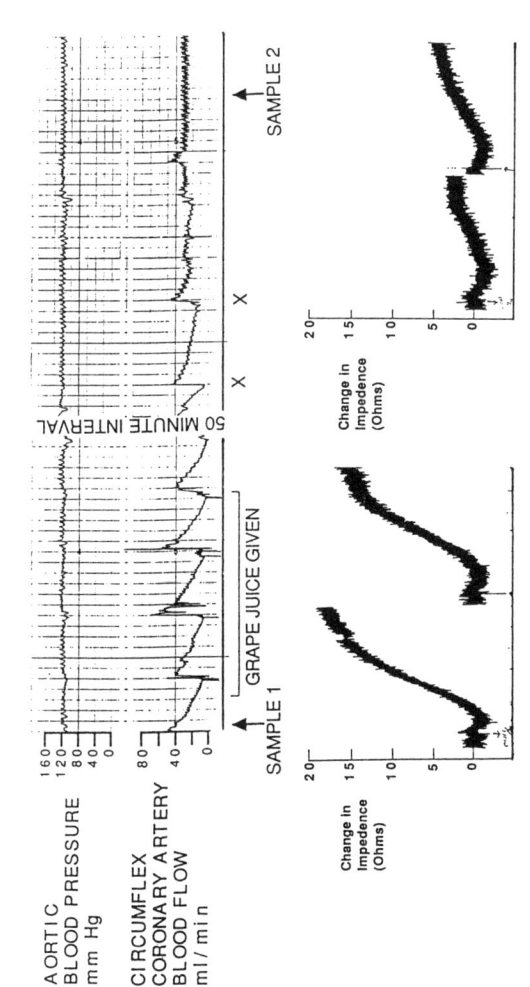

Figure 4. Top tracing shows a representative tracing of the hemodynamic effects of intragastric grape juice. X denotes a spontaneous platelet thrombus embolization that did not require the manual shaking of the occluding cylinder. Bottom tracing shows whole blood aggregation tracings from the animal in the top tracing. Sample 1 was taken before the animal was given the grape juice and sample 2 was taken when the CFRs were eliminated. The decrease in collagen induced aggregation corresponds to the decrease of the CFRs' slopes (Reproduced with permission from ref. 67. Copy-right 1995 Am. Heart Assoc.).

collagen before the grape juice administration was compared to the response when the CFRs were eliminated. The studies showed a 67.6±19.7% decrease in aggregation to the same concentration of collagen (p<0.01).

Discussion

The "Folts Coronary Thrombosis Model" is an on-line in vivo bioassay for platelet activity producing cyclic flow reductions (CFRs) in coronary blood flow (*10*). The CFRs were abolished by both the red wine and the grape juice when administered intragastrically. The white wine did not show significant results in eliminating the CFRs and decreased the slope of the CFRs only slightly. These results suggest that there are compounds present in red wine and grape juice that are not present, or present in a lower concentration, in white wine that may be anti-thrombotic and platelet inhibitory.

Pure ethanol has been shown to inhibit platelet aggregation in vitro, ex vivo, and in vivo although a blood alcohol content of 0.25 g/dl or more is required (*14,15,51*). We previously demonstrated in this model that an average of 1.0 ml/kg of pure ethanol given intravenously eliminates the CFRs, producing an average peak BAC of 0.24 g/dl (*14*). The BAC of the dogs given the red wine was 0.036 g/dl, 14% of the BAC of the dogs given pure ethanol. Since the amount of ethanol necessary to eliminate the CFRs is greatly reduced when red wine as opposed to pure ethanol was given, there must be other active platelet inhibitors in the red wine in addition to the ethanol. These compounds may be the same anti-platelet compounds that give grape juice it's anti-thrombotic activity.

Antioxidant Effect of Flavonoids. It has been proposed that the protective effects of wine, specifically red wine, are possibly due to a large number of naturally occurring constituents in the beverage. Wine contains a wide variety of compounds including naturally occurring fungicides, tannins, anthocyanins, and phenolic flavonoids (flavonols and flavones) (*68*). The phenolic antioxidant phytochemicals in wines may be partly responsible for the lower rates of cardiac disease mortality. Frankel studied the activities of 20 selected California wines in inhibiting the copper catalyzed oxidation of human LDL. The relative antioxidant activity correlated with total phenol contents of wines (*69*). He reported that wine based antioxidants, flavonoids, are more powerful protectors against heart disease than alpha-tocopherol (*70*). Whitehead used a chemilumenescent essay of serum antioxidant capacity to study the effect of the ingestion of red wine, white wine and high doses of vitamin C. The in vitro study showed a high antioxidant capacity of red wine in addition to its ability to increase the antioxidant capacity in vivo (*71*). Teissedre studied the in vitro inhibition of LDL oxidation by phenolic antioxidants from grapes and wines. He found that the more active fractions contained the components of the catechin family. The catechin oligomers and the procyanadin dimers (B2, B3, B4, B6, B8) and trimers (C, C2) were extracted, isolated and purified from grape seed. The procyanadin dimers, B2 and B8, the trimer C1, and the monomers catechin, epicatechin and myrecetin had the highest antioxidant activity. The procyanadin dimers B3, B4 and C2 and the monomers gallic acid, quercetin, caffeic acid, and rutin had the least antioxidant activity (*72*). Studies have also shown that the fungicide resveratrol lowers overall cholesterol levels (*73*), increases HDL cholesterol levels (*50*), and inhibits the oxidation of LDL cholesterol (*74*).

Antiplatelet Effect of Flavonoids. The naturally occurring flavonoids found in wine, grape juice and other foods have been shown to decrease platelet aggregation in vitro (*75-78*), inhibit platelet aggregation on blood-superfused collagen strips in vivo (79), and cause platelet disaggregation of pre-formed platelet thrombi in vitro (79). Our group has shown that the flavonoids quercetin and rutin inhibited platelet activity, eliminating the CFRs in the Folts *in vivo* model (80). There is also evidence that flavonoids inhibit the production of thromboxane A2 perhaps by inhibiting platelet cyclooxygenase activity (75,77). Flavonoids have been shown to inhibit the release of serotonin from human platelets (76,81). Especially interesting are the studies demonstrating that quercetin raises platelet cAMP levels (78,82), and that myricetin (75), morin (54), and quercetin (54,57,61) potentiate the increase in cAMP induced by PGI2. Flavonoids (particularly quercetin, kaempferol, apigenin, and amentoflavone) have been shown to inhibit cAMP and cGMP phosphodiesterases (83-87). The studies of Ferrel suggest that flavonoids compete with cAMP for a nucleotide binding site (83). The inhibition of cAMP or cGMP phosphodiesterases would raise the platelet levels of cAMP or cGMP. This in turn would lower platelet cytosolic calcium levels, and decrease the level of in vivo platelet activity (86).

Flavonoids in Clinical Studies. In the Zutphen study middle aged men were followed for eight years. Their diet was examined and a calculation made of the quantity of flavonoids consumed. There was a clear inverse relationship between the intake of dietary flavonoids and heart attacks (87). In other words, those with the lowest intake of flavonoids had the highest incidence of heart attacks. This concept of protection with flavonoids was also confirmed in the Seven Countries Study (88). The predominant flavonoid consumed in the diet of the subjects was quercetin, with quercetin intake giving essentially the same relative risk as overall flavonoid intake (89). More recently, a cohort study of 552 men aged 50 to 69 reported that the dietary intake of flavonoids (mainly quercetin) was inversely associated with stroke incidence (90).

Conclusion

It is therefore possible to speculate that the cardio-protective effects of red wine consumption observed in the French and other populations may be attributed, in part, to the ethanol content of the wine and, in part, to the antioxidant and platelet inhibitory properties of flavonoids in the wine. Since platelet adhesion to damaged endothelium and subsequent platelet aggregation are major steps in both thrombosis and atherogenesis, the chronic inhibition of platelet activity by the daily consumption of flavonoid-containing foods and beverages may retard atherogenesis and prevent thrombosis. Red wine offers cardio-protective platelet inhibition to drinkers whereas grape juice (and perhaps other flavonoid-rich foods) extend platelet inhibition to non-drinkers as well. The potentially beneficial effects of alcoholic beverages and fruit juices on CAD warrants further study.

References

1. Food and Agriculture Organization of the United Nations. *Food and Agr. Org. of the United Nations* **1991**,*109-111*, 360-362.
2. World Health Organization. The WHO Monica Report : a world-wide monitoring system for cardiovascular diseases In: *World Health Statistics Annual*. Geneva, Switzerland: World Health Organization, **1989**, 27-59.
3. Ulbright, T.L.V.; Southgate, D.A.T. *Lancet.* **1991**,*338*, 985-992.
4. Ferro-Luzzi, A.; Sette, S. *Eur. J. Clin. Nutr* **1989**, *43(2)*,13-29.
5. Cabot, R.C. *JAMA.* **1904**,*43*, 774-775.
6. Moore, R.D.; Pearson, T.A. *Medicine.* **1986**, *65(4)*, 242-267.

7. Fuster, V.; Badimon, L.; Badimon J.J.; Chesebro, J.H. *N. Engl. J. Med.* **1992**, *326(4)*, 242-250.
8. Davies, M.J.; Thomas, A. *N. Engl. J. Med.* **1984**, *310(18)*, 1137-1140.
9. Antiplatelet trialists' collaboration. *BMJ.* **1988**, *296*:,320-331.
10. Bush ,L.R.; Shebuski, R.J. *FASEB J* **1990**, *4*, 3087-3098.
11. Folts, J.D.*Circulation.* **1991**, *83 [suppl IV]*, IV-3-IV-14.
12. Bertha, B.G.; Folts, J.D. *J. Lab. Clin. Med.* **1984**, *103*, 204-214.
13. Rovin, J.D.; Stamler, J.S.; Loscalzo, J.; Folts J.D. *J. Cardiovsc. Pharm..* **1993**, *22*: 626-631.
14. Keller, J.W.; Folts, J.D. *Cardiovasc. Res.* **1988**, *22(1)*, 73-78.
15. Keller, J.W.; Saltzberg, M.; Folts, J.D. *Cardiovasc. Res.* **1990**, *24(3)*, 191-197.
16. Demrow, H.; Jackson, D., Folts, J. *Thromb. Haemostas.* **1993**, *69(6)*, 587.
17. Gronbaek, M.; Deis, A.; Sorensen, T.I.A.; Becker, U.; Schnohr, P.; Jensen, G. *BMJ*, **1995**, *310*, 1165-1169.
18. Gronbaek, M. *BMJ* **1994**, *308*, 302-306.
19. Doll, R.; Peto, R. *BMJ*, **1994**, *309*, 911-918.
20. Fuchs, C.S.; Stampfer, M.J.; Colditz, G.A.; Giovannucci, E.L.; Manson, J.E.; Kawachi, I.; Hunter, D.J.; Hankinson, S.E.; Hennekens, C.H.; Rosner, B.; Speizer, F.E.; Willet; W.C. *N. Engl. J. of Med.* **1995**, *33(19)*, 1245-50.
21. Friedman, L.A.; Kimball, A.W. *Am. J. Epidemiol.1986*, *124(3)*, 481-489.
22. Boffetta, P.; Garfinkel, L. *Epidemiology.* **1990**, *1*, 342-348.
23. Ducimetiere, P.; Guize, L.; Marciniak, A.; Milon, H.; Richard J.; Rufat, P. *Eur. Heart J.* **1993**, *14*, 727-733.
24. Klatsky, A.L.; Armstrong, M.A.; Friedman, G.D. *Ann. Intern. Med.* **1992**,*117*, 646-654.
25. Rimm, E.B.; Giovannucci, E.L.; Willett, W.C.; Colditz, G.A.; Ascherio, A.; Rosner, B.; Stampfer, M.J. *Lancet.* **1991**, *338*, 464-468.
26. Stampfer, M.J.; Colditz ,G.A.; Willett, W.C.; Speizer, F.E.; Hennekens, C.H. *N. Engl. J. Med.* **1988**, *319(5)*, 267-273.
27. Gaziano, J.M.; Buring, J.E.; Breslow, J.L.; Goldhaber, S.Z., Rosner, B.; VanDenburgh, M.V., Willet ,W.; Hennekens, C.H. *N. Engl. J. Med.* **1993**, *329*, 1829-1834.
28. Gaziano, J.M. *Am. J. of Med.* **1993**, *97(3A)*, 18S-28S.
29. Renaud, S.; DeLogeril, M. *Lancet.* **1992**, *339*, 1523-1526.
30. Nanji, A.A. *Int. J. of Cardiol..* **1985**, *8*, 487-489.
31. St. Leger, A.S.; Cochrane, A.L.; Moore, F. *Lancet.* **1979**, *12*, 1017-1020.
32. Hennekens, C.H.; Willett, W.W.; Rosner, B.; Cole, D.S.; Mayrent, S.L. *JAMA.* **1979**, *242(18)*, 1973.
33. Klatsky, A.L.; Armstrong, M.A. *Am. J. of Cardiol..* **1993**, *71*, 467-469.
34. Criqui, M.H.; Ringel, B.L. *The Lancet* **1994**, *344*, 1719-1723.
35. Coate, D. *Am. J. of Public Health*, **1993**, *83(6)*, 888-890.
36. DeLabry, L.O. *J. of Studies of Alcohol* **1992**, *53(1)*, 25-32.
37. Lazarus, N.; Kaplan, G.; Cohen, R.L. *BMJ* **1991**, *303*, 553-6.
38. Woodward, M.; Tunstall-Pedoe, H. *J. of Epidemiology* **1995**, *11*, 9-14.
39. Jepson, R.G.; Fowker, F.G.R.; Hously, E. *Eur. J. of Epidemiology* **1995**, *11*, 9-14.
40. Camargo, C.A.; Stampfer, M.J.; Gaziano, J.M. *Am. J. of Epidemiology* **1995**, *141(11 Suppl)*, S57.
41. Klatsky, A.L. *Alcoholism: Clin. and Exp. Res.* **1994**, *18(1)*, 88-97.
42. Klatsky, A.L.; Armstrong, M.A.; Friedan, G. *Ann. of internal Med.* **1992**, *117*, 456-564.
43. Camargo, C.A.; Hennekens, C.H. *Am. J. of epidemiolog* **1994**, *sup. 139*, abstract 99.

44. Anderson, P.; Cremona, A.; Paton A.; Turner, C.; Wallace, P. *Addiction* **1993**, *88*, 1493-1508.
45. Lavy, A.; Fuhrman, B.; Markel, A.; Dankner, G.; Ben-Amotz, A.; Presser, D.; Aviram, M. *Ann. of Nutrition and Metabolism* **1994**, *38*, 287-294.
46. Clevidence, B.A; Reichman, M.E.; Schatzkin, A. *Arteriosc. Thromb. and Vasc. Biol.* **1995**, *15*, 179-184.
47. Langer, R.D.; Criqui, M.H.; Reed, D.M. *Circulation.* **1992**, *85*, 910-915.
48. Langer, R.D.; Criqui, M.H.; Reed, D.M. *Am. J. Epidemiol.* **1988**, *128(4)*, 916.
49. Razay, G. *JBM* **1992**, *304,* 80-83.
50. Seigneur, M.; Bonnet, J.; Dorian, B.; Benchimol, D.; Drouillet, F.; Gouverneur, G.; Larrue, J.; Crockett, R.;Boisseau, M.R.; Ribereau-Gayon, P.; Bricard, H. *J. Appl. Cardiol..* **1990**, *5*, 215-222.
51. Mikhailidis, D.P.; Barradas, M.A.; Jeremy J.Y. *Alcohol* **1990**, *7(2),* 171-180.
52. Pikaar, N.A.; Wedel, M.; Van der Beek, E.J.; Van Dokkum, W.; Kempen, H.J.M.; Kluft, C.; Ockhuizen, T.; Hermus, R.J. *Metabolism.* **1987**, *36(6)*, 538-543.
53. Renaud, S.C.; McGregor, L.; Martin, J.L. In *Diet, Diabetes, and Atherosclerosis*; Pozza, G., Micossi, P,, Catapano, A.L., Paoletti R, eds; Raven Press: New York, NY; **1984**; pp 177-87.
54. Criqui, M.H. *Alcohol Clin. Exp. Res.* **1986**, *10(6),* 564-569.
55. Criqui, M.H.; Cowan, L.D.; Tryoler, H.A.; Bangdiwala, S.; Heiss, G.; Wallace, R.B.; Cohn, R. *Am. J. Epidemiol.* **1987**, *126(4)*, 629-637.
56. Struck, M.; Bierenbaum, M. *Nutrition Res.* **1994**, *14(12)*, 1811-1819.
57. Renaud, S; De Lorgeril, M. *Lancet* **1992**, *339*, 1523-6.
58. McGarry, G.W.; Gatehouse, S.; Vernham, G. *Clinical Otolaryngology* **1995**, *20(2),* 174-7.
59. Rubin, R.; Rand, M.L. *Alcoholism, Clin. and Exp. Res.* **1994**, *18(1),* 105-10.
60. Renaud, S.C.; Beswick, A.D.; Fehily, A.M.; Sharp, D.S.; Elwood, P.C. *Am.J. of Clin. Nutrition.* **1992**, *55(5),* 1012-7.
61. Mehta, P.; Mehta, J.; Lawson, D.; Patel, S.*Thrombosis Res.* **1987**, *48(6),* 653-61.
62. Ridker, P.M.; Hennekens, C.H. *JAMA* **1994**, *272(12),* 929-933.
63. Chabielska, E.; Malinowska, B.; Buczko, W. *Pharmacology* **1990**, *40 (5),* 288-92.
64. Latta, E.K.; Packham, M.A.; DaCosta, S.M.; Rand M.L.*Arteriosclerosis and Thomb.* **1994**, *14(8),* 1372-7.
65. Kitagawa, S.; Hirata, H. *Biochemica and Biophysica Acta* **1992**, *111*, 14-8.
66. Smith, C.M.; Tobin, J.D. Jr.; Burris, S.M.; White, J.G. *J. of Lab & Clin. Med.* **1992**, *120(5),* 699-706.
67. Demrow, H.S.; Slane P.R.; Folts, J.D. *Circulation* **1995**, *91*, 1182-1188.
68. Singleton, V.L.; Esau P. *Phenolic Substances in Grapes and Wine, and Their Significance.*; Academic Press: New York, NY, **1969**; pp 8-41.
69. Frankel, E.N.; Waterhouse, A.L.; Teissedre. *J. of Agr. and Food Chem.* **1995**, *43*, 890-894.
70. Frankel, E.; Waterhouse, A.; Kinsella, J. *The Lancet* **1993**, *341*, 454-457.
71. Whitehead, T.P.; Robinson, D.; Alaway, S.; Syms, J.; Hale, A. *Clinical Chemi* **1995**, *41(1),* 32-5.
72. Teissedre, P. *J. of Sci. and Food Agr.* ,(in press).
73. Siemann, E.H.; Creasy, L.L. *Am. J. Enol. Vitic.* **1992**, *43 (1),* 49-52.
74. Frankel, E.N.; Waterhouse, A.L.; Kinsella, J.E. *Lancet* **1993**, *341*, 1103-1104.

75. Landolfi, R.; Mower, R.; Steiner, M. *Biochem. Pharmacol.* **1984**, *33(9)*, 1525-1530.
76. Corvazier, E.; Maclouf, J. *Biochim. Biophys. Acta* **1985**, *835*, 315-321.
77. Mower, R.; Landolfi, R.; Steiner, M. *Biochem.Pharmacol.* **1984**, *33(3)*, 357-363.
78. Beretz, A.; Stierle, A.; Sutter-Bay, A.; Landry, A. *Proc. from the Inter. Bioflavonoid Symp*, Munich, FRG, **1981**.
79. Gryglewski, R.; Korbut, R.; Robak, J.; Swies, J. *Biochem. Pharmacol.* **1987**, *36(3)*, 317-322.
80. Slane, P.R.; Qureshi, A.A.; Folts, J.D. *Clin. Res* **1994**, *42(2)*, 162A.
81. Beretz, A.; Cazenave, J.P.; Anton, R. *Agents Actions* **1982**, *12(3)*, 382-387.
82. Beretz, A.; Stierle, A.; Anton, R.; Cazenave, J.P. *Biochem. Pharmacol.* **1981**, *31(22)*, 3597-3600.
83. Ferrell, J.E.; Peter, D.G.; Sing, C.; Loew, G.; King, R.; Mansour, J.M.; Mansour, T.E. *Mol. Pharmacol.* **1979**, *16*, 556-568.
84. Ruckstuhl, M.; Beretz, A.; Anton, R.; Landry, Y. *Biochem. Pharmacol..* **1979**, *28*, 535-538.
85. Beretz, A.; Anton, R.; Stoclet, J.C. *Experientia* **1978**, *34*, 1054-1055.
86. Loscalzo, J. *Am. J. Cardiol.* **1992**, *70*, 18B-22B.
87. Hertog, M.G.L.; Feskens, E.J.M.; Hollman, P.C.H.; Katen, M.B.; Kromhout, D. *Lancet* **1993**, *342*, 1007-11.
88. Hertog, M.G.L.; Kromhout, D.; Aravanis, C.; Blackburn, H.; Buzina, R.; Fidanza, F. *Arch. Intern. Med.* **1995**, 155, 381-386.
89. Hertog, M.G.L.; Feskens, E.L.M.; Hollman, P.C.H.; Katan, M.B.; Kromhout, D. *Lancet* **1993**, *342*, 1007-1011.
90. Sirving, O.K. *Arch. Intern. Med.* **1996**, *154*, 637-642.

Chapter 20

California Wine Use Leads to Improvement of Thrombogenic and Peroxidation Risk Factors in Hyperlipemic Subjects

Tom R. Watkins and Marvin L. Bierenbaum

Kenneth L. Jordan Heart Foundation, 48 Plymouth Street, Montclair, NJ 07042

Recently, protective benefits have been attributed to moderate wine consumption, particularly in the case of cardiovascular disease. To test the efficacy of wine on known risk factors, 180 ml/d of either a California Chardonnay or Cabernet was given to twenty hyperlipemic subjects. In this three-month cross-over design, serum lipids, peroxidized lipid, selected vitamins and platelet aggregation were compared before and after red and white wine consumption. No major change occurred in serum lipids as a result of daily wine usage, though Chardonnay consumption led to a mild decrease in serum LDL cholesterol fraction that approached significance ($p<0.08$). Serum thiobarbituric acid reactive substances, an indicator of peroxidation declined during the Chardonnay period ($p<0.05$), though not during the Cabernet period. Serum α-tocopherol levels did not change significantly during these short-term studies. Similarly, serum ascorbic acid data did not change for either red or white wine alone, though the combined data showed a modest decline ($p<0.05$). In these hyperlipemic subjects, both antithrombogenic and antioxidant benefits resulted from daily use of either white or red California wine, Chardonnay being more efficacious. The benefits were attributed, in part, to wine phenols.

Coronary artery disease (CAD) has been attributed to several environmental risk factors. Roles for serum cholesterol, elevated blood pressure and cigarette smoking have been well documented (1). Gey (2) in a multi-center study, has observed that serum α-tocopherol has greater predictive power than any of these three factors. More recently, in this laboratory we have reported that scorched, i. e. peroxidized, material in the blood serum which reacts with, hence can be identified and measured (with thiobarbituric acid, TBARS), represents another potent risk factor. Such peroxidation of the so-called 'bad' cholesterol (mainly in the LDL particle) has been associated by Steinberg (3) with increased foam cell deposition, plaque build up and eventually clogged arteries, a disease well known as atherosclerosis. Adequate intake of dietary antioxidants *per se* like vitamins E (4; 5), C (6) and others have been shown to retard peroxidation and inhibit development of clogged arteries, and other characteristics known to be associated with atherosclerosis.

Regular, moderate intake of alcohol has been correlated inversely with the risk of CAD. Moderate alcohol users have lower rates of heart disease, in general, than abstainers (5). Moore (7) has reviewed data consistent with the notion that moderate alcohol intake reduced one's risk of developing CAD by 20 - 30%. This held true for both smokers and non-smokers (5; 8), women (4) and the elderly (9).

Use of alcoholic beverages was thought to benefit one by way of increased HDL cholesterol levels, a notion not inconsistent with current thinking (10). In terms of haemostatic factors, moderate drinkers have lower fibrinogen levels and elevated fibrinolytic and anti-thrombin III activity (11; 12), which would lead to decreased clotting activity.

Subsequent reports have shown convincing evidence of the potential importance of aspirin. After aspirin ingestion, fewer coronary events occur, implicating the platelet as an important risk factor (Antiplatelet Trialists' Collaboration, 13). Later, Elwood (14) reported an inverse relationship between myocardial ischemia and thrombin-induced platelet aggregation and moderate alcohol intake.

An apparent anomaly has focussed attention recently on yet another dietary factor. Renaud (15) has reported that the incidence of coronary artery disease is unexpectedly low in Toulouse, France (a component center of the MONICA Study), though the dietary (& serum) cholesterol levels are high, fat intake is relatively high, the smoking incidence is high and the inhabitants are not particularly fond of regular exercise. In contrast to these French, their counterparts in Ireland sharing most of these life style features have a much higher rate of CAD. On the basis of this "French paradox," he has implicated regular intake of wine, since the French consume about twice as much wine as the Irish, 45 versus 20 g/d.

Thrombosis is yet another face of heart disease in general and may be a more important consideration in China. These scorched fats have been associated directly with increased thrombogenic risk in hypercholesterolemic subjects (16). As the scorched fats increase the stickiness of the blood, an indirect measure of its viscosity or resistance to flow, the risk of a thrombus--a plug of small blood cells called platelets--rises. Dietary conditions leading to increased risk would be those abundant in fat, especially scorched fat (as from fried, fast food), contaminated water, and smoggy air, and at the same time limited in antioxidants. Antioxidants are nature's first line of defense in stopping the scorching. When the intake of fresh fruit and vegetables is limited, as in America, insufficient antioxidants are present to stop the scorching peroxidation of tissues. We presently experience very high risk and incidence of heart attack and stroke. In addition to the natural antioxidant vitamins and minerals provided by fruit and vegetables in the diet, other antioxidant substances are present in food, especially fruit and vegetables, and beverages such as grape juice and wine. Wine, rich in these potent antioxidant flavonoids, taken on a regular basis should prevent the scorching of blood fats like cholesterol and triglycerides, thereby diminishing the risk of atherosclerosis via the 'bad' LDL cholesterol, and also decrease the tendency of the blood platelets to become sticky. Would it?

Unbound iron has been known to promote free radical generation (17). Should constituents in wine effectively bind metals like iron, they might enhance absorption of iron and other metals. Since elevated serum iron has been implicated as a cardiovascular risk factor, possibly via platelet activation, were such binding of metals to occur in serum, one would expect attenuated platelet aggregation. We recruited five hyperlipemic subjects for a preliminary trial with tannic acid. We prepared blood drawing tubes with tannic acid to compare platelet activity in the presence of citrate versus tannic acid. We next drew blood samples from these hyperlipemic subjects as a pilot study, and measured platelet aggregation in response to collagen as agonist. The platelet response was about one-tenth as great in the presence of tannic acid as in the presence of citrate, despite the fact that a 20-fold more dilute solution was used, Table I. On the basis of these data, we decided to expand the study.

Table I. Platelet Aggregation Response to Collagen Agonist in Citrate Treated & Tannic Acid Treated Venous Blood Samples of Hypercholesterolemic Subjects

Subject/gender	*Citrate*, Ω	*T. A.*, Ω
TERI/m	18.0	3.5
COPR/m	18.5	4.2
IRWG/m	22.0	0.4
LEVC/f	17.0	2.3
STIA/f	31.5	1.2
Means	21.4 ± 5.9	2.3 ± 1.6[a]

Individual and group data. Citrate: 0.105 M; T. A.: Tannic Acid: 5.0 mM. N = 5. [a] $P \ll 0.01$. Data in ohms (Ω). Conditions: Whole blood diluted in sterile saline, v/v; doped with human collagen, 2 μg/mL, the mixture incubated for six minutes.

The aim of this study, then, was to extend the pilot study and examine the influence of moderate California wine intake, both red and white, on known risk factors of CAD, serum lipids, peroxidation products, serum vitamins and platelet activity in the whole cohort.

Materials & Methods.

Twenty hypercholesterolemic subjects (serum cholesterol >5.7 mM/L), aged 36-72 years (57.5 ± 10), both men (16) and women, and free of other know disease, were selected for this crossover study, Table II. All were normotensive. Only two smoked cigarettes. All wine was provided by the Research Foundation, Chardonnay (WHITE, Sutter Home, St. Helena, CA) and Cabernet Sauvignon (RED, Inglenook Vineyards, Madera, CA). Subjects discontinued all alcohol intake for two weeks prior to baseline readings for all parameters studied. None of the cohort had been previously heavy drinkers (*i.e.*, consumed less than three drinks daily). Half of the subjects were randomly assigned to consume 180 ml/day of either RED or WHITE wine for a four-week period while continuing to eat a self-selected diet.

Repeat blood sampling was done at the end of four weeks and another two weeks of alcohol abstinence ensued. Blood was then sampled after this abstinence period and the second four weeks of crossover wine consumption started. Upon completion, repeat blood sampling was done. A 24-hour dietary recall was recorded at the start of each wine period. They were analyzed by the Nutritionist III program (N^2 Computing, Medford, OR). The calculated diet showed an average of 37% of calories derived from fat, with 18% saturated, 13% monounsaturated and 6% polyunsaturated. Cholesterol content was 430 mg/day and vitamin E 10 mg. Thirteen of the group were on vitamin supplementation. This was continued unchanged throughout the study.

Table II. Subjects' characteristics

Age, years	36-72
Gender, M/F	16/4
Body weight, kg	79.4 ± 3.6
Blood pressure, mm Hg	
Systolic	131 ± 10
Diastolic	83 ± 8
Serum cholesterol, mM/L	5.7 ± 0.25
Smoking habit	2/20

N = 20.

Subjects' vital parameters included weight (initial weight was 79.4 ± 3.6 kg), blood pressure and blood values. Blood specimens were drawn by venipuncture into evacuated citrate containing Vacutainer™ tubes for aggregation analysis, except in the comparative study when they were drawn into tannic acid (Sigma Chemical Co., St. Louis, MO), and a serum separator tube containing silicone gel and a clot activator for other analyses.

Blood was spun at 3400 rpm for 10 minutes and serum analyzed immediately, or stored frozen (-20° C.) overnight before analysis. Butylated hydroxytoluene in ethanol was added to final concentration of 5 μM, keeping the final ethanol concentration <1%, v/v. A lipid profile was measured on each subject, including serum cholesterol, triglycerides, high density lipoprotein cholesterol (HDL) and low density lipoprotein cholesterol (LDL) by difference (18), using standard chemical methods. All analyses were done under amber light to reduce photo-induced oxidation. To assess the effect of usual dietary habit upon peroxidation, the level of malondialdehyde equivalent substances (TBARS) was measured to quantitate fragments of lipid peroxidation by the method of Mihara, *et al.* (19). TBARS was quantitated in μM of 1,1,3,3-tetramethoxy-propane. In addition, plasma fatty acyl hydroperoxides were measured with a commercial kit. [These were measured by following the equimolar release of methylene blue when fatty acid hydroperoxide reacts with 10-N-methylcarbamoyl-3,7-dimethylamino-10H-phenothiazine in the presence of catalytic amounts of hemoglobin at 675 nm, according to Ohishi, *et al.* (20). Cumene hydroperoxide was used as the standard.]

Serum ascorbic acid, vitamin C, was measured spectrophotometrically using 2,4-dinitrophenylhydrazine as chromagen by Roe's method (21). Serum α-tocopherol was separated and quantitated by the HPLC method of Bieri, *et al.* (22). The separation was done on a C18 surface in a 5 cm. column with 3 μm mean diameter, using dl-α-tocopheryl acetate as internal standard.

The platelet response was measured with an impedance aggregometer (Chronolog, Havertown, PA 19108) by the method of Mackie, et al. (23) after six minutes of incubation at 37° C. Thrombin and collagen were was as agonists to initiate aggregation. Reagents were obtained from Sigma Chemical Co., St. Louis, MO, except luciferin-luciferase and collagen, which were obtained from Chronolog and dl-α-tocopheryl acetate (Roche, Nutley, NJ 07110), unless otherwise indicated. Solvents, double distilled ('HPLC grade') were purchased from EM Science (Gibbstown, NJ 08027).

Group means and standard errors were determined and compared using Student's paired t test. Differenced data were sequentially analyzed.

The Human Study Scientific Review Committee of the K. L. Jordan Heart Foundation reviewed and approved the protocol. Subjects had the option to withdraw at any time during the study.

Results.

Repeat analyses of the self-selected diet during the second wine period showed no difference, except for the change of wine. In addition, patients experienced no significant change in body weight or blood pressure level during the study. The average change in blood pressure during the RED period was: systolic, -0.8 mm Hg, diastolic, -1.7 mm Hg; and for the WHITE period: systolic, -1.5, diastolic, -2.25 mm Hg. Similarly, the pulse rate did not change significantly, either, decreasing by 1.0 beat per minute in the RED period, and increasing by 0.6 beat per minute in the WHITE period.

The *in vitro* data in Table I show a powerful anti-thrombogenic effect of tannic acid compared with citrate on whole blood. This blood was taken from hyperlipemic subjects who were eating self-selected diets as a pilot study. In the presence of tannic acid, platelet aggregation was about one-tenth the response seen in the presence of citrated blood. Note that the tannic acid concentration was 5 mM, whereas the citrate concentration was about 100 mM. The rest of the results were measured ex vivo after subjects had consumed wine as described.

The data of Table III show the serum lipid values of subjects after they had consumed the RED wine daily over a four-week period. No significant changes were seen in these measurements. In the table we see similar results for the WHITE wine period. Again, no significant change occurred in these serum

Table III. **Subjects' Serum Lipid Levels after Four Weeks' Wine Addendum**

mM/L	Red Base	Red Final	White Base	White Final	Combined Base	Combined Final
Chol	5.65 ±0.21	5.79 ±0.24	5.85 ±0.28	5.63 ±0.24	5.76 ±0.18	5.66 ±0.16
Trig	0.11 ±0.01	0.13 ±0.01	0.13 ±0.01	0.13 ±0.01	0.12 ±0.01	0.13 ±0.01
HDL Chol	1.11 ±0.05	1.12 ±0.07	1.13 ±0.08	1.11 ±0.07	1.12 ±0.05	1.11 ±0.05
LDL Chol	4.05 ±0.19	4.03 ±0.22	4.31 ±0.24	4.01 ±0.19[a]	4.18 ±0.15	4.02 ±0.14

Data presented as means ± s.e.m. N = 20. [a] $P<0.08$. Chol: cholesterol; Trig: triglyceride; HDL chol: high density lipoprotein cholesterol; LDL chol: low density lipoprotein cholesterol. Source: Reproduced with permission from reference 42.

lipids, though the decrease in LDL cholesterol values approached significance, changing from 4.31 to 4.01 mM/L, p<0.08. In the table we also see displayed the combined data for all subjects. No change was observed in these hyperlipemic subjects after daily wine use for four weeks.

Platelet responses to various agonists appear in Table IV. In the case of each wine, ATP release after a challenge of thrombin (EC 3.4.21.5, from human plasma), consumption of either wine resulted in decreased ATP release, being 0.81 initially and 0.68 finally for RED and 0.98 initially and 0.81 finally for

Table IV. Platelet Responses after Consumption of Wine for Four Weeks

Agonist	Red Base	Red Final	White Base	White Final	Combined Base	Combined Final
ATP*, μM/L	0.81 ±0.08	0.68 ±0.05	0.98 ±0.09	0.81 ±0.06[a]	0.91 ±0.06	0.75 ±0.04[a]
Coll, Ω	14.3 ±1.4	15.5 ±1.3	14.8 ±1.9	17.1 ±1.7	14.6 ±1.2	16.3 ±1.1
ATP, μM/L**	0.40 ±0.06	0.60 ±0.11	0.51 ±0.07	0.45 ±0.06	0.46 ±0.05	0.52 ±0.06

Data as means ± s.e.m. N = 20. ATP: release of adenosine triphosphate; Coll: stimulation by collagen, 2 μg/ml. * ATP release to thrombin agonist, 1 NIH unit/mL; collagen, human, 2 μg/mL. ** ATP release to collagen stimulus. [a] p<0.05. Source: Reproduced with permission from reference 42.

Table V. Peroxidation Products in Serum after Wine Consumption for Four Weeks

μM/L	Red Base	Red Final	White Base	White Final	Combined Base	Combined Final
TBARS	0.96 ±0.10	0.80 ±0.10	1.16 ±0.02	0.77 ±0.01[a]	1.05 ±0.01	0.79 ±0.06[b]
LOPS	1.26 ±0.14	1.29 ±0.12	1.24 ±0.13	1.21 ±0.14	1.25 ±0.09	1.25 ±0.09

Data as means ± s.e.m. N = 20. TBARS: thiobarbituric acid reactive substances; LOPS: fatty acid hydroperoxides. [a] p<0.05; [b] p<0.01. Source: Reproduced with permission from reference 42.

WHITE. The combined data for both wines showed a significant decrease in platelet ATP release, values decreasing from 0.91 to 0.75, p<0.05. No significant changes occurred in the aggregation response to collagen for either wine. Likewise, no noteworthy change was observed in ATP release when the platelet was challenged with collagen.

Consumption of either the RED or WHITE wine resulted in an antioxidant effect, as shown in Table V. After regular consumption of the RED wine, TBARS values decreased to 0.80 from 0.96 μM/L, though not significant. In contrast, after daily drinking the WHITE wine, values decreased markedly from 1.16 to 0.77 μM/L, p<0.05. Combining the data for all subjects for both wines, the mean TBARS values changed from 1.05 to 0.79 μM/L, p<0.01, a highly significant decrease. No change was measured in the hydroperoxides values during either wine period.

The baseline and final values for two antioxidant, ascorbic acid, a water-soluble vitamin, and α-tocopherol, an oil-soluble vitamin, appear in Table VI. The values are expressed in μM/L. Values of circulating ascorbic acid did not change during either wine period, though a modest decrease was seen for the combined data, changing from 88.6 to 80.1, p<0.05. No change was observed in the serum vitamin E levels, though they, too, tended to decrease somewhat.

Table VI. Serum Vitamin Levels after Consumption of Wine for Four Weeks

Vitamin	Red Base	Red Final	White Base	White Final	Combined Base	Combined Final
Ascorbate, μM/L	88.0 ±5.1	78.9 ±2.8	89.1 ±4.5	80.6 ±4.5	88.6 ±2.8	80.1 ±2.8[a]
α-Toco, μM/L	38.3 ±2.8	35.1 ±4.6	52.5 ±6.5	46.9 ±6.0	46.0 ±3.9	41.6 ±3.9

Data as means ± s.e.m. N = 20. [a] p<0.05. α-Toco: α-tocopherol.
Source: Reproduced with permission from reference 42.

Analyses of phenolics of the test wines appear in Table VII. The RED contained 47 ppm of total benzoic acid moieties, the WHITE, 2. Though total flavan-3-ols was about the same in both wines, being 49 ppm in the RED and 45 ppm in the WHITE, the
WHITE contained 9 ppm catechin versus 3 in the RED. Total hydroxycinnamates was similar, being 19 ppm in the RED and 15 in the WHITE, though the WHITE contained 3 ppm of caffeic acid, and the RED none detected. In terms of total flavonols, the RED contained 12 ppm, the WHITE 9 ppm; quercetin was not detected in either sample. Anthocyanins were present at 3 ppm in the RED.

The relative responses of heart and liver enzymes to the addendum of wine in the diet revealed that despite a significant increase in serum SGOT in the RED wine group from 17.6 ± 0.84 to 19.8 ± 1.17, p<0.05, all heart and liver function studies remained within normal limits. In regard to kidney function, RED wine use resulted in a significant decrease in BUN from 17.3 ± 0.76 to 15.2 ± 0.78, p<0.05. All values, however, remained within normal limits. Additionally, all serum mineral and uric acid concentrations remained within normal limits, even though serum calcium levels decreased during both wine periods; RED: 9.54 ± 0.06 to 9.39 ± 0.08, p<0.07; WHITE: 9.58 ± 0.08 to 9.39 ± 0.08, p<0.05; and combined wines: 9.58 ± 0.08 to 9.39 ± 0.08, p<0.01.

No significant changes were seen in serum phosphorus or uric acid levels. Finally, fibrinogen levels showed slight but insignificant increases for all categories, (mg/dL): RED: 277.5 ± 6.29 to 278.1 ± 11.17; WHITE: 272.1 ± 8.20 to 282.2 ± 10.34; and combined wines: 275.1 ± 5.00 to 280.0 ± 7.59.

Table VII. **Phenolic Composition of Test Wines**

	Red (CS, nv)	White (CH, '90)
Gallic acid	42	2
Total benzoic acid	47	2
Catechin	3	9
Epicatechin	0	0
Total Flavan-3-ols	49	45
Caffeic acid	0	3
Total Hydroxy-cinnamates	19	15
Quercetin	0	0
Total Flavonols	12	9
Anthocyanins	3	0

Data in ppm. CS: cabernet sauvignon; CH: chardonnay; NV: non-vintage. Analyses kindly provided by Dr. Andrew Waterhouse, University of California, Davis, CA.

Discussion.

Over the past twenty years, moderate use of alcohol has been associated with attenuation of heart disease risk, compared with non- or heavy drinking. In terms of the lipid etiology of heart disease this decreased risk was associated with modestly increased HDL cholesterol levels (Criqui, 24; Castelli, 25). Others have disagreed (Moore, 7; Renaud, 15), suggesting that the differences were too small to be important. Others have suggested that the decreased fibrinogen levels along with associated fibrinolytic and antithrombin III acitivity in users of alcohol may account for the apparent protection (11; 12). Renaud, et al. (15) have focussed our attention on wine, particularly red wine, for its beneficial effects on attenuating platelet activity. Siegneur's (26) further work with wine, platelet and serum lipids has added additional support to the importance of wine in a healthy diet. Folts (27) has demonstrated the kinetic character of this effect of wine upon platelet activity both in a dog model and more recently in human subjects, noting a more potent response in the case of red wine. This has been attributed to several phenolics (28) as well as the resveratrol content of wines (29; 30; 31). In addition, Fitzpatrick (32) has demonstrated that red wine usage also modulates vascular tone, leading to relaxation of the endothelium, suggesting the potential importance of wine in improving hypertension.

In these hyperlipemic subjects regular wine consumption of 180 ml/day did not lead to improved serum lipid changes. Seigneur et al. (26) have reported that use of 500 ml/day of wine led to increased levels of LDL cholesterol. At the modest levels we administered, no such elevation of serum lipids was measured. In fact, a modest, nearly significant ($p<0.08$) decrease in LDL cholesterol was seen in our subjects during the WHITE period.

The results here presented have shown that both red and white California wines lead to improved platelet in as little as four weeks. In particular, the response to thrombin led to significantly attenuated thrombin response of the platelets of these hyperlipemic subjects.

On the other hand, the data here presented have shown that a regular addendum to the diet of as little as 180 ml/day of either RED or WHITE California wine resulted in significantly decreased levels of peroxidation products circulating in the serum as malondialdehyde equivalent material, here labelled TBARS. The actual level reached significance ($p<0.05$) only during the WHITE period. However, TBARS values also decreased during the RED period. Since the subjects diets remained stable during the test periods, it is inferred that the wine contributed substance(s) which inhibited peroxidation. Frankel, et al. (33) have reported the potent, antioxidant potency of red wine in inhibiting peroxidation in vitro of LDL lipoprotein lipid. In a more recent paper from their laboratory (34) they have surveyed many wines, testing both reds and whites in this bioassay system. Though the reds outperformed the whites, the white also contained phenolics which demonstrated antioxidant potency. Sharpe, et al. (35) have reported that 200 ml/day of red wine (French, Ardeche region) resulted in decreased LDL cholesterol levels in young (mean age 37.2 years), normolipemic subjects. These positive results with a white wine addendum also corroborate earlier results obtained by Klurfeld, et al. (36), who fed rabbits hypercholesterolemic diets with water, beer, whiskey, white or red wine. Though pure alcohol resulted in just 75% the incidence of atherosclerosis, whiskey, 83%, white wine, 67%, and red wine, merely 40% the incidence of water drinking mates.

Since white wines bear very limited levels of trans-resveratrol (30), we infer that catechin--and possibly caffeic acid--play an important role in the beneficial antioxidant effects observed in the white over the red wine here tested in these human subjects. Other yet unidentified substances may also be implicated in the antioxidant protection here observed. We have not precluded the possible importance of a substance inadvertently present from wine processing (e. g., ellagic acid, V. Singleton, personal communication). We have shown in this laboratory (7) an inverse relation between the tendency of platelets to aggregate and serum α-tocopherol levels: with supplementation of vitamin E, TBARS, hydroperoxides and platelet aggregation decreased in hypercholesterolemic subjects.

Membrane dynamics may be enhanced by flavanoids in wine, and other foods. Decreased thrombin response for the combined wines suggested that sufficient phenolics are present in the white wine to influence platelet membrane dynamics. Throughout the RED and WHITE periods, levels of vitamin E did not change significantly, though platelet membrane stability was apparently enhanced, since the thrombin response was attenuated, Table 4. The modest decrease in ascorbic acid values observed suggested that it may have been used to recycle phenols (37), or its turnover may have been decreased in the presence of wine flavonoids. Uptake and metabolism of phenolics may distinctly differ, such that some present in the WHITE may have been preferentially bioavailable. In recent uptake studies Maxwell, et al. (38) have reported that in serum antioxidant potential increased significantly above baseline for at least four hours after red wine (5.7 ml/kg) taken with a meal. Whitehead, et al. (39), have recently reported a study in which serum antioxidant potential was increased in the serum of nine human subjects after taking 300 ml of red wine, with an average increase of 18% at one hour and about 10% at two hours; in comparison, a modest effect was observed with white wine, 4% at one hour and 7% at two hours. Such changes in serum total antioxidant capacity do not necessarily correlate directly with a functional test, such as platelet aggregation tendency.

With the data available in this study no means exists to assign a mechanism to explain the apparent advantage of WHITE over RED here presented with certainty. Klatsky (40) has aptly pointed out using a very large cohort that wine did not necessarily confer greater protection than other forms of alcohol. Further, even ethanol itself in modest doses also exerts potent membrane effects, as common experience testifies. As we noted in studies with polyunsaturates (41) in membrane systems, even modest levels of 5 mole% markedly modify membrane functions, such as respiration. We have reported tests of actual *in tissue* functional capacity, platelet performance. It is presumed that publication of absorption and metabolism studies from the Davis group and others will shed further light on this point in due season.

Literature Cited.
1   Kannel, W. B., Dawber, T. R., Kagan, A., Revotskie, N., Stokes, J. *Ann. Intern. Med.* **1961**, *55*, 33-52.
2   Gey, K. F., Puska, P., Moser, U. K. *Am. J. Clin. Nutr.* **1991**, *53*, 326S-334S.
3   Steinberg, D., Parthasarathy, S., Carew, T. E., Khoo, J. C., Witztum, J. L. *New Engl. J. Med.* **1989**, *320*, 915-924.
4   Stampfer, M. J., Colditz, G. A., Willett, W. C., Speitzer, F. E., Hennekens, C. H. *N. Engl. J. Med.* **1988**, *319*, 267-273.

5 Rimm, R. B., Giovannucci, F. L., Willett, W. C., et al. *Lancet* **1991**, *338*, 464-486.
6 Riemersma, R. A., Wood, D. A., Macintyre, C. C. A., Elton, R., Gey, K. F., Oliver, M. F. *Ann. New York Acad. Sci.* **1989**, *570*, 291-295.
7 Moore, R. D., Pearson, T. A. *Medicine.* **1986**, *65*, 242-267.
8 Friedman, L. A., Kimball, A. W. *Am. J. Epidemiol.* **1986**, *24*, 481-489.
9 Colditz, G. A., Branch, L. G., Lipnick, R. J., et al. *Am. Heart J.* **1985**, *109*, 886-889.
10 Corti, M. C., Guralnik, J., Salive, M., et al. *J. Am. Med. Assoc.* **1995**, *274*, 539-544.
11 Meade, T. W., Chakrabarti, R., Haines, A. P., Morth, W. R. S., Stirling, Y. *Br. J. Med.* **1979**, *1*, 153-156.
12 Rogers, S., Yarnell, J. W. G., Fehily, A. M. *Eur. J. Clin. Nutr.* **1988**, *42*, 197-205.
13 Antiplatelet Trialists' Collaboration: Secondary prevention of vascular disease by prolonged antiplatelet treatment. *Br. J. Med.* **1988**, *296*, 320-331.
14 Elwood, P. C., Renaud, S., Sharp, D. S., Beswick, A. D., O'Brien, J., Yarnell, J. W. G. *Circulation* **1991**, *83*, 38-44.
15 Renaud, S. de Lorgeril, M. *Lancet* **1992**, *339*, 1523-1526.
16 Bierenbaum, M. L., Reichstein, R. P., Bhagavan, H. N., Watkins, T. *Biochem. Intl.* **1992**, *28*, 57-66.
17 Halliwell, B. & Gutteridge, J. M. C. *Free Radicals in Biology & Medicine*, 2d ed., Clarendon Press: Oxford, 1989, pp 18-19.
18 DeLong, D. M., DeLong, R., Wood P. D., Leppel, K., Rifkind, B. M. *J. Am. Med. Assoc.*, **1986**, *256*, 2372-2377.
19 Mihara, M., Uchiyama, M., Fukizawa, K. *Biochem. Med.* **1980**, *23*, 302-311.
20 Ohishi, N., Ohkawa, H., Miike, A., Tatano, T., Yagi, K. *Biochem. Intl.* **1985**, *10*, 205-211.
21 Roe, J. H. Chemical determination of ascorbic, dehydroascorbic and diketogulonic acids. *Methods of Biochem. Analysis*. Wiley & Sons: New York, 1954, 115-139.
22 Bieri, J. G., Tolliver, T. J., Catigniani, C. L. *Am. J. Clin. Nutr.* **1979**, *32*, 2143-2149.
23 Mackie, I. J., Jones, R., Machin, S. J. *J. Clin. Pathol.* **1984**, *37*, 874-878.
24 Criqui, G. A., Cowan, L. D., Tyroler H. A., et al. *Am. J. Epidemiol.* **1987**, *126*, 629-637.
25 Castelli, W. P., Gordon, T., Hjortland, H. A., et al. *Lancet* **1977**, *2*, 2153-2155.
26 Seigneur, M., Bonnet, J., Dorian, B., et al. *J. Appl. Cardiol.* **1990**, *5*, 215-222.
27 Demrow, H., Slane, P., Folts, J. *Circulation* **1995**, *91*, 1182-1188.
28 Waterhouse, A. L., Frankel, E. N. In: *Proc. OIV 73rd General Assembly*, San Francisco, August 29-September 3, 1993. OIV: 11 Rue Roquepine, 75008 Paris, France, pp. 1-15.
29 Siemann, E. H. & Creasy, L. L. *Am. J. Enol. Vitic.* **1992**, *43*, 49-52.

30 Goldberg, D., Yan, J., Ng, R., Diamandis, E., Karumanchiri, A., Soleas, G., Waterhouse, A. *Am. J. Enol. Vitic.* **1995**, *46*, 1-7.
31 McMurtrey, K. *J. Ag. Food Chem.*, **1995**, *42*, 2077-2080.
32 Fitzpatrick, D., Hirschfield, S. L., Coffey, R. G. *Am. J. Physiol.* **1993**, *265*, H774-778.
33 Frankel, E. N., Kanner, J., German, B., Parks, E., Kinsella, J. E. *Lancet* **1993**, *341*, 454-457.
34 _____, Waterhouse, A. L., Teissedre, P. L. *J. Ag. Food Chem.* **1995**, *43*, 890-894.
35 Sharpe, P. C., McGrath, L. T., McClean, E., Young, I. S., Archbold, G. P. R. *Q. J. Med.* **1995**, *88*, 101-108.
36 Klurfeld, D. M., Kritchevsky, D. *Exp. Mol. Pathol.* **1981**, *34*, 62-71.
37 Miki, M., Motoyama, T., Mino, M. *Ann. New York Acad. Sci.* **1989**, *570*, 474-477.
38 Maxwell, S., Cruickshank, A., Thorpe, G. *Lancet* **1994**, *344*, 193-194.
39 Whitehead, T. P., Robinson, D., Allaway, S., Syms, J., Hale, A. *Clin. Chem.* **1995**, *41*, 32-35.
40 Klatsky, A. L., Armstrong, M. A. *Am. J. Card.* **1993**, *71*, 467-469.
41 Eletr, S., Williams, M. A., Watkins, T., Keith, A. *Biochem. Biophys. Acta* **1974**, *339*, 190-204.
42 Struck, M., Watkins, T., Tomeo, A., Halley, J., Bierenbaum, M. *Nutrition Res.* **1994**, *14*, 1811-1819.

INDEXES

Author Index

Alonso, E., 69
Anderson, J. L., 230
Archier, P., 6
Baldi, Alessandro, 166
Bierenbaum, Marvin L., 261
Bills, Nathan D., 215
Bisson, Linda F., 180
Bononi, M., 94
Cheynier, Véronique, 81
Clifford, Andrew J., 215
Coen, S., 6
Coffey, Ronald G., 237
de la Torre-Boronat, M. C., 56
Demrow, H. S., 247
Desimoni, E., 94
Diamandis, E. P., 24
Ebeler, John D., 215
Ebeler, Susan E., 215
Fitzpatrick, David F., 237
Folts, John D., 247
Frankel, Edwin N., 196
German, J. Bruce, 196
Ghiselli, Andrea, 166
Goldberg, David M., 24
Guyot, Sylvain, 81
Hahn, S. E., 24
Hansen, Robert J., 196
Hinrichs, Steven H., 215
Jantzen, Paul T., 237
Karumanchiri, A., 24
Klatsky, Arthur L., 132
Kovac, V., 69
Lamuela-Raventós, Rosa M., 56
Lloret, M., 56
Maalej, N., 247
Maxwell, Simon R. J., 150
McMurtrey, Kenneth D., 44
Monetti, A., 113
Moutounet, Michel, 81
Mulinacci, Nadia, 166
Munson, L., 230
Prieur, Corine, 81
Reniero, F., 113
Revilla, Eugenio, 69
Rigaud, Jacques, 81
Roggero, Jean-Pierre, 6
Romani, Annalisa, 166
Romero-Pérez, A. I., 56
Slane, P. R., 247
Soleas, G. J., 24
Stoewsand, Gilbert S., 230
Tateo, Fernando, 94
Teissedre, Pierre-Louis, 12
Versini, Giuseppe, 113
Vincieri, Franco F., 166
Walzem, Rosemary L., 196
Waterhouse, Andrew L., 12,56,196
Watkins, Tom R., 2,261

Affiliation Index

Andres Wines Limited, 24
Cornell University, 230
Istituto Agrario di San Michele all'Adige, 113
Istituto Nazionale della Nutrizione, 166
Kaiser Permanente Medical Center, 132
Kenneth L. Jordan Heart Foundation, 2,261
Leicester Royal Infirmary, 150
Liquor Control Board of Ontario, 24
Tehnoloski Fakultet, 69
Unité de Recherche Polyméres et Techniques Physico-Chimiques, 81
Universidad Autónoma de Madrid, 69
Universidad de Barcelona, 56
Università degli Studi di Firenze, 166
Università degli Studi di Milano, 94
Université d'Avignon, 6

University of California—Davis, 12,56,180,196,215
University of Nebraska Medical Center, 215
University of South Florida, 237
University of Southern Mississippi, 44
University of Tennessee, 230
University of Toronto, 24
University of Wisconsin, 247

Subject Index

A

Acetic acid, role in chromatography of phenolics in wine, 8
Acquired immune deficiency syndrome, role of visual latency, 211
Agroecological factors, role in catechin and procyanidin content in grapes and wines, 71–75
Alcohol
  nutritional value and therapeutic potential, 4–5
  role
    in cardiac dysrhythmias, 144f,145–147
    in cardiomyopathy, 132–133,145–147
    in cardiovascular diseases, 132–147
    in coronary artery disease, 137–143,145–147
    in hypertension, 133–137,145–147
    on lipids, 249
    on platelets, 250–251
  See also Ethanol, Wine
Alcoholic cardiomyopathy, 132–133
Anthocyan–tannin interaction compounds, antioxidant potencies, 169,171–178
Antioxidant(s)
  balance of oxidation with prooxidants, 203–204,205t
  biological containment of inappropriate oxidation, 199
  countering of toxic oxygen radical, 5
  description, 4,199
  flavonoids in wine, activity in vivo, 150–162
  fruit in diet as source, 3
  impact on antioxidant activity in vivo, 150–162

Antioxidant(s)—Continued
  plant phenolics, 207–208
  protective strategies, 199,201–202
  role in peroxidation of tissue, 262–263
  role of flavonoids in red wine, 256
Antioxidant potencies of polyphenols in grapes and wines
  experimental description, 167–170
  grapes, 170,172t
  role in prevention of cardiovascular disease, 237
  wine
    low-molecular-weight polyphenols, 170–171
    tannin–anthocyan interaction compounds
      2-deoxyribose assay, 177,178f
      EPR spectroscopy, 171–172,174t
      platelet aggregation assay, 177,178f
      TRAP assay, 173,175–176f
Antiplatelet, role of flavonoids in red wine, 256–257
Antithrombotic activity of flavonoids in red wine
  antioxidant phytochemicals, 256
  platelet aggregation, 256–257
  cardioprotective benefits, 248–251
  in vivo studies, 251–255
Asbestosis, role of phagocyte activation, 210–211
Asthma, role of leukotrienes, 210
Atherosclerosis
  association with low-density-lipoprotein oxidation, 204,206
  risk factors, 150–151
Authenticity monitoring of wines, natural stable isotope ratio analysis, 113–128

B

Beer, role in cardiovascular disease, 56
Biological properties, trihydroxystilbenes in wine, 24–42
Breast cancer, model, 224

C

Caffeic acid
  levels in California varietal wines, 21
  role in carcinogenesis inhibition, 230–235
California varietal wines, levels of phenolics, 12–22
California wine use related to thrombogenic and peroxidation risk factors in hyperlipemic subjects
  antioxidants in wine, 210–211,267–268
  ascorbic acid levels, 268
  blood pressure changes, 265–266
  experimental description, 264–265
  phenolic composition of wines, 268–270
  platelet aggregation response to agonist, 263,266
  tannic acid compared to citrate, 266
Cancer
  association with oxidation, 208–209
  role of fruits and vegetables, 215
Carbohydrate, interaction with ethanol, 185,187
Carbon, natural stable isotope ratio analysis for monitoring authenticity and regional origin of wines, 113–128
Carcinogenesis inhibition, induced by ethyl carbamate, 230–235
Cardiac dysrhythmias, associated with alcohol ingestion, 144f,145–147
Cardiac heart disease, potential of wine to improve health, 12–13
Cardiomyopathy, alcohol-associated, 132–133,145–147
Cardioprotective role of wine
  platelets aggregation, 250–251
  relationship between mortality and alcohol consumption, 248–249
Cardiovascular disease
  and alcohol consumption, 132–147
  cause of premature death and disability, 150
  impact of wine antioxidants on antioxidant activity in vivo, 150–162
Catechin(s)
  chromatography in wine, 9
  protective effect in atherosclerosis, 70
Catechin content
  agroecological factors, 71–75t
  experimental description, 70
  in California varietal wines, 18–19
  technological practices, 75–78
Catechin hydrate, role in carcinogenesis inhibition, 230–235
Chemiluminescent assay, antioxidant activity in biological fluids, 150–162
Chromatographic peak-shape analysis, 95–96
Chromatography of phenolics in wine
  assay, 10–11
  catechins, 9
  flavonols and flavonol glycosides, 9–10
  phenolic acids and esters, 9
  proanthocyanidins, 9
  setup, 7–8
L-Citrulline, production, 238
Colon carcinoma, multiple intestinal neoplasia model, 223–224
Condensed tannins, See *Proanthocyanidins*
Coronary artery disease
  alcohol and blood pressure, 137–143,145–147,262
  environmental risk factors, 261–262
  wine consumption, 248–249
Cultivar, role in catechin and procyanidin content in grapes and wines, 71–72,73t
Cyanidin-3-glucoside, levels in California varietal wines, 21
Cyclic guanosine monophosphate mediated relaxation of vascular smooth muscle, role of wine, grapes, and plant products, 237

INDEX

D

2-Deoxyribose assay
  antioxidant potencies of polyphenols in grapes and wines, 166–178
  procedure, 169–170
Destemming of grape clusters, role in catechin and procyanidin content in grapes and wines, 75–76
Diabetic individuals, increases risk of development of coronary heart disease, 180
Dietary factors that delay tumor onset, in vivo experimental protocol for identification and evaluation, 215–227
Diseases associated with oxidation
  DNA damage and cancer, 208–209
  French paradox, 204
  low-density lipoprotein oxidation and atherosclerotic cardiovascular disease, 204,206
DNA polymer, damage by oxygen radicals, 3

E

Eicosanoid, metabolism, 40f,41–42
Electron paramagnetic resonance spectroscopy, antioxidant potencies of polyphenols in grapes and wines, 166–178
Electrospray MS, antioxidant potencies of polyphenols in grapes and wines, 166–178
Enantiomeric analysis of linalool for Muscat wine flavorings composition
  experimental description, 95–97
  high-resolution GC, chiral analysis, 97–105
  peak-shape analysis, 105–109
Endothelium-dependent vasorelaxing activity of wine, grapes, and plant products
  aortic rings by grape skin extract, 239–244
  aortic tissue by plant extracts, 243,245f

Endothelium-dependent vasorelaxing activity of wine, grapes, and plant products—*Continued*
  cyclic guanosine monophosphate levels, 239
  experimental description, 238
  mechanism, 243,245
Epicatechin, levels in California varietal wines, 19
Ethanol
  consumption, 190–191
  factors affecting interplay with macronutrient energy, 187
  interaction
    with carbohydrate, 185,187
    with ethyl carbamate, 231
    with fatty acids, 184–185,186f
  metabolism, 183
  role in human diet, 181
  use as energy source, 183–184
  See also Alcohol, Wine
Ethyl carbamate induced carcinogenesis, role of wine in inhibition, 230–235

F

Fatty acids, interaction with ethanol, 184–185,186f
Fermentation, resveratrol evolution, 59,62f
Fining of wines, role in catechin and procyanidin content in grapes and wines, 76
Flavonoid(s)
  antithrombotic activity in red wine, 247–257
  protection against cardiovascular disease, 154–162
  source in wine, 4
Flavonol(s), chromatography in wine, 9–10
Flavonol glycosides, chromatography in wine, 9–10
Folts coronary thrombosis model of platelet aggregation and thrombus formation, 248

French paradox
  association with oxidation, 204
  description, 4,69,153–154,181,247
  hypotheses, 247–248
Fruit, source of antioxidants in diet, 3

G

Gallic acid
  levels in California varietal wines, 20f,21
  role in carcinogenesis inhibition, 230–235
Grape(s)
  antioxidant potencies of polyphenols, 166–178
  endothelium-dependent vasorelaxing activity, 237–245
  phenolic composition, 207–208
  structures and protein interactions of proanthocyanidins, 81–91
Grape cultivars, classifications, 70

H

Heart disease
  protection by flavonoids and red wine, 153–154
  role of diet, 56
Hemangioendotheliomas, role of wine in inhibition, 232–233,235
Hepatocellular adenomas, role of wine in inhibition, 232–233,235
High-performance liquid chromatography
  analysis of linalool, 94–109
  antioxidant potencies of polyphenols in grapes and wines, 166–178
  piceid levels in wines, 56–65
  resveratrol levels in wine, 44–54,56–65
Human T-lymphotropic virus type 1 model, 222t,223
2-(p-Hydroxyphenyl)ethanol, identification in wine, 10
Hydrogen, natural stable isotope ratio analysis for monitoring authenticity and regional origin of wines, 113–128
Hydroxyl radical, risk factor, 3
Hyperlipemic subjects, effect of California wine on thrombogenic and peroxidation risk factors, 261–271
Hypertension, related to alcohol consumption, 133–137,145–147

I

In vivo experimental protocol for identification and evaluation of dietary factors that delay tumor onset
  administration of test compounds, 224–225
  chemical carcinogen models, 219
  chemically defined diet, 224–225
  diet, 217t,218
  experimental description, 216,218
  growth vs. wine solid supported diet, 219,220f
  red wine solids vs. tumor onset, 225–227
  time of tumor onset vs. wine solid supplemented diet, 219,221f
  transgenic mouse models, 222t–224
Ion-spray high-performance liquid chromatography–mass spectrometry, antioxidant potencies of polyphenols in grapes and wines, 166–178

L

Leukotrienes, role in asthma, 210
Linalool, enantiomeric analysis for Muscat wine flavoring composition, 94–109
Lipid levels, role of alcohol, 249
Lipid peroxy radicals, risk factors, 3
Low-density-lipoprotein, protection using natural antioxidant mechanisms, 151
Low-density-lipoprotein oxidation, association with atherosclerotic cardiovascular disease, 204,206
Low-molecular-weight polyphenols, antioxidant potencies in grapes and wines, 167–168,170–171
Lung alveolar adenomas, role of wine in inhibition, 234t,235

INDEX

M

Macronutrient energy, factors affecting interplay with ethanol, 187
Malvidin-3-glucoside, levels in California varietal wines, 20f,21
Mediterranean diet, health, 56
Metabolic syndrome X
  associated diseases, 180
  definition of moderate ethanol consumption, 190–191
  ethanol as macronutrient, 183–184
  glucose utilization in affected cells, 181,182f
  interactions of macronutrient energy sources, 184–187
  role of ethanol, 187–189
Millésime, description, 70
Multiple intestinal neoplasia model, colon carcinoma, 223–224
Muscat wine flavorings composition, enantiomeric analysis of linalool, 94–109
Myrecitin, levels in California varietal wines, 21

N

Natural stable isotope ratio analysis for monitoring authenticity and regional origin of wines
  experimental materials, 115
  identification of wine geographical origin, 123,125–128
  isotopic ratios correlated with latitude, 117
  samples by region, 115–116
Nitric oxide, production, 238
NMR spectroscopy of site-specific natural isotope fractionation of deuterium, 113–115

O

Oxidant-induced cell activation, associated diseases, 210–211

Oxidant signaling, associated diseases, 209–210
Oxidation
  balance between prooxidants and antioxidants, 203–204,205t
  biological containment via antioxidants, 199
  chemistry, 197–199,200t
  definition, 196
  diseases, 204
  of low-density lipoprotein, protection using natural antioxidant mechanism, 151
  processes within organisms, 203
Oxidative stress
  damage caused, 197
  occurrence, 151
  role in development of chronic diseases, 196
Oxidized low-density lipoprotein particle, role in cardiovascular disease, 3–4
Oxygen
  natural stable isotope ratio analysis for monitoring authenticity and regional origin of wines, 113–128
  toxic forms, 2
Oxygen radicals, damage to DNA polymers, 3

P

Peroxidation
  of tissue, role of antioxidants, 262–263
  risk factor in hyperlipemic subjects, role of California wine, 261–271
Phagocyte activation, role in asbestosis, 210–211
Phenolic(s)
  chromatography in wine, 6–11
  correlation with reduced cardiac heart disease mortality, 13–14
  flavonoids identified, 14–15
  in California varietal wines
    absorption, 16
    caffeic acid levels, 21

Phenolic(s)—*Continued*
  in California varietal wines—*Continued*
    catechin levels, 18–19
    cyanidin-3-glucoside levels, 21
    epicatechin levels, 19
    experimental description, 17–18
    gallic acid levels, 20f,21
    key issues, 211–212
    malvidin-3-glucoside levels, 20f,21
    myrecitin levels, 21
    plant, *See* Plant phenolics as antioxidants
    quercetin levels, 19–20
    resveratrol levels, 22
    role in chronic disease, 196
    sinapic acid levels, 21
    total phenolic levels, 21–22
  mechanisms of action, 16
  nonflavonoids, 15
Phenolic acids and esters, chromatography in wine, 9
Piceid in wine production and in finished wines
  experimental description, 58–59
  identification in wine, 10
  red wines, 59,60f
  resveratrol evolution during fermentation, 59,62–65
  role in decrease in cardiovascular disease, 57
  rosé wines, 59,61f
  structures, 56,60f
  white wines, 59,61f
Plant phenolics as antioxidants
  atherosclerotic cardiovascular disease, 207
  composition of grapes, wines, and foods, 207–208
Plant products, endothelium-dependent vasorelaxing activity, 237–245
Platelet(s)
  aggregation inhibition test, antioxidant potencies of polyphenols in grapes and wines, 166–178
  in atherosclerosis and coronary artery disease, 248
  levels related to alcohol consumption, 250–251

Polyphenol(s), antioxidant potencies in grapes and wines, 166–178
Polyphenolic antioxidants, source in wine, 4
Proanthocyanidins in grapes and wines
  chromatography, 9
  characterization, 83–84,86f
  enzymatic inhibition studies, 87,89,90f
  experimental description, 82
  grape seed procyanidin fractions with poly(vinylpyrrolidone), 87,88f
  interactions with proteins, 87–90
  methods of structure determination, 83
  procyanidin oligomers, 87
  properties, 81
  structures, 82–83
  study methods, 85
  wine tannin composition, 84–85,86f,88f
Procyanidin(s), 70
Procyanidin content
  agroecological factors
    cultivar, 71–72,73t
    degree of maturity, 74,75t
    site of production, 73–74
    year of production, 72–73
  experimental description, 70
  technological practices
    addition of supplementary quantities of seeds during fermentation, 76–78
    destemming of grape clusters, 75–76
    fining of wines, 76
    length of maceration, 75
Prooxidants, balance of oxidation with antioxidants, 203–204,205t
Prostaglandins, role in thrombosis, 210
Proteins, interactions with proanthocyanidins in grapes and wines, 81–91

Q

Quercetin
  identification in wine, 9–10
  levels in California varietal wines, 19–20

INDEX

R

Recommended dietary allowances of vitamin and minerals, 2
Red wine
 antithrombotic effect of flavonoids, 247–257
 flavonoid protection against cardiovascular disease, 154–162
 potential positive effects on human cardiovascular health, 44
 resveratrol and piceid levels, 56–65
 See also Alcohol, Ethanol, Wine
Red wine solids, in vivo experimental protocol for identification and evaluation of delay of tumor onset, 215–227
Regional origin of wines, natural stable isotope ratio analysis, 113–128
Resveratrol
 analytical conditions, 47–51
 biological properties, 24–42
 eicosanoid metabolism
  platelets, 40*f*,41
  neutrophil leukotriene production, 41–42
 enological procedure, 31,33,35
 experimental description, 24–25,44, 58–59
 identification, 24–42
 in vitro studies
  lipid metabolism, 34–39
  platelet aggregation, 37,41
 levels
  California varietal wines, 22
  red wines, 52–54,59,60*f*
  rosé wines, 59,61*f*
  white wines, 51–52,59,61*f*
 method comparison, 28
 regional differences
  cis-resveratrol concentrations, 30
  trans-resveratrol concentrations, 28–29
  resveratrol glucoside concentrations, 30–31,32*f*

Resveratrol—*Continued*
 resveratrol assay procedures
  derivatization GC–MS, 25,27
  direct-injection GC–MS, 25
 resveratrol evolution during fermentation, 59,62–65
 resveratrol glucoside assay procedures
  normal-phase HPLC, 26*f*,27
  reversed-phase HPLC, 27
 structures, 56,60*f*
cis-Resveratrol, identification in wine, 10
trans-Resveratrol
 identification in wine, 10
 role in decrease in cardiovascular disease, 56–57
Reversed-phase high-performance liquid chromatography analysis of structures and protein interactions of proanthocyanidins, 81–91
Rosé wines, resveratrol and piceid levels, 56–65

S

Sinapic acid, levels in California varietal wines, 21
Solid-phase microextraction, analysis of linalool, 94–109
Stable isotope ratios of elements, detection of adulterations in fruit juices and derivatives, 113
Superoxide dismutase enzymes, function, 2
Superoxide theory of disease, 2–3
Syndrome X, *See* Metabolic syndrome X

T

Tannin(s), 81–82
Tannin–anthocyan interaction compounds, antioxidant potencies, 169,171–178
Thiolysis, analysis of structures and protein interactions of proanthocyanidins, 81–91

Thrombogenic risk factor in hyperlipemic subjects, role of California wine, 261–271
Thrombosis, role of prostaglandins, 210
Tocopherol, antioxidant activity, 202
Total phenolics, levels in California varietal wines, 21–22
Toxic oxygen radical, 5
Toxic oxygen stress, causation of disease, 2
Transgenic mouse models, 222–224
TRAP assay
  antioxidant potencies of polyphenols in grapes and wines, 166–178
  procedure, 169
trans-3,4',5-Trihydroxystilbene, See Resveratrol
Tryptophol, identification in wine, 10
Tumor, in vivo experimental protocol for identification and evaluation of dietary factors that delay onset, 215–227
Tyrosol, identification in wine, 10

U

Unbound iron, promotion of free radical generation, 263
Urate, role in antioxidant activity, 161–162

V

Vasorelaxing activity of wine, grapes, and plant products, See Endothelium-dependent vasorelaxing activity of wine, grapes, and plant products
Visual latency, role in acquired immune deficiency syndrome, 211
Vitamin E, risk modification of chronic diseases, 2

W

White wine
  flavonoid protection against cardiovascular disease, 154–162
  resveratrol and piceid levels, 56–65
Wine
  antioxidant potencies of polyphenols, 166–178
  cardioprotective effect, 248–249
  chromatography of phenolics, 6–11
  content in ethyl carbamate, 230
  endothelium-dependent vasorelaxing activity, 237–245
  interaction with ethyl carbamate, 231–235
  levels of phenolics, 12–22
  natural stable isotope ratio analysis for monitoring authenticity and regional origin, 113–128
  nutritional and therapeutic potential, 4–5
  phenolic composition, 207–208
  potential to improve health, cross-cultural studies, 12–13
  protein interactions of proanthocyanidins, 81–91
  resveratrol levels, 44–54
  role in decrease in cardiovascular disease, 56
  source of flavonoids and polyphenolic antioxidants, 4
  structures of proanthocyanidins, 81–91
  therapeutic potential, 4
  See also Alcohol, California varietal wines, Ethanol
Wine antioxidants
  experimental description, 151
  role in antioxidant activity in vivo, 150–162